D1174545

College Psychotherapy

College Psychotherapy

Edited by

PAUL A. GRAYSON, Ph.D.
State University of New York
at Purchase

KATE CAULEY, Ph.D.
Iona College

THE GUILFORD PRESS
New York   London

© 1989 The Guilford Press
A Division of Guilford Publications, Inc.
72 Spring Street, New York, NY 10012

All rights reserved

No part of this book may be reproduced, stored in a retrieval system, or transmitted, in any form or by any means, electronic, mechanical, photocopying, microfilming, recording, or otherwise, without written permission from the Publisher.

Printed in the United States of America

Last digit is print number: 9   8   7   6   5   4   3   2   1

Library of Congress Cataloging-in-Publication Data

College psychotherapy / Paul A. Grayson, Kate Cauley, editors.
     p.   cm.
   Bibliography: p.
   Includes index.
   ISBN 0-89862-747-8
   1. College students—Mental health.   2. Psychotherapy.
I. Grayson, Paul A.   II. Cauley, Kate.
RC451.4.S7C65 1989
616.89'0088375—dc19   88-24589
                                                                      CIP

Contributors

GERALD AMADA, Ph.D., Co-director, Mental Health Program, City College of San Francisco, San Francisco, California.

ROBERT L. ARNSTEIN, M.D., Chief Psychiatrist, Health Services, Yale University, New Haven, Connecticut; Clinical Professor, Department of Psychiatry, Yale University School of Medicine, New Haven, Connecticut.

KATE CAULEY, Ph.D., Director, Counseling Services, Iona College, New Rochelle, New York.

SHEILA CUMMINGS, Ph.D., Associate Chief, University Health Service, Mental Health Section, University of Rochester, Rochester, New York; Assistant Professor, Department of Psychology, University of Rochester School of Medicine and Dentistry, Rochester, New York.

CHARLES P. DUCEY, Ph.D., Director, Bureau of Study Counsel, Harvard University, Cambridge, Massachusetts; Lecturer, Department of Psychology, Harvard Graduate School of Education, Cambridge, Massachusetts.

SAM EDWARDS, JR., M.S.W., Social Worker, Counseling and Psychological Services, Cowell Student Health Center, Stanford University, Stanford, California.

MICHAEL S. GAYLOR, M.D., Director, Office of Counseling and Human Development, and Associate Professor, Departments of Psychiatry and of Community and Family Medicine, Dartmouth College, Hanover, New Hampshire.

MARVIN H. GELLER, Ph.D., Director, Counseling Services, McCosh Health Center, Princeton University, Princeton, New Jersey; Faculty, Washington University School of Psychiatry, Washington, D.C.

PAUL A. GRAYSON, Ph.D., Director, Counseling Services, State University of New York at Purchase, Purchase, New York.

GEORGE C. HIGGINS, Ph.D., Director, Office of the College Counselors, and Professor, Department of Psychology, Trinity College, Hartford, Connecticut.

KAREN H. C. HUANG, Ph.D., Psychologist, Counseling and Psychological Services, Cowell Student Health Center, Stanford University, Stanford, California; Lecturer, Department of Psychology, San Francisco State University, San Francisco, California.

ELIZABETH A. JOHNSON, Ph.D., Staff Psychologist, Medical Arts Clinic, Appleton, Wisconsin.

SAMUEL D. JOHNSON, JR., Ph.D., Dean of Students, Baruch College, City University of New York, New York, New York; Adjunct Associate Professor, Department of Psychology and Education, Teachers College, Columbia University, New York, New York.

RICHARD P. KEELING, M.D., Director, Student Health Service, and Associate Professor, Department of Internal Medicine, University of Virginia, Charlottesville, Virginia; President, American College Health Association, and Chairman, Task Force on AIDS, American College Health Association, Rockville, Maryland.

RANDOLPH M. LEE, Ph.D., Associate Director, Office of the College Counselors, and Associate Professor of Psychology, Trinity College, Hartford, Connecticut.

GARY MARGOLIS, Ph.D., Director, Center for Counseling and Human Relations, and Associate Professor, Department of English, Middlebury College, Middlebury, Vermont.

ALEJANDRO M. MARTINEZ, Ph.D., Psychologist, Counseling and Psychological Services, Cowell Student Health Center, and Affiliate Faculty, Department of Psychology, Stanford University, Stanford, California.

JOANNE D. MEDALIE, Ed.D., Senior Psychologist, Columbia College Counseling Service, and Lecturer, Department of Human Development, Columbia University, New York, New York.

PHILIP W. MEILMAN, Ph.D., Chief of Consultation-Liaison Services, Office of Counseling and Human Development; Coordinator, Alcohol and Drug Programs; and Assistant Professor, Department of Psychiatry, Dartmouth College, Hanover, New Hampshire.

W. J. KENNETH ROCKWELL, M.D., Staff Psychiatrist, Counseling and Psychological Services, Duke University, Durham, North Carolina; Assistant Professor, Department of Psychiatry, Duke University Medical School, Durham, North Carolina.

ALLAN J. SCHWARTZ, Ph.D., Chief, University Health Service, Mental Health Section, University of Rochester, Rochester, New York; Associate Professor, Department of Psychiatry, University of Rochester School of Medicine and Dentistry, Rochester, New York; Consulting Editor, *Journal of American College Health*.

PAUL A. WALTERS, JR., M.D., Director, Cowell Student Health Center, Stanford University, Stanford, California; Assistant Professor, Department of Psychiatry and Behavioral Sciences, Stanford University School of Medicine, Stanford, California.

LEIGHTON C. WHITAKER, Ph.D., Director, Psychological Services, Swarthmore College, Swarthmore, Pennsylvania; Clinical Professor, Department of Health Sciences, Hahnemann University School of Medicine, Philadelphia, Pennsylvania; Editor, *Journal of College Student Psychotherapy*.

Acknowledgments

Various people have assisted us in the preparation of this book. JoAnne Medalie, Bonnie Tyler, Irma van Dam, and especially Julie Grayson have reviewed and improved versions of the introduction and Chapter 1. Fran and Nancy Cauley, David Grayson, Catherine Luongo, and Rick Wilson have helped in other, equally important ways. Our colleagues, both within the counseling centers and in the larger college communities at the State University of New York at Purchase and Iona College, have provided the kind of supportive work environment that has enabled us to dedicate ourselves to this undertaking. We would especially like to acknowledge our clients, the college students we work with, who are the inspiration for this book and the source of abiding professional satisfaction. We also wish to salute ourselves for maintaining a successful collaboration through the inevitable ups and downs of this kind of project. For our next joint venture, we plan to write a manual on couples therapy for coeditors!

Contents

Introduction

PAUL A. GRAYSON
KATE CAULEY

College and university psychotherapists are an unusual combination—partly generalists and partly specialists. Like old-fashioned general practitioners, they must respond to every problem that comes up in their community: "My girlfriend just broke up with me"; "I don't feel like studying anymore"; "Can you cure panic attacks?"; "Last night I almost cut my wrists again"; "I have a secret I haven't told anyone here: I'm a bulimic [child of an alcoholic, gay, manic–depressive]." The problems are diverse, and so are the persons who present them. College students vary greatly in underlying issues, personality style, degree of impairment, family and cultural background, and receptiveness to psychotherapy. At the same time, college psychotherapists also must be specialists. Their area of expertise is partly the college student population, which, for all its variety, has certain distinctive characteristics that require modifications in treatment. College psychotherapists also must be specialists on the college or university setting, because the conditions under which they work have an effect on their practice. The collegiate clinical setting particularly raises concerns regarding the purity of the therapist's role, confidentiality and privacy, time constraints on treatment, and potential distractions for the therapist—concerns we return to shortly.

In *College Psychotherapy*, we have attempted to address both components of our field—its comprehensiveness and its particularity—in a practical, down-to-earth volume that should be useful to anyone who practices or wants to understand the counseling of college students. In this book, nearly two dozen prominent college psychotherapists from a cross-section of institutions—colleges and universities, large and small schools, private and public institutions—explain how they handle common problems within our subspecialty. They tell us about the difficulties college students have, the conclusions therapists may draw about these difficulties, and the exchanges that take place in the client–therapist relationship; they bring these themes to life with liberal use of case studies and brief examples. Although a one-volume collection can hardly anticipate every therapeutic problem, this book suggests approaches to some of the most typical of the difficult challenges that college psychotherapists encounter.

Our contributors are among the most respected and experienced members of our profession. Each has been chosen for general authoritativeness and for familiarity with his or her chapter's subject. The authors do not speak with one voice or hew to a single party line. Though they pay most attention to psychoanalytic and developmental theories, stressing different aspects of these broad theories, they also (where they deem appropriate) recommend cognitive therapy, drug therapy, group therapy, behavioral approaches, and a miscellany of other strategies and interventions. Perhaps not all our contributors would agree, but we take this diversity as an endorsement of our own recommended treatment approach: discriminating eclecticism. College students are too heterogeneous to be fitted to a standardized treatment regimen.

Since we are mainly concerned with practical problems, not theoretical matters, we have not agonized in these pages about such terminological distinctions as "psychotherapy" versus "counseling," "patient" versus "client," or "counseling center" versus "mental health service." Though the functions of psychotherapy and counseling can usefully be differentiated (see May, 1986, and Ducey, Chapter 9, this volume), our impression is that in practice most college professionals use one or the other of these terms not because of their differing functions, but because of public relations considerations ("therapy" sounds more exalted, "counseling" more welcoming) or because of therapists' professional affiliations (clinical psychologists, psychiatrists, and social workers like to say they do "psychotherapy"; counseling psychologists and educational and pastoral counselors prefer to say that they do "counseling"). Similarly, for all practical purposes, one therapist's "patient" is another therapist's (or counselor's) "client." As for the psychotherapy office's name, although "counseling centers," "mental health services," "human development centers," and "psychological service centers" all carry their own connotations, the problems they face and services they provide are essentially the same, regardless of the sign on the door.

Let us briefly consider four main concerns the collegiate setting raises that may influence the therapeutic process. First, the setting jeopardizes the purity of clinicians' traditional, noninvolved therapeutic role.

This is because college psychotherapists do not work in an environment removed from the lives of their clients. Rather, therapists and students belong to the same community, and therefore therapists are in a position to wield direct, extratherapeutic influence on students' lives. The impetus to do so may come from students, who want therapists to plead for them with other persons on campus; from parents, faculty, student affairs personnel, or administrators, who want therapists to offer opinions or make decisions that affect students; or from the therapists themselves, who see opportunities to act as students' advocates. The opportunities to wield influence are manifold. Therapists may involve themselves in the academic arena by trying to arrange extensions, incompletes, or reduced course schedules for students. They may cast a vote in housing decisions regarding room changes or permission for students to live on or off campus. They may participate in decisions regarding financial aid, full-time or part-time student status, or dismissal from school for psychological reasons or suitability for return after psychological withdrawal or leave.

The problem is that all such moves may damage the traditional therapeutic relationship. Clients may be tempted to slant material so that therapists make decisions in their favor. Indeed, students may originally come to the counseling center in order to persuade therapists to intervene on their behalf. Clients may have less incentive to take responsibility for their own lives and solve their own dilemmas, and they may have less motivation to understand the source of their problems. Consider a freshman who is acutely unhappy about living with a roommate and threatens to leave school unless the therapist helps her to get a single room. Why, her therapist might ask, does she view living with another person as unbearable? What has she done to contribute to the current impasse, or to find a solution? To what extent is the immediate problem a repetition of past crises, an expression of larger issues? But questions like these, central to a normal therapeutic inquiry, may seem irrelevant to the student if the therapist accedes to her request.

In order to preserve the purity of therapists' function, there are counseling centers that refuse to involve themselves in students' lives except during severe, life-threatening emergencies; even then, the responsibility for managing the crisis may pass over into other hands. On one campus we know of, the director of the counseling center prides himself on running an independent office, like an off-campus group practice, and on having virtually no contact with the rest of the college community (particularly the administration). But most college counseling centers and most college therapists occasionally do use their influence to intervene in students' lives, either because doing so is officially a part of their duties or because they believe that the plight of certain students calls for such action. In their judgment, students who have reality-based problems, or suffer from severe anxiety or depression, or are at risk of dropping or flunking out—to say nothing of planning to commit suicide—may need to be bailed out, even if this means temporarily stepping outside psychotherapists' usual noninvolved role. Our own position on this matter is that there is no easy answer, only relative costs and benefits. Every college counseling center must be guided by both a general philosophy and an assessment of the particular case in order to decide whether to wield direct influence in a student's life.

The second set of concerns—confidentiality and privacy—is closely connected to the first. As members of the college community, who interact professionally and perhaps socially with administrators, student affairs personnel, and faculty, college psychotherapists have plenty of opportunities to breach confidentiality and disclose privileged information about clients. There are two reasons why they may be tempted to do so. For one thing, requests for information often have a legitimate basis, at least in the minds of questioners. Thus persons who refer students to the counseling center may quite understandably expect information in return to assuage their anxieties. "I know you can't tell me anything," they may say, paying lip service to confidentiality, "but I'm worried about Roger. Is he okay?" A variant on this theme is the appeal for advice on the grounds that the therapist has information that will help the appealer to help the student: "Can Ron be left alone in his room tonight?" "Should I give Martha an extension on her term paper?" The chief student affairs administrator—to whom, not incidentally, the director of counseling may report—may also ask about a student's attendance and progress in therapy in order to make disciplinary, housing, or other administrative decisions. Parents may call for advice or evaluations of their children. These calls sometimes represent meddling, but often do not; parents who are legitimately concerned about their sons and daughters may feel that therapists are in the best position to help them. Besides the plausibility of these requests, the other reason why therapists may be tempted to breach confidentiality is the wish to gain acceptance for the counseling center, as well as the normal human desire to be liked and fit in. Satisfying questioners can help therapists and their service to find acceptance and belonging within the college community. Withholding information, on the other hand, may mark therapists as unhelpful, priggish, or snobbish—elitists who feel that no one else is qualified to know what they know. Holding secrets is not a good way to gain popularity or generate referrals.

Related to the problem of confidentiality is the challenge of protecting the privacy of the therapeutic relationship. Unlike therapists in other settings, college psychotherapists, particularly on small campuses, routinely come across their clients outside the therapy office, whether through chosen roles (e.g., teacher, speaker, or workshop leader) or informally in the library, gym, or parking lot. Some students welcome these contacts; they make therapists appear accessible and human. But other students find that therapists' public visibility damages the atmosphere of exclusiveness and "otherness" that they feel is essential to the therapeutic relationship. It is uncomfortable for these students to make personal disclosures to someone who later may sit at the next table in the school cafeteria; it may even feel uncomfortable simply to walk to and arrive at the counseling center, where teachers or friends may observe them. Adding to the problem of privacy in a college setting are "entangling therapeutic relationships" (Arnstein, 1972), in which therapists have clients who are socially or romantically involved with each other. Instead of viewing the therapeutic interchange as a private and exclusive dialogue, clients may wonder what their friends and lovers are saying about them, and what their therapists must be thinking.

College psychotherapists can take various measures to protect the confidentiality and privacy of the therapeutic relationship. To protect confidentiality, they can educate members of the community and parents about what they can reveal, what they cannot reveal, and why. They can set up clear and consistent procedures, such as routinely obtaining written consent from clients prior to divulging information about a case. They can also learn the art of satisfying others' needs for guidance without disclosing what these persons originally felt they had to know. To protect privacy, they can keep a low profile, and try to refer close friends and lovers of their clients to other therapists within the counseling center. But despite these precautions and despite therapists' upholding the highest ethical standards, students' concerns about confidentiality and privacy may intrude on the therapeutic relationship and require responsiveness on the part of the therapists.

The third issue at a college setting concerns time constraints on treatment. Because of the academic calendar, there is a maximum of 14 continuous weeks available when students start therapy at the beginning of the term, and correspondingly less time when treatment begins later in the semester. Thus, quite apart from therapists' theoretical convictions or the developmental needs of college students, college psychotherapists must learn to work within the confines of brief (or very brief) psychotherapy. Furthermore, on many campuses the supply of therapists is insufficient to meet the demands for psychotherapy, especially during periods of peak usage. Counseling centers may respond to client overloads by imposing a limit on sessions, setting up waiting lists (which inevitably discourage some clients), or spacing out appoint-

ments to perhaps every 10 days, 2 weeks, or more (which also may discourage students and can reduce the effectiveness of treatment). The
strategy of spacing out appointments also may entail scheduling clients
at the next available time slot, often at a different day and hour from
the last appointment; the therapy therefore lacks the rhythmic regularity
of a standing weekly appointment. Another constraint on appointments
is the occasional need to delay or postpone students' sessions because
of psychological crises or other pressing events, or (more often) because
students themselves, for various reasons, are late, cancel appointments,
or do not show up. All in all, college psychotherapists must master the
art of working with students when and as often as conditions permit.
They do not have the luxury private practitioners enjoy of scheduling
clients solely on the basis of therapeutic need.

The final issue concerns potential distractions for therapists. These
may come about if therapists play other roles within the counseling
center or on campus, such as those of crisis manager, supervisor,
administrator, researcher, course instructor, workshop leader, and com-
mittee member. It may be hard after handling a crisis, for example, to
"switch gears" and fully attend to the next client's regular therapy
appointment. Political or financial currents on campus may also distract therapists, who may find themselves more closely involved in the
fate of their service or institution than in the lives of their clients. Other
potential distractions are the responses that other campus personnel
may have to the counseling center. Every campus in the land, for example, has a few faculty members or staff persons who have unrealistic
expectations about what therapists can do. These persons may collect
chronically troubled students, even when the students are not in crisis, and deposit them at the counseling center's doorstep, as if to say,
"Here, do something about this."

Another familiar campus type who presents a much different problem is the skeptic who is dismissive of psychotherapy. One professor
liked to tell his introductory psychology class that outcome studies
negated the value of psychotherapy; every year after this lecture, a student currently in treatment would start questioning the commitment.
Even supporters of the counseling center may favor a de-emphasis of
psychotherapy, arguing that college therapists' time should be turned
over to outreach and "prevention" rather than individual appointments.
(Of course, so-called "prevention" generally results in increased demand
for individual psychotherapy.) Still another figure familiar to counseling centers is the amateur counselor—often a troubled student's
classmate—who would rather handle the student's problem alone than
make a referral to the counseling center.

As with the other issues we have discussed, college therapists can take steps to alleviate this set of problems. They can arrange their schedules so as to minimize intrusions of other activities on their therapy hours. They can educate various sectors of the campus about the purposes, values, and limitations of psychotherapy in order to minimize others' misunderstanding and opposition. Ultimately, however, college therapists have to learn to "tune out" the distractions. Part of the expertise of their position consists of the ability to put aside outside concerns so that when they are with clients they can fully concentrate on the task at hand.

In the chapters that follow, these themes appear as background motifs. We turn now in Chapter 1 to an overview of college psychotherapy clients and their responses to college psychotherapy. Chapters 2 through 16 are devoted to particular problem areas and appropriate therapeutic responses.

REFERENCES

Arnstein, R. L. (1972). College psychiatry and community psychiatry. *Journal of the American College Health Association, 20,* 257–261.
May, R. (1986). Boundaries and voices in college psychotherapy. *Journal of College Student Psychotherapy, 1*(2), 3–28.

1

The College Psychotherapy Client: An Overview

PAUL A. GRAYSON

It is no wonder that college students feel the need to come to the counseling center. Most of them are in late adolescence, a stage of life when they are expected to accomplish key developmental tasks. The strains from these tasks are sufficient in themselves to cause psychological symptoms. At the same time, many college students also evidence abnormalities in thinking, mood, and behavior that are "deeper" and more chronic than maturational struggles. These psychopathological tendencies interact with the emerging developmental strains, together leading to almost certain difficulties at college. Furthermore, college students confront reality-based challenges from the college environment, which is a stressful place to live. Environmental pressures can intensify developmental strains and catalyze psychopathological reactions; conversely, these latter, internal elements can impair students' ability to cope with the pressures at college.

All in all, there is a lot for college students to deal with. The first half of this chapter examines these three factors—developmental, psychopathological, and environmental—showing their points of overlap as well as their distinctive features. The purpose is to give an overview

This chapter contains passages adapted from "College Time: Implications for Student Mental Health Services" by Paul A. Grayson, 1985, *Journal of American College Health, 33,* 198–204. Copyright 1985 by Heldref Publications. Adapted by permission of the Helen Dwight Reid Educational Foundation.

of the sources of college students' maladjustment, the reasons why they seek psychological assistance.

The second half of the chapter moves from etiology to treatment. The same elements that account for students' problems, it turns out, also influence the process of psychotherapy. Three broad questions about therapy are addressed here: (1) What decides the length and course of therapy? (2) How do students relate to therapists (and how do therapists feel in return)? (3) How well do college students make use of psychotherapy, and why?

DEVELOPMENTAL STRUGGLES

College students who fall within the traditional age range (18–22 years) are in a transitional stage between adolescence and adulthood. They are moving away from dependency on their families and the familiar routine of home and high school, and entering a new, uncharted, more independent, and freer way of life. As they make this transition, they confront and are expected to master basic developmental tasks. Unlike academic expectations, however, these tasks are not clearly defined. Students must somehow glean from their parents' example and teachings, observations of friends, their own sense of need, and trial and error how to reach maturational goals. Confusion and missteps are inevitable. Seen from this perspective, students' psychological concerns are, in part, normal growing pains. Problems of adjustment are to be expected during such periods of rapid developmental change.

The first basic task is to separate from parents and home—or rather, to further the process of separation that has been going on since toddlerhood. Accomplishment of this task ordinarily consists of living away from home for the first prolonged period (and, in a sense, leaving home forever), and correspondingly relying less on parents in managing day-to-day affairs. College students who do not separate enough from parents cannot fully invest in undergraduate life or, more importantly, acquire the skills needed later to live as independent adults in society. Yet while greater separation is necessary, so, as a rule, is a measure of ongoing attachment. Unless the family situation is intolerable, most college students need from families a fund of emotional support as well as a foundation of financial support. Ideally, therefore, separation is a gradual process, proceeding at a pace that students are mature enough to handle, and a flexible process, in which students pull away and come back as needed. This is not only a difficult course for students to navigate, but it also places difficult demands on the family. Parents or siblings may not understand students' shifting needs or may have needs of their own in conflict with those of students. They may then complicate students' struggles with separation by binding students to the home, prematurely pushing them away, or sending contradictory signals. In one typical case, a student felt obligated to spend weekends at home consoling her lonely, bitter, divorced mother, and even during the school week she held herself back from her studies and the campus social scene. Separating from home meant, to both her mother and her, abandoning her mother as her father had done years before.

Closely intertwined with separation is identity formation (Arnstein, 1984; cf. Blos, 1946). According to Erikson's (1950, 1968) famous schema, the formation of identity is the central adolescent developmental issue; it is a complex process that requires integration of childhood identifications, libidinal drives, basic aptitudes, and social opportunities. Identity formation, like separation, is a continuation and intensification of a childhood maturational process. Although children acquire a sense of who they are, it increasingly falls to the late adolescent—the college student—to make critical identity-related choices and commitments (e.g., to decide on a college, an academic major, a career direction, political and religious values, sexual standards, and a preferred type of social network). College students betray identity concerns when they are unable to make or stand by critical decisions, or are chronically dissatisfied with their choices, or defend against uncertainty and self-doubt through overidentification with (in effect, losing themselves in) another person, a group, or a cause. The root causes of identity problems vary. Students may lack the core of self-confidence necessary to overcome the obstacles in a given path, or they may resist choosing a direction because it means foreclosing all the others and giving up childhood dreams of omnipotence.

A third developmental theme, again bound up with the other two, is achieving intimacy with peers. Although Erikson assigns this task to early adulthood, after identity formation has been accomplished, the Group for the Advancement of Psychiatry (1983) places intimacy alongside separation and identity formation as a critical task of the college years. College students have had close peer relationships before college, but now, as they turn away from the family, they are increasingly expected to satisfy their intimacy needs in friendships and romances. Like identity formation, intimacy involves making commitments, as students single out congenial others for a special bond. Ongoing difficulties with this task can be seen in patterns of isolation, noncommitment, and overdependency. An immediate difficulty associated with intimacy is the romantic breakup, among the most stressful undergraduate experiences, which can escalate into academic paralysis and suicidal risk.

Additional developmental tasks have been cited by developmental theorists. Farnsworth (1966), for example, states that students must learn to deal with authority; cope with uncertainty and ambiguity; and find security, feelings of adequacy, and self-esteem. Arnstein's (1984) survey of a number of writers adds the tasks of genital primacy, sexual identity, stability of character structure, development of a time perspective, and commitment to a set of life goals. Though these tasks are important, and self-esteem in particular stands out as a paramount concern for college students, by and large they can be subsumed under the main three: separation, identity, and intimacy.

In considering developmental tasks, we must be mindful of the influence of the college environment, our third etiological factor. Though "developmental" implies strictly age-related processes, changes set in motion solely by internal maturational forces, in reality, of course, developmental tasks are linked to a person's living situation. The college student's living situation, which has been called a moratorium or prolonged adolescence (Blos, 1946; McArthur, 1961), "pulls" for late adolescent developmental changes. One consequence of this environmental influence is that older, returning students may separate belatedly from their families of origin, or may free themselves from unsatisfactory marriages. Older students face identity challenges too, as they decide on academic majors and career paths, and re-examine themselves in light of their academic and social experiences at school. The impact of developmental tasks on a student's adjustment depends, therefore, on his or her participation in the college experience. Regardless of age, full-time, residential students are more likely than part-timers and commuters to be caught up in developmental struggles that are traditional for 18- to 22-year-olds.

Another aspect of the college experience is that different developmental challenges arise at different times, so that developmental strains—especially those pertaining to separation and identity formation—tend to come up in a sequence. Recent writings (e.g., Arnstein, 1984; Grayson, 1985; Margolis, 1976, 1980, and Chapter 4, this volume; Medalie, 1981) portray students as passing through four yearly stages, each with its own demands and potential pitfalls, from freshman year to senior year. Thus we can chart the course of normal development, and predict the periods when problems are most likely to occur, over the course of a student's college career.

Freshman year is a time for separation. Students (again, particularly residential students) must distance themselves from parents, siblings, other relatives, friends, pets, home, and community. From a broader perspective, they must part with the status and way of life of childhood. At the same time, freshmen must learn how to fit in within a radically new environment. Many of them share a bedroom with another person for the first time in their lives, and, also for the first time, find themselves in close daily contact with dozens of other persons who come from many diverse backgrounds. Freshmen must take increased responsibility for study habits, finances, diet, health, and housekeeping. They must cope with an intensified academic workload and perhaps heightened academic competition; with new temptations and expectations regarding sex, dating, and drug and alcohol usage; and with challenges to political and religious beliefs. Overall, the developmental work of freshman year emphasizes "both *divestment* of the past and *investment* in a new life" (Medalie, 1981, p. 75). Difficulty in managing these sweeping tasks surfaces directly in homesickness and social isolation, and also may be inferred from other problems freshmen have (e.g., academic underachievement).

Sophomore year introduces a new set of conditions that shifts the emphasis to self-examination and choice—in other words, to identity formation. By now, most students are accustomed to being away from home and living in the campus environment. Their familiarity with the college experience encourages sophomores to step back from day-to-day existence and ask questions about themselves and their lives. Introspection is further sparked by the requirement to begin choosing a direction in life, most immediately by concentrating on a few academic areas and preparing to declare an academic major. Those who have succeeded up to now simply by carrying out academic assignments face the new challenge of setting their own goals. On the social front, too, self-examination and choice are emphasized, since sophomores typically plan their own living arrangements rather than accepting assigned roommates and dormitory rooms. Some are unsettled by all these pressures to establish an identity. The challenges of identity formation associated with the second year is linked by Arnstein to the "sophomore slump," characterized by apathy and lack of interest or a sense of meaninglessness unattached to a specific cause (Arnstein, 1984; Margolis, 1976).

The junior year continues to emphasize identity concerns, but with a subtle difference. No longer is it sufficient simply to make choices and set goals. Now, past the midpoint of college, students are more and more expected to show commitment and meet goals; they are measured not by what they plan, but what they achieve. Like unaccomplished 50-year-olds, those college juniors who perceive themselves as academic, social, or romantic disappointments may feel a sense of urgency to do better, or already they may have internalized a sense of failure. During this year concerns about graduation also begin to come up (Margolis, 1980). The prototypical identity-related question, "Who am I?", is joined and given focus by the query, "What will I do after college?"

Finally, the last year ushers in another cluster of developmental challenges. Seniors, like freshmen, must separate all over again—this time from college friends, lovers, and the undergraduate lifestyle. Separation from families may also resurface as an interpersonal and intrapsychic issue, especially if parents either cut financial ties or, conversely, try to reassert a dependent relationship (Arnstein, 1984). At the same time, seniors further their identity formation as they review their accomplishments in college, prepare for life after college, and start committing themselves to adult careers and lifestyles. Though ambivalence about finishing college is as normal as ambivalence about entering, some students are terrified by the prospect of leaving, which they may express through academic decline, last-minute switches in academic majors, unfinished work, frantic efforts to cram in sexual and social experiences, or specific or generalized anxiety (Margolis, 1976; Medalie, 1981; Roulet, 1976). All in all, senior year is as stressful as the first year: "Data suggest ... the highest levels [of psychological disturbance] occur at the times of transition into and out of college" (Schwartz & Reifler, 1984, p. 685).

This stage theory for the college career can help therapists to identify the source of college students' presenting problems. For example, surprisingly poor grades by an apparently capable freshman may signify underlying conflict about separating from home; bad grades by a senior may point to fears about graduating and establishing an adult identity. A freshman may cling to an unsatisfactory romantic relationship in order to stave off homesickness; a junior may do so in the belief that "it's now or never" to find a partner. The stage model is also a useful gauge to measure the seriousness of a problem. Just as bedwetting is considered more serious for 8-year-olds than 4-year-olds, so is failure to commit oneself to an academic major more serious in the last year of college than the second. In general, any problem that surfaces later than expected in the college cycle should sound a warning signal to the therapist that psychopathology may be involved.

PSYCHOPATHOLOGICAL TENDENCIES

While college students wrestle with developmental issues, many are also struggling with deeper, more chronic (i.e., psychopathological) problems. Students bring to college tendencies toward self-defeating and frankly self-destructive behaviors, disturbances of mood and thought, and impairments of self-concept and capacity to relate interpersonally. Though their defensive styles tend to be less "hardened" and their symptoms less entrenched, compared to those of an adult population (Blaine, 1961; Hanfmann, 1978; McArthur, 1961), some do manifest such crystallized patterns of disturbance; others have a succession of changing symptoms that add up to chronic disturbance; and still others have acute, intensely disruptive symptoms. This psychological profile contrasts with college students' generally robust physical health. "Students are a boring population to treat medically," a college physician once remarked to me. "You people in counseling get all the action."

The boundary between normal developmental issues and psychopathological tendencies is fuzzy; depth and chronicity are relative, somewhat subjective criteria. The differentiation is best made in conjunction with corroborating evidence. If a student reports a history of family problems—abuse, neglect, an emotionally ill parent, extreme family conflicts, or reversal of parent–child roles—then the current difficulty may well have a psychopathological basis. The same can be said when students' self-presentation in therapy is extreme—unusually distant, confused, indirect, suspicious, confrontational, or self-abasing. Seasoned therapists acquire a sixth sense to detect emotional disturbance from students' behavior within the first minutes of the opening session. Therapists' assessment of psychopathology also depends on their own theoretical orientation. Those of a psychoanalytic bent, for example, may see emotional disturbance where humanistically oriented therapists may discern struggles of development. Finally, therapists' familiarity with the college scene is still another consideration. Off-campus practitioners, one will notice, often interpret students' odd statements, impulsive behaviors, and emotional swings as signs of disturbance, whereas college therapists, accustomed to students' excesses and belonging to a community that tends to tolerate them (Schwartz & Kahne, 1977), tend to be more cautious about labeling a student as emotionally disturbed.

Reflecting this diagnostic complexity, experts disagree about the extent of psychopathology within the college student population. Several early studies (Selzer, 1960; Smith, Hansell, & English, 1963; Whittington, 1963) found psychological disorders to be commonplace on campus, prompting Selzer to comment that users of college mental health services are typically underdiagnosed. Similarly, a more recent study (Dunn, Lanning, Patch, & Sturrock, 1980) found that 70% of college psychotherapy clients had a neurotic disorder and 17% had a personality disorder. But Rimmer, Halikas, and Schuckit (1982) concluded that roughly one-third of students in treatment had a diagnosable psychiatric problem—a still sizable but much lower figure. Offer and Spiro

(1987) estimate that one-fourth of entering college students are disturbed and in need of mental health care.

Whatever the true statistical picture, psychopathological tendencies are clearly not rare for college students, and often lurk behind their seemingly normal concerns of homesickness, academic problems, and relationship difficulties. When a student has psychopathological tendencies, the psychopathology and developmental strains potentiate each other. Emotionally disturbed students find it particularly hard to separate from home, form an identity, and relate well with peers. Having failed to resolve earlier developmental challenges, they lack the resources—basic trust, basic sense of autonomy, ego strength—to master these fresh challenges. Conversely, the pressure to accomplish these developmental tasks activates their latent psychopathological tendencies, upsetting whatever tenuous psychological equilibrium they have managed to maintain prior to college.

For example, Estelle, a freshman, came to the counseling center because of depression, flagging academic effort, and suicidal ideas. On the surface, her current difficulties were a recent development, since throughout high school she had excelled as a student and an actress, and, compared to her two sisters, had manifested the fewest problems. The immediate cause of her symptoms was a developmental challenge. Other students in her highly competitive college acting class were obviously more talented than she was—a realization that caused her to wonder who she really was, if not a talented actress, and what she could become. But this rather typical late adolescent issue also triggered a reaction on a more profound personality level. Estelle had always stifled her drive toward selfhood, squelching her own ideas and wishes, in an effort to be perfect and please her emotionally ungiving parents. She had cultivated a false self while neglecting genuine personality development. Now that she was no longer the best, she felt that she had forfeited her parents' approval—she was lost. It seemed futile to continue trying to be perfect, yet inconceivable to start trying to be anything less. Thus the challenge of constructing a realistic identity provoked a crisis in this young woman who had very little sense of self to build on; the combination of developmental tasks and pre-existing psychological vulnerability caused the symptoms that brought her, as they do many students, into treatment.

ENVIRONMENTAL PRESSURES

The conditions at college are a third factor contributing to the timing, form, and intensity of students' problems. Environmental concerns are usually what students notice first when, worried or frightened or distraught, they make their way to the counseling center. Though these concerns are less central, less enduring, and less important for students in the long run than developmental and psychopathological issues, reality-based pressures are not trivial. Who among us, if we had to live again in a crowded dormitory and take final exams, would not feel the psychological repercussions?

Certain aspects of the college environment have already been mentioned. This section expands on these topics and addresses additional aspects of the undergraduate experience.

The Changing Semester

The college experience contains a sequence within a sequence. Not only does a progression of events take place from freshman year through senior year, but a similar process unfolds during the semester. If, then, the 4-year college career represents a "mini-life cycle" (Medalie, 1981), the semester constitutes a mini-college career. It too advances from a disorienting beginning to an abrupt end, and it too, like a steeplechase, presents an obstacle course along the way. Both the content and the pace of these changes have a powerful effect on students.

The semester, like the college career, can be divided into four stages. The first stage, covering roughly the initial 2 weeks of school, resembles freshman year as a time of separation and orientation. Students must leave their prior living situation and adjust to their lodgings and their roommates, hallmates, or housemates. They also must either select or confirm their course schedules, depending on the institution, and adjust to these courses. Because of its transitional character, this first period elicits the most homesickness and indecision about courses, as well as the most psychiatric emergencies requiring hospitalization (Perlmutter, Schwartz, & Reifler, 1984). Next comes the relatively uneventful second stage, lasting until roughly the midpoint of the term. With separation from home and re-entry to school completed, and with academic pressure not yet consistently mounting, the emphasis shifts, as in a miniature sophomore year, to issues of identity. Students are most free to take stock and explore personal issues, set goals, and make choices—and suffer a mini-sophomore slump. The third stage, approximately from the midpoint to the weeks before final examinations, witnesses a gradual increase in academic pressure. Daily routines are not disrupted and social and extracurricular activities continue, but a sense of duty shadows these pursuits. Procrastination and poor study habits are on many therapy clients' minds. Finally, in the fourth stage, during the last 2 weeks of the term, nonacademic concerns are eclipsed as final examinations and term papers monopolize students' attention. Students may dramatically alter sleeping, eating, and study habits; feelings of anxiety and fatigue may predominate. Meanwhile, the upcoming vacation looms as another sudden transition, and in that sense the fourth stage parallels senior year as a time to anticipate and plan for life outside the college.

As important as the content of these changes is the *pace* of change, dizzying by the standards of adult living. Because of the kaleidoscopic conditions, certain vulnerable students are almost perpetually in crisis, as they struggle to find a response for each new stressor. Yet because stressors also pass by quickly, the symptoms students develop may not have time to "set." Consider a tendency toward indecisiveness. Whereas an adult who is indecisive about changing jobs can postpone taking action indefinitely, until vacillation about the matter becomes virtually a habit, the college student who is indecisive about a course schedule cannot delay too long. The semester deadlines force a decision, like it or not, and the student must move along.

Unstructured Time

The orderly sequence that characterizes the semester breaks down on the more immediate level of students' day-to-day existence. Although during the semester events and deadlines take place according to schedule, students' daily routines—particularly for persons who do not hold jobs—are comparatively unscheduled (Boyer, 1987). With the exception of class hours, which are by no means a sacred commitment to everyone, students' time tends to be their own, neither supervised by parents nor bound by a 9-to-5, Monday-through-Friday routine.

Having a relatively free schedule challenges students to manage their time wisely and to exercise self-discipline. On the academic front, they must plan their daytimes and evenings with an eye on deadlines that are weeks and months away. Many understandably err by going to an extreme—studying too little, too late, or practically every waking moment. Free time also can present a challenge on the psychodynamic level, confronting certain students with anxiety or depression, which they then may ward off through escapist behaviors—abnormal sleep habits, overemphasis on leisure activities, irresponsible spending of money, binge eating, or substance abuse. One chronically depressed student who felt particularly bad during his free afternoons escaped by taking long naps; these predictably brought on a new problem, nighttime insomnia. Another student assuaged anxiety during the empty evenings by endlessly playing video games. A bulimic woman passed lonely afternoons in her apartment fighting the temptation of the refrigerator. Tellingly, such symptoms often disappear during summer vacations when students hold full-time jobs. Required to work, eat, play, and sleep at set times, according to a schedule, students then manage these activities with consistency and moderation.

Living with Peers

Students help one another develop. Feldman and Newcomb (1973) assert that peer groups assist separation from home, support the academic goals of the college, offer emotional support, teach getting along with different kinds of people, and support old and new values. But living with peers can also be stressful and create psychological difficulties. Consider the implications for residential students of belonging to such a close, self-contained, largely self-governing society, not unlike that of the stranded children in *Lord of the Flies*. One consequence is that late adolescents, whose incomplete identities make them ripe for peer influence anyway, are further stimulated to follow one another's lead. The peer society and its constituent activity and friendship networks establish norms and mores that are hard for the individual student to resist. Sometimes the end result is substance abuse, an eating disorder, or ill-considered sexual experimentation.

Although college students in recent years increasingly come from diverse backgrounds (Hersh et al., 1981), students' peer society still constitutes a narrow social universe. Sometimes students feel trapped inside their tiny rooms; they cannot get away from one another. If a suitemate is loud, a roommate is obnoxious, or an ex-lover rooms down the hall, the college student literally has to live with the source of suffering. This sense of confinement may cause students to feel that parts of themselves are unappreciated and unexpressed; nobody treats them here like a son or daughter, a grandchild, a big brother or sister. The homogeneous environment can touch off developmental concerns centered around self-esteem and identity. Individuals may find it hard to maintain positive feelings about themselves when everyone else is more or less doing the same things, and some, inevitably, are doing them better.

It may seem odd that college students can also feel isolated and lonely. Certainly campus housing facilities and college functions offer unparalleled opportunities to meet people and make friends. Yet some students, shy or lacking social skills, fare poorly in the social marketplace. Even if they manage to make a few friends, their usual experience is to be blackballed by a fraternity or snubbed by a clique or roommate— to be reminded of their low social position. Loneliness and the pain of being an outsider are magnified in such an intense social climate, where everyone seems to be judged and ranked, and it is clear to all who does and does not fit in.

Academics

College can be an uncongenial setting in which to learn. Like high school, it calls on students to compete with their classmates for grades and to try to impress their professors, who assign the grades. This arrangement, which essentially recapitulates family themes of sibling rivalry and parental authority (G. Amada, personal communication, 1988), may cause unconscious conflicts that lead to academic paralysis. Some students back off from the competitive challenge; others rebel rather than submit, as they see it, to professors' authority. Though they may remain avid readers or writers or painters in their spare time, these students do not, or feel they cannot, complete their coursework. Ducey's chapter in this volume examines these issues in detail (see Chapter 9).

We should not forget, furthermore, that college work is for many students intrinsically difficult. College texts, class lectures and discussions, oral presentations, term papers, exams, laboratory classes, and performance classes (e.g., painting or dance) demand skills that not all students possess. Thus, not every academic problem is a psychological conflict in disguise. On the contrary, some seemingly nonacademic concerns have their origin in academic pressures. The student who expounds on the meaninglessness of life may really be troubled, more than anything, by the history midterm he or she just failed. A useful therapeutic rule regardless of students' presenting complaints is to check periodically on their standing in all their courses, just as one would routinely check for substance abuse or suicidal ideation.

The Environment in Context

The college environment has many components, and all of them, large and small, contribute to students' psychological adjustment. Students react to the quality of food served in the cafeteria, the warmth of the campus grounds and the architecture, the strength of the varsity and intramural sports programs, the availability of clubs and activities, and—yes—the existence of a well-regarded counseling center. An overcrowding problem that causes students to "triple" in rooms designed for two persons can lead to a rash of roommate clashes and psychological symptoms. Community resources surrounding the college or university also affect students' adjustment. A student body that cannot easily get to off-campus pizza parlors and movie theaters will develop a collective cabin fever.

We should also bear in mind that individual students help shape their college environment, just as infants through their temperamental makeup influence the parenting they receive. A socially introverted student who majors in biochemistry and a "party animal" who takes the easiest possible course schedule inhabit different collegiate worlds.

IMPLICATIONS FOR THERAPY

Students respond to treatment in characteristic ways, and their treatment, in turn, must be adapted to their special needs. We turn now to consider three broad treatment issues within the college context.

The Length and Course of Therapy

One of the important questions within college psychotherapy, particularly in light of the academic calendar and therapists' heavy caseloads, is the appropriate length of treatment for a client. Generally speaking, a strong psychopathological component calls for open-ended, long-term assistance, either at the counseling center or, if time constraints make this impossible, through a referral to an off-campus therapist. The aims of treatment then depend on the student's area of need. Students who have lacked a close attachment to a parent may need, above all else, a supportive relationship with the therapist—a "reparative relationship," as Medalie and Rockwell explain in Chapter 5 of this volume. Those who evidence entrenched patterns of disturbance consistent with a neurosis or personality disorder need therapeutic support as well, but probably within the context of a more traditional, insight-oriented approach. For clients who are in acute crisis or whose symptoms do not remit with psychotherapy alone, psychotherapy needs to be supplemented with pharmacotherapy and/or stays at the infirmary or a hospital, as Arnstein explains in Chapter 2. The chief point is that long-term treatment, provided either continually or during times of special need, is often necessary for the more troubled student to make it through college.

When the psychopathological component is less prominent, long-term treatment may be contraindicated. Since late adolescents normally need to loosen the dependent bond with their parents, it is usually inadvisable for them to form another dependency on an adult through a long-term relationship with their therapist. Brief therapy supports "normal" students' need to develop into autonomous adults (Blos, 1946; Bragan, 1980; Haggerty, Baldwin, & Liptzin, 1980; Pinkerton & Rockwell, 1982)—and also, of course, fits in well with the academic calendar. Some counseling centers employ the strict brief therapy model that Mann (1973) espouses, which fixes the number of sessions—usually at 8, 10, or 12—and predetermines the end point (Bragan, 1980; Podolnick, Pass, & Bybee, 1979). Whether or not treatment follows this format, therapy of 10 sessions or so, though brief by the standards of long-term therapy, is still long enough for a sustained, focused investigation, making it ideal for exploring developmental concerns. Meanwhile, students whose problems are predominately reality-based or situational—who are perhaps reacting to a feud with a roommate or a romantic breakup or a run of bad grades—may need even less time, a "very brief" therapy. Often a few sessions are sufficient, like jump-starting a fundamentally sound car, to help them surmount the immediate crisis and proceed successfully on their own.

The length of therapy is an unreliable indication of students' level of satisfaction. Some students come to the counseling center merely wanting a "mental health clearance" attesting to their normality (Rockwell, 1984), or they have scheduled a session just to satisfy an insistent parent, friend, or dean. Many other students do want therapeutic help, but they see their problems as strictly situational. (Therapists and clients often have different views on this point; see Schwartz & Kahne, 1977.) When their situation changes, they see no reason to keep coming. Students who come to the counseling center for any of these limited purposes may be satisfied with a very brief contact of three or fewer sessions (Dorosin, Gibbs, & Kaplan, 1976; Haggerty et al., 1980; Rockwell, Moorman, Hawkins, & Musante, 1976). On the other hand, sometimes very brief contacts betoken client dissatisfaction. According to Hanfmann (1978), students give up on therapy when therapists are incompetent, do not encourage clients, do not give an adequate explanation of how therapy helps, or have a derogatory manner. Brief therapy in these cases is treatment that has failed.

In my own experience, the length of therapy cannot be assumed in advance; one is too often surprised by who stays and who drops out. This places a burden on therapists to make the most of the opening sessions, since they may not get a second chance. Ideally, the opening sessions should be geared toward encouraging doubtful students who need therapy to come back; yet the opening should stand on its own as a useful experience, in case students do not return. The art for therapists lies in judicious pacing. Therapists do not want to move too quickly or probe too deeply with fearful, defensive students, but they also must not be too cautious with impatient students; the typical late adolescent is not long on patience. Sensitive use of active therapeutic methods—asking for students' own hypotheses, testing their receptiveness to other interpretations, identifying connections across situations, prompting passive clients with questions, collaboratively working toward a focus—may reassure students that therapy is effective but is not too threatening.

When therapy does extend for half a dozen sessions or more, its course is typically less steady than at other settings. Even when students are motivated to work on underlying issues, not just situational difficulties, the focus of therapy may blur and shift as students become distracted by the succession of stressors they encounter. For college students, last session's issues may seem as remote as last week's newspaper headlines. Therapy also does not necessarily follow the stages one would expect from psychodynamic theory. Termination, in particular, tends to be diminished as a focal point of treatment, especially when therapy extends into the fourth stage of the semester. By this time previously motivated clients show up for appointments deprived of sleep, or say that they have been thinking only about studies, or discontinue sessions altogether. Instead of the healing resolution predicted by Mann's (1973) theory, therapy closes in these cases on an anticlimactic note, not with a bang but a whimper.

Of course, so long as a student remains in school, one can never say for certain that therapy has come to a close. Many clients schedule sets of sessions at different points in their college careers, and, in effect, end up in long-term treatment. Such intermittent courses of therapy have the advantages of meshing well with the academic calendar, discouraging undue dependency on the therapist, capitalizing on students' times of peak motivation, and allowing reluctant students to enter therapy in stages. In addition, intermittent therapy permits students to work on *different* concerns when they arise (e.g., leaving home, choosing a major, and preparing to graduate), or the *same* concern whenever it comes up (e.g., preparing for final exams). Theoretically, students then can use time off from therapy to assimilate gains, so that each time they re-enter treatment with a greater level of maturity. On the negative side, intermittent courses of therapy may signify resistance to therapeutic involvement, a series of false starts rather than incremental gains, especially when each time students request a change of therapists.

The Therapeutic Relationship

The relationship between college students and college therapists is influenced, up to a point, by the college setting. Generally speaking, students associate college therapists with the institution and therefore see them as less mysterious, less removed, less "different" than off-campus therapists. This perception is reinforced when college therapists are visible in roles such as those of instructor, workshop leader, or speaker. How students feel about therapists' institutional connection depends on the individual. Some, as explained in the introduction to this volume, feel that the privacy of the therapeutic relationship is compromised and that confidentiality is jeopardized. Others react to college therapists as if they are not fully professional and offer an inferior product. "I want," said one student who requested a referral for private treatment, "to see a *real* therapist." On the other hand, some students feel reassured; they feel that college therapists are accessible and easy to talk to, since they are part of the familiar college scene.

Another factor within the college setting affecting college therapists and private practitioners alike is the abundance of potential confidants, on and off campus, that college students can draw on. For every student who confides only in the therapist, there is another, it seems, who freely airs personal problems and even recaps therapy sessions with roommates, friends, lovers, resident assistants, student affairs personnel, or faculty advisors, not to mention parents, friends, and maybe therapists from home too. When this happens the college therapist's role is reduced to that of one counselor among many. This role may be further diminished by the limitations of time caused by the academic calendar and therapists' heavy caseloads.

But more critical for the therapeutic relationship than the setting are the personal issues of college students, especially their developmental position. Some students feel the need to attach themselves strongly to college therapists, like children seeking support, guidance, and approval from parents; these students may be searching for a nurturant relationship to make up for past deficits in parenting. Students at a more advanced developmental level, whose needs and transference responses are different, tend to be more conflicted about dependency. They may grow attached to the therapist but feel ashamed of the bond, explaining that they should be able to get by without the assistance of an adult. Or they may actively resist a close therapeutic relationship. Engaged in an internal (and sometimes external) struggle to separate from their parents, they may unconsciously transfer the battleground to the therapist's office, where they keep their distance or challenge the therapist's opinion, as if by staying aloof or arguing they can protect their fragile sense of identity. (These tactics also unconsciously protect certain clients from the rejection and loss that they have learned dependency brings.) Finally, there are others, at a still higher level of development, who are able to relate to a therapist more as one adult to another, without feeling a threat to their sense of autonomy.

Students may keep maneuvering to find a developmentally comfortable level of closeness to the therapist. Sometimes their stances toward the therapist follow a developmental progression, as the therapeutic relationship and students themselves mature. An initially child-like, dependent posture may be succeeded by an uncertain, somewhat wary position *vis-à-vis* the therapist, which may, finally, evolve into a collaboration between equals. Such shifts may be detected through subtle cues, such as students' form of address for therapists. One sophomore, at the beginning stages of therapy, deferentially called me "Dr. Grayson," then for a long while never referred to me by name; finally, nearing graduation, he started to call me, politely but more assertively, "Paul."

College students also use the therapeutic relationship for the identity-building purpose of testing who they are. Thus students may be flirtatious or seductive with the therapist to establish that they are attractive and lovable. They may show off their vocabularies or reasoning ability to prove the power of their minds and the force of their personalities. The therapist's office is a safe place to experiment with ways of being.

This brings us to the difficult question of when a therapist should bring up the subject of a student's feelings and behaviors toward the therapist. Clearly, if a basic rapport is lacking, or if a student acts toward the therapist in consistently off-putting or self-defeating ways that also presumably contaminate other relationships, then it may be necessary to raise these issues in therapy. Just as certainly, strong feelings of anger, fear, hurt, or disillusionment in relation to the therapist also need to be brought out into the open. But there are reasons for college therapists to be hesitant about making numerous "transference interpretations." For one thing, students who anticipate a short-lived therapy contact to work on immediate problems may balk at questions about their feelings toward the therapist, just as they would object to an in-depth inquiry into their dreams or their childhood. "I came here to work on my problem," they may feel, "not to talk about you and me." More importantly, negative or seemingly inappropriate feelings and behaviors that students display toward the therapist may have a more adaptive, less psychopathological significance than they would coming from an adult population. Distancing or oppositional tactics may not represent "hardened" character defenses, but may be developmentally appropriate resistances against feelings of dependency; seductiveness or showing off may not be defenses against genuine relating, but may represent valid attempts at self-discovery. By not calling into question students' reactions within the therapy hour, therapists implicitly endorse students' right to try on different relating styles for size.

Therapists' countertransference responses also enter into the therapeutic relationship, and of course need to be closely monitored. College therapists may feel frustrated or saddened when students terminate because of semester endings and graduation; good treatment is rarely carried through to its completion. More unsettling still are cases where students unexpectedly drop out after a seemingly promising start or ask to be referred to another therapist on the service. The danger here is that instead of engaging in constructive self-scrutiny, asking themselves candidly what might have gone wrong, therapists begin to lose faith in themselves or blame clients. Dropouts are inevitable in college psychotherapy, and therefore college therapists have to remain sensitively open to the students who can work with them without being thin-skinned about the students who do not.

Therapists may find themselves reacting in complementary ways as clients play out in treatment their developmental themes or psychopathological issues. An aloof or competitive student may elicit corresponding aloofness or competitiveness in the therapist. Needy clients "pull" for parental feelings; therapists must watch out, as Medalie and Rockwell observe in Chapter 5, for rescue fantasies. Therapists must also be aware of anger or disapproval or feelings of helplessness when students ask for more than the therapists can or feel they should give. College therapists also may be charmed, even aroused romantically or sexually, by the youth, attractiveness, verbal skills, intelligence, and bright prospects for success of their clients, who epitomize the "YAVIS" patient. Alternatively, these qualities may bring a pang of wistfulness or envy to therapists who no longer feel quite so young, attractive, and ambitious themselves. Despite their charms, college students occasionally can be boring, especially on those days when every one of them seems to be ruminating about term papers or housing selection. Sometimes it is a challenge for college therapists, who are progressing through adulthood in their own lives, to find excitement and growth from clients who are forever wrestling with the same late adolescent issues.

Lastly, and fortunately, college therapists often feel gratified in their relationship with college students for the compelling reason that students benefit from the service therapists provide.

Students' Potential for Progress

Although some college students prematurely drop out and others seem to be spinning their wheels in treatment, a sizable segment make good use of psychotherapy. Blaine (1961) extols college clients as "remarkably vulnerable [but] remarkably treatable" (p. 380), and Hanfmann (1978) expresses "joy at seeing how fast and how far many counseling students [are] able to move" (p. 1). Let us conclude our overview of the college psychotherapy client by briefly considering, in light of earlier observations, why this should be true.

A main asset students bring to therapy is their developmental stage; they are at an age that is ripe for self-exploration. College students are old enough to use reason, apply perspective, and—to a certain extent—control impulses. Naturally reflective and introspective, they have cognitive tools lacking in earlier stages of development to consider their experience and learn from it. Yet college students are not so old as to have strong resistances to change. Still rapidly developing, still making major decisions, their characters, to borrow William James's metaphor, have not yet set like plaster. Adding to this advantage of age is students' situation. Because students are moving away from home, the family's influence is diminished. College students can question what they have been taught by parents, who no longer have absolute authority over them. Meantime, the new living situation they have entered, though stressful, is also an opportunity to learn, a laboratory in living. Here they can observe and try out new behaviors, make new relationships, formulate new ways of thinking, develop an identity. In short, two of the factors that account for college students' problems—their developmental stage and environmental pressures—are the same ingredients that go into their therapeutic success.

Sometimes these advantages can lead to remarkable therapeutic progress. Ellen, for example, was referred to me at the counseling center by an academic dean after she had failed several courses during her first semester at college. She described herself as "ugly and stupid" (she was neither) and said that she was too obsessed by thoughts of her home life to concentrate on schoolwork. For roughly the first 8 weeks of therapy, her memories poured out in a torrent as she told of incessant criticisms and neglect by her divorced, alcoholic parents and of threats and beatings by an older brother. As she recounted episode after episode of horrific experiences, such as the time her drunken mother stormed through the home throwing dishes at the children, I, who mostly listened and occasionally validated her perceptions, wondered whether short-term therapy could make a difference. Could such despair and self-condemnation, rooted in a lifetime of traumatic experiences, actually be alleviated by these few hours of emotional release? Yet toward the end of the term Ellen somehow turned a corner, and the sessions began to take on a surprising character—lighter, more topical, with touches of humor and self-confidence. The family history seemed to relax its hold on her imagination, and she turned her attention to friends, personal strengths, and studies. She got straight B's in her courses. She showed signs of liking herself.

During two follow-up sessions after the summer vacation, Ellen reported occasional setbacks of intense self-doubt and preoccupation with her family. But her grades were still strong, she was active with friends and activities, and she had about her an air of incipient self-acceptance that was so conspicuously lacking at the beginning of therapy just 6 months earlier. Though I knew she had more problems to work out, I could also understand her wanting to take a pause and enjoy the gains she had made. She was no longer someone to worry about. She would continue to grow on her own.

Though Ellen's case is by no means the norm, anyone who does therapy with college students can furnish examples of equally remarkable progress. Every year, a number of college students who come to the counseling center in pain and disability end up feeling and doing substantially better, thanks to their capacity for growth, changes in their situation, and a supportive therapeutic relationship. College students are a population of clients who improve, and therapists can ask no greater satisfaction than that.

REFERENCES

Arnstein, R. L. (1984). Developmental issues for college students. *Psychiatric Annals, 14,* 647–652.

Blaine, G. B. (1961). Therapy. In G. B. Blaine & C. C. McArthur (Eds.), *Emotional problems of the student* (pp. 364–380). New York: Meredith.

Blos, P. (1946). Psychological counseling of college student. *American Journal of Orthopsychiatry, 16,* 571–580.

Boyer, E. L. (1987). *College: The undergraduate experience in America.* New York: Harper & Row.

Bragan, K. (1980). Separation conflicts and therapeutic strategies. *Journal of the American College Health Association, 28,* 222–224.

Dorosin, D., Gibbs, J., & Kaplan, L. (1976). Very brief interventions—a pilot evaluation. *Journal of the American College Health Association, 24,* 191–194.

Dunn, R. F., Lanning, J. R., Patch, V. D., & Sturrock, J. B. (1980). The college mental health center: A report after ten years. *Journal of the American College Health Association, 28,* 321–325.

Erikson, E. H. (1950). *Childhood and society.* New York: Norton.

Erikson, E. H. (1968). *Identity: Youth and crisis.* New York: Norton.

Farnsworth, D. L. (1966). *Psychiatry, education, and the young adult.* Springfield, IL: Charles C Thomas.

Feldman, K. A., & Newcomb, T. N. (1973). *The impact of college on students.* San Francisco: Jossey-Bass.

Grayson, P. A. (1985). College time: Implications for student mental health services. *Journal of American College Health, 33,* 198–204.

Group for the Advancement of Psychiatry. (1983). *Friends and lovers in the college years* (Report No. 115). New York: Mental Health Materials Center.

Haggerty, J. J., Baldwin, B. A., & Liptzin, M. B. (1980). Very brief interventions in college mental health. *Journal of the American College Health Association, 28,* 326–329.

Hanfmann, E. (1978). *Effective therapy for college students.* San Francisco: Jossey-Bass.

Hersh, J. B., Backus, B. A., Brody, R., Forti, R., Hoffer, D. C., & Prieto, E. J. (1981). Emerging ethical issues in college mental health services. *Journal of the American College Health Association, 30,* 61–63.

Mann, J. (1973). *Time-limited psychotherapy.* Cambridge, MA: Harvard University Press.

Margolis, G. (1976). Unslumping our sophomores: Some clinical observations and strategies. *Journal of the American College Health Association, 25,* 133–136.

Margolis, G. (1980). Learning to leave: Problems of graduating—Clinical observations and strategies. *Journal of the American College Health Association, 28,* 336-338.

McArthur, C. C. (1961). Distinguishing patterns of student neuroses. In G. B. Blaine & C. C. McArthur (Eds.), *Emotional problems of the student* (pp. 52–72). New York: Meredith.

Medalie, J. (1981). The college years as a mini-life cycle: Developmental facts and adaptive options. *Journal of the American College Health Association, 30,* 75–79.

Offer, D., & Spiro, R. P. (1987). The disturbed adolescent goes to college. *Journal of American College Health, 35,* 209–214.

Perlmutter, R. A., Schwartz, A. J., & Reifler, L. B. (1984). The college student psychiatric emergency: A descriptive study. *Journal of American College Health, 32,* 191–196.

Pinkerton, R. S., & Rockwell, W. J. K. (1982). One or two session psychotherapy with university students. *Journal of the American College Health Association, 30,* 159–162.

Podolnick, E. E., Pass, H. L., & Bybee, D. M. (1979). A psychodynamic approach to brief therapy. *Journal of the American College Health Association, 28,* 109–113.

Rimmer, J. D., Halikas, J. A., & Shuckit, M. A. (1982). Prevalence and incidence of psychiatric illness in college students: A four year prospective study. *Journal of American College Health, 30,* 207–211.

Rockwell, W. J. K., Moorman, J. C., Hawkins, D., & Musante, G. (1976). Individual versus group: Brief treatment outcome in a university mental health service. *Journal of the American College Health Association, 24,* 186–190.

Roulet, N. L. (1976). Success neurosis in college seniors. *Journal of the American College Health Association, 24,* 232–234.

Schwartz, A. J., & Reifler, C. B. (1984). Quantitative aspects of college mental health: Usage rates, prevalence and incidence, suicide. *Psychiatric Annals, 14* (9), 681–688.

Schwartz, C. G., & Kahne, M. J. (1977). The social construction of trouble and its implications for psychiatrists working in college settings. *Journal of the American College Health Association, 25,* 194–197.

Selzer, M. L. (1960). The happy college student myth. *Archives of General Psychiatry, 2,* 131–136.

Smith, W. G., Hansell, N., & English, J. (1963). Psychiatric disorder in a college population. *Archives of General Psychiatry, 9,* 351–361.

Whittington, H. G. (1963). *Psychiatry on the college campus.* New York: International Universities Press.

2

Chronically Disturbed Students

ROBERT L. ARNSTEIN

It may seem ironic in a book about college psychotherapy to devote a chapter to "chronically" disturbed students. First, students are in school for a defined length of time and are expected to complete their degrees and move on, so that the issue of chronicity is often moot as far as providing psychotherapy or psychiatric support in college is concerned. Second, most counseling centers and/or student health services have limited resources; therefore, they stress short-term treatment and are usually not prepared to offer service to a student over an extended period of time.

Both these reasons on closer examination turn out to be more complex and less true than they initially appear. In regard to the first point, students may be in school for a defined length of time, but this is not necessarily short. Although this volume is entitled *College Psychotherapy*, many colleges are embedded in universities, and counseling centers at these institutions offer services to graduate and professional students as well as to undergraduates. Thus, the number of years a person is in student status may range from 2 years (a junior college or associate degree program) to 11 years (4 undergraduate years and 7 years of doctoral work). Moreover, although some graduate schools impose limits, others allow extensions. Although the United States does not officially have an occupational category of "permanent student" (as seems to have existed in 19th-century Russia), if one considers part-time programs with extensions for special circumstances, the time period as "student" may be very long. And because there is no institutional rule against multiple degrees, someone, assuming that he or she has a source of financial support, could reasonably prolong studying almost indefinitely.

Furthermore, regardless of length of stay, there will be a certain number of students with chronic problems, either because they have developed what appear to be unremitting symptoms after entering or because they have gained admission despite prior psychiatric difficulties. For example, a number of individuals currently are returning to college and to graduate study in order to change careers or to complete education that was interrupted for a variety of reasons, ranging from lack of interest in academic work to a need to earn money to a wish to devote time to child rearing. Because these individuals are usually older, some may well have developed rather entrenched emotional difficulties prior to re-enrolling in the institution and may wish to take advantage of available college therapy resources.

In regard to the second point, college counseling centers may stress short-term treatment, but they inevitably tend to respond to crises and to severity of symptomatology, so that the student who presents with chronic problems unquestionably will be an object of concern and often will elicit a heavy investment of staff resources. Sometimes other therapeutic arrangements can be made, but if these are not possible because of financial difficulties or because the college is located at some distance from a medical center, such students may place considerable strain on counseling staffs. This may either simply overtax the staff in the absolute sense, or it may cause concern that an inordinate amount of time is being devoted to a few individuals and raise issues about the allocation of available resources.

These points raise philosophical questions about the underlying mission of a college counseling or psychiatric service—questions that are often not clearly framed or answered. Is the underlying purpose to deal with psychopathology in the students? Is it to help students develop their individual potentials? Is it to help them complete whatever academic degrees they are pursuing? Or is it all three? In 1920, Frankwood Williams addressed these questions by citing four aims of a college mental health service that almost 70 years later still seem valid:

1. The conservation of the student body, so that intellectually capable students may not be forced unnecessarily to withdraw, but may be retained.
2. The forestalling of failure in the form of nervous and mental diseases, immediate or remote.
3. The minimizing of partial failure in later mediocrity, inadequacy, inefficiency, and unhappiness.
4. The making possible of a large individual usefulness by giving to each a fuller use of the intellectual capacity he [sic] possesses, through widening the sphere of conscious control and thereby

widening the sphere of social control. (cited in Farnsworth, 1957, p. 11)

The first two obviously deal with ameliorating psychopathology, and the latter two attempt to encourage maximum development of personal potential. Incorporated in the first is the aim of helping students to complete the relevant degrees. Nothing, however, is said about how one should respond if a student is making little headway toward a degree. An undergraduate usually must complete a specified number of academic credits in a specified time period in order to be promoted and to continue uninterrupted progress toward a degree. If these levels are not reached, the student is required to withdraw. In some periods of graduate study, however, little objective progress is required. If no progress is made, does the counseling service have an obligation to continue therapeutic work with the student, and, if so, for how long?

DEFINITIONS

An immediate consideration in any discussion of chronically disturbed patients involves the definition of "chronic." Standard diagnostic systems such as the *Diagnostic and Statistical Manual of Mental Disorders*, third edition (DSM-III; American Psychiatric Association, 1980) do not contain a group of chronic conditions (other than Personality Disorders, which have a somewhat different implication). The term "chronic" appears in DSM-III as a coding indicator of the length of time in certain disorders that symptoms have existed. For example, Substance Abuse Disorders may be designated (by a fifth coding digit) as "continuous," and Schizophrenic Disorders may be designated as "subchronic" (defined as from 6 months to 2 years) or "chronic" (over 2 years). The recent revision of DSM-III (American Psychiatric Association, 1987) omits the term "continuous" for Substance Abuse, but retains the use of "subchronic" and "chronic" for Schizophrenia.

In addition to the individual who displays symptoms consistently over a period of time, the person who has periodic outbreaks of symptoms between symptom-free periods may be described as having a "chronic" condition. Although linguistically this condition would be more accurately described as "recurrent," if the recurrences are frequent enough over a prolonged period, it seems reasonable to view the illness as chronic. DSM-III and DSM-III-R address this aspect of chronicity by using "episodic," "in remission," or "recurrent" for various disorders.

This latter definition of chronicity resembles the concept often applied to alcoholism. There is a general tendency to believe that "once an alcoholic, always an alcoholic," even though the individual may not currently be drinking; this implies that an alcohol problem is always subject to recurrence, no matter how long the person's period of abstinence may have been. Although the analogy of chronic disturbance to alcoholism may be inexact because of the greater volitional component in alcoholism, there are certainly types of psychiatric illness in which the concept of "cure" in the usual medical sense is problematic at best.

Further complicating the definition of chronicity, it is not clear that there is any general agreement as to the duration of illness necessary to establish it as chronic. Obviously, any rigid duration is arbitrary, but the duration of 2 years established by DSM-III for Schizophrenia seems reasonable. The nature of the illness, however, may influence criteria of chronicity. Two manic episodes in the course of a year might raise the presumption of chronicity, in which case the designation would probably be determined more by the fact of recurrence than by the time period involved, but the designation of chronicity might be abandoned if a sufficiently long period of asymptomatic functioning followed the second episode.

Finally, in defining the chronically disturbed patient, one can focus on the degree of severity and restrict the category to individuals who are quite disturbed, or one can focus on the patient's self-defined need for treatment manifested by a recurrent request for psychotherapeutic support.

In this chapter, "chronic" is defined as a general category to refer to more severely upset individuals.

TYPES OF CHRONIC ILLNESS

In considering the student as chronic patient, the setting cannot be ignored. Specific syndromes must be viewed in the context of the academic task at hand: for example, how the student's symptoms affect the ability to study. Psychotic illnesses usually interfere significantly, but they may either be in remission or sufficiently well controlled that academic work is possible. Personality disorders are often sufficiently severe that functioning is problematic, but not so severe that it is impossible. Some students display neurotic symptoms, such as depression, anxiety, or eating difficulties, that fluctuate in severity but do not in themselves preclude studying. Some present with debilitating obsessional symptoms. Finally, some suffer from neuroses that interfere directly with the academic process, such as acute exam anxiety or an inability to finish assigned papers. The latter may be chronic only in the sense that they recur consistently in the educational setting, but they become a problem because the individual wishes to complete an educational program for practical or symbolic reasons. If the student withdraws, he or she may have no difficulty whatsoever with a job (even a stressful job), but on return to student status, study difficulties recur.

Psychotic Illnesses

Psychotic illnesses come in various shapes and sizes. The two most obvious categories are schizophrenia and affective disorder. Although most individuals in the midst of acute episodes will not be able to pursue their studies, even this generalization has its exceptions. I remember one patient who, as a result of delusions that involved dormmates making fun of him, retired to his room and rarely ventured forth. Despite a thought disorder that included clear auditory hallucinations, his intellectual functioning remained unimpaired; feeling confined to his room because of his delusions, he studied more, and his already high grades rose even higher.

In general, psychotic episodes will incapacitate the student, at least temporarily. The existence of rapid treatment methods, however, including the use of medication, may allow for relatively speedy reintegration, and the individual may be able to complete course work and continue in college. For some there may be a rather complete "sealing-over" process, but for others there will be an uneasy balance between psychotic symptomatology and nonpsychotic functioning. In such cases, careful thought must be given as to how to maintain that balance or increase the tilt toward effective functioning. These individuals are at risk for recurrences. Although there are some who have a single psychotic episode and never have another, more will continue to display reactions that are on the border of psychosis, and will accurately be characterized as chronically disturbed. At the present state of knowledge, moreover, there is no way of predicting who will and will not have a recurrence, so that all must be regarded as potentially at risk.

Personality Disorders

The personality disorders represent a different type of problem and as a diagnostic group are less well defined. Severity can range from mild symptoms that may cause discomfort to quite serious pathology that essentially cripples the student's ability to function or leads to behavior that runs afoul of institutional regulations and lands the student in disciplinary trouble. By definition, personality disorders are rather stable conditions and do not easily change either as a result of time or treatment. However, when a disorder interferes significantly with a student's academic progress, the student has a right to expect that efforts will be made to help, and it is not easy to ascertain what these efforts might be. Presumably, some variety of long-term therapy is indicated, and it is just this type of therapy that may be difficult for any college to provide. If the college is located near an urban center, there may be clinics to which the student can be referred, but these may not exist for those colleges in more isolated locations.

One particular personality disorder needs comment—borderline personality disorder, because of the severity of symptoms and their tenacious resistance to change. Many years ago, I (Arnstein, 1958) did a small study on a group of students who seemed to be "borderline." Admittedly, the diagnosis was applied then to a more acute and fluid condition rather than a personality disorder, but the patients included in the study would in most instances qualify as "chronically disturbed." In one situation the student was supported through a very difficult freshman year and then was not seen again until his third year of graduate school, after which he continued to be symptomatic for several years while completing his doctorate and working in a postdoctoral capacity. It was possible to offer him therapy throughout, but if he were to appear today, it probably would not be possible to provide the same amount of support because of demand by a greater number of students for service from the counseling staff.

Neuroses

In the neurotic category, one would include certain depressive, anxiety, and obsessive–compulsive disorders. The first can frequently be quite pervasive and continue indefinitely, with periodic suicidal actions or threats and a clearly dysphoric mood. There may be events that precipitate the state, but often the events do not seem sufficient to cause the degree of upset, and when one event has been coped with, another tends to take its place. Similarly, obsessive–compulsive symptoms and panic attacks can occur with considerable persistence; not only do they cause the individual great discomfort, but they may also interfere significantly with ability to function. Obsessional states in students frequently take the form of an inability to choose courses or to decide about participation in a sport or an extracurricular activity such as a play. Although most colleges have well-defined deadlines for course choice, an obsessional individual often demonstrates a remarkable ability to stretch the deadline, to maintain the decision in flux, and simultaneously to generate a tremendous amount of anxiety that interferes with all pleasure as well as effective academic work. Similarly, the individual who participates in a sport for a period of time, but then decides it has lost its appeal or is taking too much time, may have difficulty giving it up. Such a student may develop rather severe anxiety and depression in connection with the decision. Again, this may seem to be an acute problem, and may be resolved by the end of the sport season; however, it usually occurs in an individual who is susceptible to such obsessional states, so that it may recur in a slightly altered form in an ensuing year.

Eating Disorders

A rather frequent syndrome involves eating problems. These range from life-threatening anorexia nervosa to a relatively mild case of bulimia that is troubling to the individual but is not necessarily serious. Anorexia nervosa is, of course, the most alarming syndrome. It may be a particularly difficult problem on campus, because the afflicted individual (usually a female student) is quite pleased with her thin state, and, if anything, feels that the loss of a few more pounds would enhance her attractiveness. Thus, the alarm is often sounded (at least in a residential college) by roommates and/or deans, and it may be quite difficult to convince the student even to go to the health service, let alone to participate in a program designed to increase weight. Once treatment is instituted, improvement may be slow, and it is a rare individual with severe weight loss who does not run a chronic course.

Bulimia, on the other hand, may be a less acutely severe problem, but some aspects of the institutional setting make it difficult to treat. Most students live away from home; in consequence, their eating routine is likely to be less well ordered than at home, even granting that meals in some homes may be reasonably chaotic. If the student is in a residential college, most have cafeteria-style dining halls, so that the amount of food that may be consumed is not limited. If the student is living in an apartment, he or she may eat irregularly or exist on foods that are easy to binge on. Thus, the external environment may not be conducive to any kind of orderly eating regimen, and bulimic symptoms can thrive in such conditions.

Substance Abuse Disorders

Another prevalent campus syndrome is that of substance abuse. Alcohol is currently the most widely used drug, and inevitably a number of students will develop chronic problems with alcohol. However, because drinking is a traditional and highly valued college activity, it often is difficult to convince a student that a problem exists. Further-more, it is well known that alcoholism is very difficult to treat and that relapses are frequent, so that anyone with an alcohol problem should probably be viewed as chronic.

The campus is not a remote island, so that in addition to alcohol, almost any drug that exists in the culture may make an appearance. Most recreational drugs are addictive, psychologically if not physiolog-ically, so that a student may present with a problem with any one—cocaine, heroin, marijuana, amphetamines, barbiturates, and hallucino-gens. Over the years, campus use of one or another has waxed and waned, and the likelihood of severe problems will vary somewhat with the specific drug. The problems, however, are not dissimilar, and they are very likely to be chronic.

Academic Disorders

Finally, there are chronic problems, already alluded to, that relate to the academic task. These are not included in DSM-III, so the applica-tion of the term "disorder" may be overstating the pathological aspect, but anyone who has worked as a counselor or therapist on a college campus is extremely familiar with such problems. Inability to complete assigned papers, while obviously not life-threatening, can be a symp-tom that is very difficult to modify and inevitably interferes directly with academic success. It is often self-limiting as a therapeutic chal-lenge for a counseling center: The student is required to withdraw, but the same student often returns to try again, the problem recurs, and the student presents to the counseling service in an even more desper-ate mood. Furthermore, some graduate students attempting to com-plete their dissertations may be able to postpone the final deadline almost indefinitely, and in the meantime they seek treatment in an attempt to resolve the problem. The other relatively common problem is exam anxiety, which by definition is acute, but, if recurrent, can be considered a chronic disorder.

Developmental Problems as Chronic Illness

In addition to the problems listed above, which are generally not age-specific, there are a few conditions that are age-related in nature and associated with the developmental phase of the college student. These include issues related to emancipation from the family of origin and difficulties stemming from identity problems. Although one hopes that any difficulties that arise will be resolved so that adult development may proceed smoothly, it is not impossible to see a senior who is still having separation difficulties, and such a concept as Erikson's (1980) "identity diffusion" indicates that if the identity issue is not resolved satisfactorily, it may become chronic. A version of the latter concept is currently included in DSM-III (American Psychiatric Association, 1980) as Identity Disorder, which is characterized by distress regarding long-term goals, career choice, friendship patterns, sexual orientation and behavior, religious identification, moral value systems, and group loyalties.

Sexual Problems

Problems of sexuality may not in themselves be primary in creating chronic disturbance, but they are an exceedingly common contributing factor. Because college students of traditional age are almost always in the throes of experimenting with and attempting to establish satisfactory modes of sexual behavior, uncertainties and failures in this area often add greatly to anxiety, depression, and even suicidal ideation at times. Furthermore, although some individuals negotiate the experimental stage relatively smoothly, others have repeated failures or abortive attempts, so that the sexual problems become chronic in their own right.

TREATMENT

General Principles

There are several general principles relevant to treating the chronically disturbed individual. First, a stable therapeutic relationship is desirable, whatever the treatment mode. Such a relationship with a single therapist both provides a kind of anchor for the patient, and also, because of the therapist's familiarity with the patient, facilitates the ability to change the intensity of treatment by varying the frequency of the therapeutic sessions. If therapists change, the patient must re-establish a working relationship; although this may at times be advantageous, the repetition of history may become so burdensome if changes are frequent that the patient is tempted to avoid therapy. Furthermore, having worked with the patient through prior crises, the therapist may develop greater ability to weather such periods, since he or she knows that they have been resolved in the past without drastic measures (e.g., hospitalization). Although some record of past therapeutic interaction will presumably be available to a new therapist, it is difficult to convey accurately the "feel" of an acute episode, and many record systems will not convey such information despite the excellence of the system and the best intentions of the prior therapist.

Second, the impact of the setting must be taken into account. The student role creates both opportunities and dangers for the chronically disturbed patient. In general, college allows a certain amount of flexibility, so that a missed class or a late paper is usually not so disastrous as missing work or making an error on a job. Moreover, an academic environment tends to be rather tolerant, so that eccentricity may be noted but not necessarily condemned, and a variety of behaviors may be considered more or less acceptable. On the other hand, this tolerance may be disadvantageous if the student responds to the lack of structure and becomes more depressed or suffers an increase in anxiety because the assignment remains to be done, even though not doing it has initially relieved stress. Although colleges and programs vary considerably in their academic difficulty, the relationship of the student's intellectual ability to the expected standard of performance affects the margin that a given individual has in the amount of work necessary to pass a course, and, consequently, in the amount of transient disability that can be overcome.

Third, an obvious consideration in treating the chronically disturbed student is the academic calendar. Since some institutions have a long summer vacation, the counseling service may be closed, or the student may have plans to leave the campus. Arrangements must be made for these possible gaps in the availability of therapy. In addition to vacation periods, there are clearly defined stress periods during term time (e.g., end-of-semester exams and final submission dates for assigned term papers), which may increase the student's anxiety considerably and create acute crisis points within the broader stream of ongoing disturbance.

Therapist Issues

An important factor in the treatment process is the impact of the therapist's attitude toward chronically disturbed students. This is not easy to describe and may be subtle, but must certainly be considered. First, when and how the label of "chronic" is assigned to a patient, and who assigns it, are all relevant. Some therapists have an unshakable therapeutic optimism and always feel that just a little more time in psychotherapy or a change in medication or a different behavioral approach will induce a marked improvement or "cure." Others are more impressed with the tenacity of certain types of psychopathology if a period of time has elapsed and no great improvement is noted, and thus at that point they may set very limited goals. Just how long it takes for a therapist to reach that conclusion, and what determines when it is reached, are not so clear.

Furthermore, it may be very difficult to predict how the therapist's attitude will affect the patient's therapeutic course. The subject of hope and its influence on therapy is interesting and complex, and needs further elucidation. There is now a growing realization that some psychotic individuals do not seem to respond to any therapy, whereas others respond but have recurrent relapses. This view probably does not represent a change in actual psychopathology, but results from an attitudinal change on the part of therapists. When psychotropic medications, such as lithium and neuroleptics, were first introduced, there was an upsurge of therapeutic optimism that all psychoses would now be controllable indefinitely. This euphoria gave way to the realization that, helpful as these medications may be, they are not panaceas. The therapist's beliefs about the nature of psychoses and their treatment—specifically, about the usefulness of medication, exploratory individual psychotherapy, supportive psychotherapy, group psychotherapy, environmental manipulation, and family involvement—all affect choice of treatment and in all probability the process itself. Furthermore, a therapist's convictions about treatment for nonpsychotic chronic conditions also vary and may range from a belief that psychoanalysis is indicated to a greater emphasis on behavioral therapies. If these are not available, the therapist may be pessimistic about the effectiveness of the treatment that can be offered.

When treating chronically disturbed patients, the therapist is recurrently faced with situations created by the patient that are very anxiety-producing, because they involve threats to the patient's welfare or life or possibly even danger to the community. Consequently, in treating such patients, therapists often will take risks, and they will vary in their ability to tolerate the resulting anxiety. When, for example, a patient is known to have the means for a serious suicide attempt but refuses hospitalization, the therapist is faced with a very difficult decision. What will the consequences of involuntary hospitalization be, and how does one weigh the possible negative consequences against the risk of a suicide attempt? With a chronic patient, the therapist may suffer a kind of "burnout" phenomenon: The therapist may tolerate a crisis relatively well the first few times it occurs, eventually to be overcome by a "Not again!" feeling if recurrences continue. This feeling may be even more pronounced if the new crisis occurs after a period of relatively intact functioning, during which the therapist is lulled into a sense of therapeutic accomplishment and the belief that crises are events of the past.

These considerations lead to what may be loosely (if probably inaccurately) called countertransference issues. If the anxiety mentioned above becomes too great, the therapist may find ways to terminate treatment. This may be appropriate if the anxiety causes the therapist to be paralyzed or to lose sound clinical judgment, but it simultaneously may be devastating to the patient, who feels confirmed in the inner belief that the situation is hopeless. Furthermore, a shift in therapists may cause the patient to feel abandoned, but in some cases it may be the only move to make. If so, it is probably best for the therapist to be clear about his or her feeling and to communicate this to the patient. Termination that really occurs because of the therapist's anxiety but is explained on some other basis is likely to be more confusing and upsetting to the patient.

Other feelings that a therapist may have involve rescue fantasies, either competitive (he or she will succeed where a prior therapist has failed) or Pygmalionesque (the student is brilliant, and helping him or her to complete a degree and go on to fame will give the therapist a vicarious sense of worldly accomplishment). These fantasies may be useful if they help the therapist cope with a difficult patient, who is making little progress or even undergoing a relapse. However, they run the risk of causing the therapist to be disappointed, which may not be easy to hide from the patient. The therapist may even wonder whether the effort being expended is worthwhile. Finally, when working on a college campus, the therapist's anxiety may be increased by criticisms from students or other campus personnel of the treatment being provided.

Specifics of Treatment

When treating a chronic psychotic patient, one may employ psychotherapy or medication, or more often a combination of both. At times one may arrange brief stays in the infirmary if such a facility exists on campus, or possibly even short admissions to a psychiatric ward. Group therapy may also be a beneficial adjunctive treatment mode. Psychotherapy may be exploratory and insight-oriented, or it may be supportive, using primarily techniques such as reassurance and encouragement. Although the latter are not generally considered to be effective techniques with neurotic or acute psychotic patients, they may be quite helpful with a chronic psychotic patient if the therapist has come to know the patient very well and can relate current upsetting events to previously understood patterns of emotional response.

For example, it became clear over time that the symptoms of a particular student increased whenever he achieved a notable success, because it caused him to feel guilty about achieving beyond his family. As soon as he received either an academic honor or a job offer, he would feel that the family would be angry with him, despite all objective evidence to the contrary. The patient, although highly intelligent and psychologically sensitive, frequently failed to recognize this sequence of events until the therapist, as a result of long acquaintanceship, was able to point it out. Although this could be considered "insight," it probably acted in a more supportive sense. The therapist would phrase the interpretation so that it tended to reduce anxiety, rather than stressing the insight. For example, he might comment, "You know you tend to get upset when you've had an academic success." Then the comment might or might not be linked with the patient's feelings about his family. At other times, a more directive stance might substitute for the usual nondirective therapeutic approach. Suggestions, for example, might be couched in the form of a question: "Have you thought of exercising more frequently if you find it relaxing?" These seem like simple-minded interventions, but they can have a very supportive effect.

Inasmuch as most chronically disturbed students have a rather severe underlying feeling of inadequacy, it seems important in therapy to avoid statements or questions that may be heard as criticism. Thus, many of the issues (e.g., lateness and missed or canceled appointments) that are traditionally explored in psychotherapy may be better left unaddressed. If the therapist feels that they must be addressed in order to maintain the integrity of the treatment, it is important to be alert to any reaction on the patient's part that suggests a feeling of being criticized, to identify its source, and (if possible) to explain why the behavior is being explored. Even the therapist's identification of a feeling of anger in the patient may be heard as a criticism, because many individuals grow up with the belief that anger is wrong; they may not understand that the therapist regards becoming aware of angry feelings as potentially beneficial.

Medication

Prescribing medication for chronically disturbed students does not necessarily differ greatly from prescribing medication for chronically disturbed nonstudents of similar age. The fact of chronicity, however, immediately raises questions about possible side effects from continuing use, the most alarming being tardive dyskinesia from neuroleptics. The possibility of kidney damage from long-term lithium use must also be seriously considered. Both risks, however, must be balanced against the effectiveness of the medication in correcting the symptomatology that may be interfering with a patient's functioning. In addition to the possible hazards of sustained use, there may be side effects that interfere with specific academic tasks, such as sedation that may cause falling asleep in class or while studying, and visual blurring that may interfere with reading. Although the latter may be corrected with eyeglasses, it still may cause the patient to refuse to comply with the medication regimen.

Other medications, such as the anxiolytics and the antidepressants, have their own problems. Although their side effects may be less bothersome, most anxiolytics have some addictive potential, and one inevitably thinks twice before starting a relatively young individual on a potentially addicting medication. The tricyclic antidepressants have some troublesome if not serious side effects, but they also can be lethal if taken as an overdose. Thus, one may be reluctant to prescribe such medication to a chronically depressed individual who displays relatively constant suicidal ideation. Lithium, although well tolerated by some individuals, may also have side effects, one of which is increased acne. This could be upsetting to anyone, but it is particularly likely to be upsetting to late adolescents who are still very concerned with and insecure about their physical appearance.

In addition to the physiological problems associated with psychotropic drugs, their use may be undercut by psychological obstacles. A certain number of students have strong philosophical objections to taking medication on a sustained basis. Sometimes these objections are based on a belief that one should not be taking chemicals into one's body on a regular basis, or on the feeling that one should not change oneself artificially. Some associate psychotropic medication with "the establishment," and view it as an attempt by the therapist to maintain an unacceptable status quo. Sometimes the reluctance may be partially based on reality (e.g., long-term effects), but it may be enhanced by the exhortations of a peer group that is especially vocal against the use of any psychotropic medication. Some students refuse medication because they do not like the way it makes them feel, although they cannot be more specific than that about the exact effect it has. Finally, some object to taking medication because it reminds them constantly that they have an illness.

Use of the Infirmary

The use of the infirmary can be especially helpful in dealing with chronically disturbed students. Even if there is no overall therapeutic program available for inpatients, the infirmary may be used as a haven to protect a student temporarily from the impact of dormitory life or to insure that the patient gets sufficient sleep. It may be used to start a patient on medication, to stabilize medication that the patient is already on, or to insure that a patient is actually taking the medication prescribed. It may be used preventively, for example, to protect a student with an alcohol problem from drinking on weekend nights when the temptation is great. It may at times be used for detoxification. On occasion, it may provide a more orderly environment, allowing a student to study more effectively. Finally, it makes it easy for the therapist to see the patient for brief periods on a daily basis, which may be extremely effective and supportive during a crisis period and even preferable to longer interviews. Although similar visits on an outpatient basis are possible, scheduling can often be difficult, and availability in the infirmary facilitates such a treatment program.

When a student is admitted to the infirmary, the stay may be brief or more extended. If brief, the admission usually occurs because of an acute crisis that may be resolved rather rapidly. If the crisis is less acute, the stay may be longer because the purpose is to improve the patient's overall functioning. The patient will be encouraged to keep abreast of academic work and will be given passes to attend classes and work in the library. Toward the end of such an infirmary stay, as discharge is approaching, the patient may be on pass all day and be in the infirmary only to sleep. Although the infirmary can be very useful, admission may be resisted by an individual with recurrent psychotic episodes because of a prior experience in which admission to the infirmary was followed by psychiatric hospitalization. Such a student may avoid the infirmary because of its associations and the fear that the sequence will be repeated.

Family Involvement

One problem that may arise with a chronically disturbed student is the need to involve the family. Recently, such organizations as the National Alliance for the Mentally Ill have made the point that families will inevitably be involved when a family member is chronically ill, and they have been critical of therapists who, citing confidentiality, fail to consult with families. With students, this is a particularly tricky issue, because they are often at a developmental stage when one aspect of their problem is the struggle for independence from their families. Thus, it may be difficult to balance a patient's need to separate from the family against his or her need for the family to play a supportive role. This points to the issue of the therapist's ability to predict the patient's course. If, when the student first presented, the therapist were certain that he or she were going to be chronically disturbed, as opposed to acutely ill but not chronically so, the therapist might approach the family differently from the beginning. Under these circumstances, the therapist might make immediate contact and attempt to discuss the implications, both immediate and long-term, of the patient's illness. It is frequently difficult, however, to make this judgment when the student first becomes ill, and because the therapist cannot be certain, he or she may be reluctant to be too pessimistic in speaking with the family or to force communication with the family if the student is opposed.

Involvement with Other Campus Personnel

For reasons similar to those for involvement with the family, treatment of the chronically disturbed student may require greater involvement with other campus personnel. These may include deans, instructors, resident assistants, chaplains, and coaches, as well as general medical health care providers. Although the usual concerns about confidentiality need to be observed, chronically disturbed patients tend to make themselves known to a variety of individuals on campus, and these individuals usually (and appropriately) see themselves in a caretaker role. Opening up, with a patient's knowledge and permission, lines of communication between these individuals and the therapist can be extremely helpful in the management of crises that inevitably seem to arise in the lives of such patients. Sometimes information about unusual behavior reported by an instructor or dean can be used by the therapist to convince the patient that medication is needed. In the case of one athlete who tended to become upset during games, the therapist (who for his own pleasure was in the stands) informed the team physician where he would be sitting. This allowed for occasional therapist–physician consultations between periods and led on more than one occasion to emergency postgame meetings between therapist and student. There is obviously a risk in such situations that the patient will begin to distrust communications between the therapist and other campus personnel, and this could lead to therapeutic problems or an interruption in therapy. More often, however, such patients recognize their need, and, if anything, are pleased that all involved are sufficiently concerned to consult with one another and spend time in trying to help.

Administrative Considerations

There are two types of administrative considerations. The first involves the use of staff resources. There is a very real tension between the amount of time and energy one would ideally offer a chronic patient and the time needed to meet the broader demand for service from students who have more transient or less severe problems. In the early days of college counseling, there was a clear intent to offer service not only to students who present with clear psychopathology, but also to students who wished to maximize their potential and enhance their emotional development (see the Frankwood Williams quotation above). Although budget pressures in recent years have often made the latter goal more of a well-intentioned hope than an actuality, the challenge of helping chronically disturbed students raises the philosophical and practical question of what obligation an institution has to an individual it has admitted. Does it have an obligation to offer treatment indefinitely to individuals with chronic problems, at the expense of others with real but less severe problems? Should there be any limitations on the treatment offered to those designated as chronically disturbed patients?

The second administrative problem relates to the student's enrollment status. Because chronically disturbed students frequently have periods of more or less total dysfunction, issues relating to medical leaves, withdrawals, and readmission frequently arise. Some colleges are quite liberal about letting students leave and return; others have regulations that limit the number of times a student may leave and expect to return. In the latter colleges, medical leaves or withdrawals may constitute a special category, and certain conditions are required (e.g., severity and recommendation by a college-affiliated physician) in order for a student to obtain a medical leave or withdrawal. Often, difficult questions of both an administrative and an ethical nature arise, and the therapist or someone else in the health service or counseling center may be involved. Because a medical leave may have certain nonmedical consequences (e.g., financial or academic) that the student feels are advantageous, who makes the final decision as to type of leave or withdrawal and how much that individual is swayed by student or parental pressure may all be at issue.

A medical leave or withdrawal usually leads to an application for readmission, and when the leave or withdrawal has been granted for emotional reasons, the college counselor may be asked to evaluate the individual during the readmission process and render an opinion about the student's readiness to return. This complicated evaluation involves assessing the student's functioning while away from college, judging the therapeutic response if the student has been in therapy, evaluating the individual's current emotional state, estimating the possibility of recurrence, attempting to predict the chance of academic success, and trying to decide what caused the illness and the relationship of its onset to the college tasks and environment. In other words, how likely is a recurrence? Is return to college likely to precipitate such a recurrence? Would postponing the return decrease the likelihood of recurrence? Are there any steps that can be recommended or required to demonstrate readiness to return or that can be suggested to increase the likelihood of success if readmission is granted? A recent article (Gift & Southwick, 1988) discusses the consequences of premature return after a psychotic episode.

Another difficult issue relates to the responsibility that the college has for the health and safety of the individual student. Can a student be required to withdraw for medical reasons if the college feels that the student's health is such that irreversible damage or even death may occur if the student remains in college? In most states, the college physician or psychiatrist can intervene and arrange for involuntary hospitalization, but such emergency hospitalization is usually time-limited, and at the end of the mandatory period the student may be released with only minor changes in psychological state or medical condition. If the student and the student's family wish the student to remain in college, a difficult impasse may ensue. Continuing suicidal threats or attempts, problems with alcohol manifested in drunken behavior, anorexia nervosa with life-threatening weight loss, and hypomanic episodes are examples of illnesses that may invoke this dilemma. Colleges differ in their methods of dealing with these crises, but there is no easy solution.

Variants on this theme occur when students who are probably not in major danger behave so as to distress roommates or to disrupt the community. One example is the hypomanic individual who needs little sleep, and consequently keeps roommates up or wakes them with phone calls in the middle of the night. Similarly, the bulimic individual who vomits within the hearing and smelling of roommates may occasion considerable anxiety and distress. Although sometimes the problem can be resolved by community action, the college counseling service is often asked to intervene, and chronically disturbed students are frequently the source of concern because the history of their problems may be well known to deans or residence hall advisors. The latter may feel that therapy is essential, and they may be correct, but if the student resists, a problem may arise because the counseling service may have policies against mandatory therapy. Thus, the service is unwilling to treat the student under these conditions, and considerable discussion may be necessary to work out a satisfactory solution.

SUMMARY

It is clear that a certain number of students are chronically disturbed. Although they may constitute a small minority of students, providing them with the therapeutic help that they ideally should have inevitably strains the resources of most college counseling centers or mental health services. As a result, the ability of counselors to serve students with less severe problems is reduced, or the service provided to the chronically disturbed students is less than adequate. This raises important philosophical questions about the mission of the college mental health service.

If psychotherapeutic support can be provided, chronically disturbed students may well be able to complete their studies. The support necessary, however, is frequently difficult to provide, and therapists often must be able to tolerate a rather high level of anxiety in conducting treatment. Although psychotherapy is usually the main method used, it may be combined with medication, environmental manipulation, and brief stays in the infirmary. Thus, management may commonly be a major aspect of treatment with these patients, and it must be amalgamated with "purer" exploratory or nondirective, insight-oriented psychotherapy. The therapist's task is not easy, and progress may be slow or even at a standstill for considerable periods of time, but the eventual result can make the effort worthwhile.

REFERENCES

American Psychiatric Association. (1980). *Diagnostic and statistical manual of mental disorders* (3rd ed.). Washington, DC: Author.

American Psychiatric Association. (1987). *Diagnostic and statistical manual of mental disorders* (3rd ed., rev.). Washington, DC: Author.

Arnstein, R. L. (1958). The borderline patient in the college setting. In B. M. Wedge (Ed.), *Psychosocial problems of college men* (pp. 173-200). New Haven, CT: Yale University Press.

Erikson, E. H. (1980). *Identity and the life cycle.* New York: Norton.

Farnsworth, D. L. (1957). *Mental health in college and university.* Cambridge, MA: Harvard University Press.

Gift, T. E., & Southwick, W. H. (1988). Premature return to school following a psychotic episode. *Journal of American College Health, 36,* 289-292.

3

Suicide and Other Crises

LEIGHTON C. WHITAKER

The purpose of this chapter is to convey an understanding of the major kinds of crises, including suicide threats and attempts, in terms that can prepare the college psychotherapist to prevent or minimize destructive outcomes and to maximize the opportunities inherent in crises. Crises often require that the psychotherapist be able to work effectively with many other members of the college community, including students who would not ordinarily see a psychotherapist. This chapter begins, therefore, by discussing resources for handling crises and then proceeds to address the characteristics of students who present urgent concerns, the psychotherapist's own particular contributions, and the importance of addressing the underlying issues (e.g., problems with self-esteem).

CAMPUS RESOURCES

College and university campus communities are well suited generally to anticipate and prepare for the prevention of some predicaments, the lessening of other predicaments before they reach our offices, and the supplying of community support to students we do see in psychotherapy. A constructive, psychologically sensitive campus community is a powerful asset in any attempt to prevent and ameliorate mental health hazards. However, there are also many challenges and limitations inherent in even the most ideal campus communities.

Many students are sent to college with the hope that they will prosper in the new environment, even though they have a history of severe emotional problems. And two major legal developments have promoted what some observers have called a mass migration of emotionally disturbed people onto campuses. Section 504 of the federal Rehabilitation Act of 1973 prohibits discrimination against emotionally or mentally, as well as physically, handicapped persons on the basis of their handicaps per se. One result of this law is that college and university admissions offices cannot routinely screen out students on the grounds of their emotional problems alone, just as they cannot screen out students because of physical handicaps. Another result is that institutions of higher learning are prevented in certain ways from dismissing students on the basis of their mental disorders per se. The reader is referred to an excellent book by attorney Gary Pavela, *The Dismissal of Students with Mental Disorders* (Pavela, 1985), for an understanding of the complex considerations entailed in Section 504 as well as of constitutional issues affecting mandatory withdrawal policies. In effect, institutions of higher learning must accept many emotionally handicapped students whom they would have screened out for admission before 1973, and they have more responsibility for emotionally disturbed students after they are admitted.

The second major legal development increasing the numbers of severely disturbed students on campuses relates to the prevalence of state laws requiring the discharge or "deinstitutionalization" of state mental hospital patients. The movement of mental patients out of public hospitals became extreme in the 1970s, and only a small fraction of state mental hospital patients have not been discharged. In California, for example, the population of the state's mental hospitals has decreased during the past 20 years from 37,000 to 3,000 patients (Amada, 1986). Colleges and universities, knowingly or unknowingly, have been greatly affected by the mass exodus. A major New England university, for example, received hundreds of "new students" from a nearby state hospital, greatly increasing crises on campus as well as requests for regular appointments for psychotherapy. These laws resulted often in a kind of reinstitutionalization of patients into college campus communities, as well as halfway houses and boarding homes. Together with the federal Rehabilitation Act of 1973, they in effect redefined the responsibilities of institutions of higher education, making them more accessible to and responsible for mentally disturbed persons.

Another problem is that the usefulness and continuity of campus resources are limited by the academic calendar, which restricts the times when students can use the resources. Because of graduation and the long summer break, fall break, spring break, and long winter recess to conserve energy, psychotherapy is frequently interrupted or even terminated (particularly by graduation) independently of students' emotional needs. In fact, the fear of graduation is a problem of crisis proportions for many students.

Campus resources are also challenged by the estranged nature of the population they serve. Most students leave home to live at college, where they have to establish themselves in new environments quite different from home physically and interpersonally, in addition to facing more difficult academic challenges. Leaving family, friends, and pets and having to cope with the on-again, off-again nature of the academic calendar make for a stressed migratory population whose migrations fit academic but not necessarily mental health timetables. For a comprehensive treatment of this and related concerns to students and parents alike, the reader is referred to *Parental Concerns in College Student Mental Health* (Whitaker, 1988).

Finally, campus mental health resources are limited by the financial constraints of institutions of higher learning, which are primarily in the business of formal education and only secondarily in the business of the "second curriculum" or "student support services." Most campus mental health services cannot afford to provide comprehensive or long-term services.

In response to these challenges and limitations, the psychotherapist who would make the most of campus resources supports their development and tries to establish effective work liaisons with deans, resident assistants (RAs), faculty, and other staff members, including health service personnel. It is also critically important to establish a contract with a psychiatric hospital, and perhaps even a special insurance policy for students to cover emergency and hospital expenses. At Swarthmore College, for example, we have a mandatory low-cost health insurance policy that guarantees payment for psychiatric emergency and hospital services for 3 or 4 days—time enough to make any other necessary arrangements. Otherwise, there would be no assurance that our students would be covered, since they come from nearly every state plus about 40 foreign countries.

Working relationships with other college personnel must vary with particular institutions and their personnel (Whitaker, 1986a). Practices regarding confidentiality, appropriate use of information, and the proper handling of emergencies must be the subjects not only of formal policy and procedure manuals, but of active, ongoing discourse. Perhaps the only thing worse than not having anything in writing about the handling of crises is not discussing the matter each year to insure that everyone concerned is aware of varied and changing student populations, professional staff, and local conditions, as well as of the professional literature. It may be good, for example, to have a written policy that a dean call parents rather than a psychotherapist in an emergency, but the dean and the psychotherapist will do well to think about, and perhaps discuss, the usefulness of this policy in each particular case as it comes about.

RAs can play a very great and valuable part in handling crises through their work of anticipating crises, mediating responses to crises, and making referrals to psychotherapists (Boswinkel, 1986). The process of referral to a psychotherapist must often be a fine art, requiring cooperation between therapist and RA, if it is to be effective. The majority of students may tend to utilize mental health services only for acute, crisis-like situations (Offer & Spiro, 1987), and many will be extremely resistant to seeing a psychotherapist even then. The psychotherapist's time is well spent in consulting with staff or students who may be able to learn the fine art of referral, especially in crisis cases.

MAKING CRISES MANAGEABLE, UNDERSTANDABLE, AND BENEFICIAL

Although crises themselves cannot be scheduled, we can allot time for them so that they can be made manageable, understandable, and beneficial. Practically, we can plan staff time and availability by having an emergency on-call system and allowing enough time to intervene. In that way, both student and therapist can begin to arrive at an understanding of the meaning of the crisis, so that the crisis, in accord with the Chinese definition of the word, can be realized as an opportunity to be creative (Tabachnik, 1973). In addition to making the mental health or counseling service highly accessible generally, and perhaps providing an especially accessible walk-in clinic (Hersh & Lathan, 1985; Johnson, Whitaker, & Porter, 1980; Love, 1983), it is important to make sure that there is no rigid limit on the amount of time available to handle a crisis. We cannot schedule 20-minute crises for students; they may need much longer to tell us their problems and to begin finding ways to solve them.

Failure to allot at least a 45- or 50-minute evaluation session has been known to result in lawsuits based on the premise that the psychotherapist or clinic fell below the average level of professional practice in the community. For example, in the case of *Thomas Speer, Administrator v. State of Connecticut* (1985), which involved a 26-year-old man's death and was ultimately decided by the Connecticut Court of Appeals, "The trial court determined, on the basis of the testimony of the sole expert witness for the plaintiff, a psychiatrist, that the intake history was inadequate to ferret out patients with suicidal tendencies" (p. 734). The appellate court agreed with the trial court that the single most important factor in determining whether a health care facility is negligent in failing to prevent a suicide is whether its agents knew or should have known that the patient in their care was suicidal. Similarly, a large university was sued after a student committed suicide following a brief walk-in clinic evaluation. Standard or average practice at the vast majority of colleges and universities is to provide at least a 45-minute session for an "initial evaluation," regardless of whether it is called an "intake" or simply a first session. Falling below this "average standard of practice" therefore would seem to leave us open to lawsuits in cases of suicide or other seriously destructive occurrences; it would also put staff members under undue pressure to make quick judgments.

Any students that *anyone* thinks may be suicidal, homicidal, or having a psychotic breakdown ought to be evaluated initially at least for the standard 45- or 50-minute hour, and seen at least for a follow-up appointment within the next couple of days—provided, of course, that the student is cooperative. In cases where the therapist's initial evaluation reveals a probability of imminent threat to life, the psychotherapist also needs to consider psychiatric hospitalization or a careful plan of continuous accompaniment of the student.

Since psychotherapists for students in crisis must relate often to persons other than the students, it is essential to have in mind the kinds of clinical, ethical, and legal problems that will inevitably be encountered. The challenge is greatest when a student is both uncooperative and severely disturbed. For examples of practical approaches to these problems, the reader is referred to the articles by Amada (1986), Rockwell (1983), and Wagener, Sanders, and Thompson (1983).

Beyond allotting enough time to evaluate risk and to provide adequate follow-up in terms of crisis management, the therapist needs time with the student to begin understanding not only the precipitant but also the underlying basis for the crisis. There is usually a specific precipitant that will become apparent during the initial evaluation, in part by interviewing persons who are concerned about the student. In addition, there needs to be enough discussion for both the therapist and student to begin to comprehend the influences of the student's orientation, background, and circumstances on the dangerous behavior, and for the student to be informed about the limits of confidentiality. For clinical, ethical, and legal purposes, the therapist has a duty to inform others of an imminent threat to life when such other persons might help to reduce the threat (e.g., *Tarasoff v. Regents of the University of California*, 1976).

The student who begins to realize that the therapist is taking the threat seriously *and* delving into its basis, and not just dealing with the manifestation of distress and its immediate precipitant, will begin to experience the therapist as a helpful ally, notwithstanding the fact that helpful allies are often not easily accepted by people in crises. By providing adequate time for evaluation and an initial understanding, which will be accompanied by the development of some rapport and hope for resolution, the therapist provides the student with greater perspective. Being caught up in the crisis itself limits the student to the here-and-now, whereas the therapist gives attention not only to the immediate crisis but to its meaning. Quite often, for example, a suicide threat is a bid for attention that the student has assumed cannot be attained, at least legitimately, without having a crisis. The therapist legitimizes the need for attention, making the crisis an opportunity to provide the kind of serious attention that is really needed. Thus the crisis is an opportunity to develop new and more effective possibilities for resolving conflict.

TYPES OF CRISES

The crises encountered by the college psychotherapist are of several types that often appear in combination. Threats of and attempts at suicide, drug overdoses, psychotic breakdowns, and assaultive behaviors occur singly or in combination every year on virtually all college and university campuses. These are the principal types of crises one can expect and plan to encounter. No rigorous and comprehensive account of mental health crises on campuses is presently available, though there are important pioneering efforts to provide such data (Perlmutter, Schwartz, & Reifler, 1984). But we do have a sense of the nature of the hazards to life among college students.

The leading form of death among college-age persons is automobile accidents, which are quite often (if not usually) associated with the number one problem drug in the United States, alcohol. The second leading form of death is obvious or deliberate suicide. The combined lethality of auto accidents, alcohol and other drug use, and outright suicidal behavior is enormous among college-age persons. No fewer than 50% of serious and fatal auto accidents involve drivers who have been drinking excessively, and these drivers account for approximately 30,000 deaths annually in the United States, as well as vast numbers of serious and crippling injuries (Selzer, 1980). College students who use psychoactive drugs, including alcohol, tend to be more often involved in traffic violations (Nicholi, 1985). Altogether, the greatly overlapping behaviors of driving, use of alcohol and other drugs, outright suicide threats and actions, and psychotic reactions account for the vast majority of life-threatening campus crises. Physical health crises—other than psychologically induced health problems—are probably fewer in number than mental health crises. However, AIDS and worry about

AIDS are also rapidly becoming a type of campus crisis that needs the psychotherapist's attention (Keeling, Chapter 13, this volume; Widen, 1987).

Hazardous drug use clearly includes prescription drugs, in terms of overdose, their combination with alcohol, and other nonprescribed uses (e.g., combining two or more prescribed drugs that are dangerous when used together). Some of this hazardous use is caused by ignorance on the part of the user, but much hazardous use is deliberate or at least half-intentional. Though the student may not know it, or sometimes *because* the student knows it, alcohol used together with a prescribed or "street" drug (e.g., sedatives) greatly increases the potency of the drugs through their synergistic action and therefore multiplies the potentially lethal effects. Since psychoactive drugs are commonly prescribed for emotionally disturbed students, all health professionals should be as aware of their hazardous potentials as of the danger of street or illicit drugs.

It is particularly worth noting that tricyclic antidepressants, commonly prescribed for depressed and suicidal persons, are especially hazardous, even without the use of alcohol. Kathol and Henn (1983) have shown that tricyclic antidepressants are used in about 50% of potentially lethal overdoses.

College psychotherapists and all health professionals, on and off campus, should be alert to the hazards of psychoactive drugs. It is a wise precaution to limit the availability to prescribe these drugs to a psychiatrist on the staff of the college or university who, in consultation with a campus psychotherapist, can evaluate and monitor the hazards involved and ascertain the meaning to the student of taking drugs. The more such strict guidelines are followed, the smaller the chances are that overdoses will occur. One college, which had previously allowed any physician to prescribe psychoactive drugs, found that the rate of near-lethal overdoses in its student population was cut in half after instituting such strict guidelines. Not only does such strictness serve to control access to dangerous prescribed drugs, but it gives the message to potentially suicidal and drug-abusive students that the hazards of all drugs are taken seriously by the college and its health professionals. For example, the student who is casually given drugs by a parent—drugs that were actually prescribed for the parent or another family member—will think twice on hearing about how carefully the college or university safeguards the use of drugs through its conservative policies and the explanations given by psychotherapists, psychiatrists, and other staff.

Since various forms of substance abuse play such an overwhelmingly important part in the development of crises, as well as emotional problems in general, every college psychotherapist should become familiar with all aspects of substance abuse among college and university students. Psychotherapists should do this even though they are not often inclined to pursue students who "act out" their problems in various antisocial ways; they are more used to waiting in their offices for students to approach them. But many, if not most, crises will be associated with students' harmful use of drugs, especially alcohol. Psychotherapists who would deal with crises most effectively, through both prevention and amelioration, will learn a great deal about how to help both through reading the professional literature and through studying their own campus substance abuse problems. The reader is referred particularly to two current publications designed especially to meet this need (Burns & Sloane, 1987; Rivinus, 1988), as well as to Meilman and Gaylor's chapter in this volume (see Chapter 10).

Probably the clearest prototype of a campus mental health crisis, as well as a frequently encountered crisis in its own right, is the threat of suicide, which is therefore treated in detail within the next two sections.

GENERAL CONSIDERATIONS IN PREVENTING SUICIDE

The college psychotherapist should be aware of information about suicide rates and probabilities, overall prevention strategies, specific methods of working collaboratively with other staff members, assessment of the suicidal student, and various therapeutic methods of intervention. This section provides a general overview of these considerations, and the next section specifically addresses psychotherapeutic approaches.

Actual suicide among college- and university-age persons has increased about threefold since 1950, according to the best available data. However, difficulties in achieving accurate reporting of suicide and variations in operational definitions of suicide—for example, in coroners' reports—suggest that one should be somewhat cautious in interpreting the data. U.S. Census Bureau data and the reports of the Centers for Disease Control of the U.S. Department of Health and Human Services probably provide the best suicide data (e.g., see Centers for Disease Control, 1985, 1986). In all probability, we can say that suicide in the 16- to 24-year age group has increased greatly since 1950 (at least until 1980), especially among males and particularly among white males. It is likely that most, if not nearly all, of the increase is accounted for by the suicides of young males. Outmoded and destructive role models may help to explain why the current generation of males engage in so much lethal and near-lethal behavior (Dickstein, 1987; Whitaker, 1987).

Although females attempt suicide three times as often as males, males' attempts are three times as likely to succeed. Similarly, males' suicide threats have a far greater likelihood of leading to actual suicide. Males generally employ more lethal methods, such as using firearms and jumping from buildings.

College and university students probably differ significantly from their noncollege peers in terms of both suicide methods and rates of actual suicide. Perhaps 80% of suicide attempts on campuses involve students' taking pills, with or without the use of alcohol—a relatively high percentage—whereas the use of firearms on campus is less than it is off campus. Accessibility of suicide methods is a major factor in the incidence of attempts and actual suicides; one can observe on most campuses that students rarely possess firearms, but alcohol and other drugs, including prescription drugs, are usually quite readily available. Although programs to teach "responsible drinking" have demonstrated no benefit in terms of reducing alcohol abuse, and may actually increase alcohol abuse, it is probable that making alcohol and other dangerous drugs less available will help reduce the rates of all of the most lethal behaviors, including car accidents, drug overdoses, and suicide.

It was claimed some years ago that suicide was 50% more frequent among college students than among their noncollege peers (Ross, 1969), but it is more likely that suicide is less frequent among college students, though presently available data have not been adequate to prove the point conclusively (Schwartz & Reifler, 1980, 1984). For example, there was a 17.3 rate of suicides per 100,000 for the entire 20- to 24-year-old United States white male and female population in the 1970s, whereas the rate for the portion of this population enrolled in colleges and universities was significantly lower (Schwartz & Reifler, 1984). Similarly, more recently available data, on a limited sample of campuses, would suggest that the rate of college and university suicides is lower than for same-age nonstudents (Schwartz & Reifler, 1988).

Overall prevention strategies should take into account the largely negative attitudes that prevail toward suicidal individuals. In general, people are reluctant to get involved with a suicidal individual, for several related reasons. Fully admitting to the distress of the suicidal person arouses great anxiety in would-be helping persons, so that even serious threats and attempts may be ignored or minimized. Persons who empathically confront the suicidal student will find themselves resonating with the student's suicidal drive in terms of their own tendencies to self-destructiveness, even if these tendencies exist merely to the extent of "the average person who limits and denies [himself or herself] life in the face of death anxiety" merely by not investing fully in life (Firestone & Seiden, 1987, p. 31).

There is also a stigma on suicidal and other manifestly disturbed people that discourages associating with them. And getting involved may seem, or actually be, far more involving and distressing than most people can tolerate. Often, the suicide threat or attempt is just the outer manifestation of quite profound problems, including severe depression and real-life problems, that require intense, long-term helping involvements. Although emergency interventions, including psychiatric hospitalization, are usually brief forms of treatment, adequate resolution of suicidal crises often takes many months or even years. Furthermore, college staffs may not be able to summon help from families because of a variety of logistical and psychological impediments. Families of students may be distant geographically, insensitive to cries for help, or unwilling or inadequate to take responsibility.

What is usually needed to prevent suicide is quite active intervention, especially on the part of the campus mental health service (e.g., Dasheff, 1984). The importance of the active approach and some of students' resistances to it are illustrated in the following example. A woman student was reported to be poised halfway out of her fourth-floor dormitory room window, threatening to jump. She was momentarily restrained by her roommates, but threatened again to jump. The mental health service therapist on emergency on-call status was notified, but was told that the student refused to see him or any staff person. The mother, who lived in a city 100 miles away, was notified and was asked to speak with her daughter, but she minimized the threat, saying that the matter could wait until the morning. Meanwhile, the therapist told the student that her threat was being taken seriously and got her to agree finally to be seen by another therapist at the mental health service a couple of hours later.

The student kept the appointment, but expressed rage at being compelled to do so and claimed that her mother's attitude of relative indifference was more appropriate. She went so far as to say that she felt like killing the emergency on-call therapist for intervening. Several months later, she ran into the same on-call therapist unexpectedly, whereupon he had a quick image of being killed on the spot. But the student, standing there in a public hallway among many other students, enthusiastically and rather loudly expressed her gratitude at being taken seriously and enabled to get the help she needed. Suicidal persons' initial reactions to active intervention—active in the sense of taking them seriously and strongly encouraging them to accept help and support—may be antagonistic. However, I have yet to know even one suicidal person who has not eventually responded quite positively to this kind of respect and caring.

Emergency room treatment and psychiatric hospitalization have essential roles in any comprehensive suicide prevention program, though they are only temporary measures. The suicide risk may be considerably reduced after even a brief hospitalization, but in some cases it may be actually greater, especially if the suicidal student is not engaged in adequate psychotherapy after discharge. Of course, the "improved" suicidal individual may be even more ready to succeed at suicide, once he or she is more energetic and able to think effectively about suicide methods. A common but potentially tragic mistake is to take the suicidal person's denial of suicidal intent at face value; concluding that there is "no suicidal ideation" simply because the student says so is naive. For example, a student who had made a quite serious suicide attempt with a large quantity of alcohol plus psychotropic drugs prescribed for a relative was virtually unconscious all night but was released from the hospital just a few hours later. She put the matter this way: "Of course, I knew what to tell the psychiatrist who saw me that morning, in order to get out of the hospital." After another student's near-fatal attempt, a psychiatric nurse instigated a quick discharge, concluding that "there wasn't any suicidal ideation at the time she took the overdose" as evidenced simply by the student's saying, "I didn't want to kill myself." The fact that the presumably unintentional overdose had nearly killed the student was thereby discounted. All mental health professionals should be made aware that most suicidal persons are of two minds about accepting help and that a rapid shift from one mind-set to the other is common.

Discharge from a hospital should *never* occur before there is a carefully orchestrated plan of follow-up care, partly because the student needs to know that people are still going to care and that there are practical plans to provide this care. If referral to a new therapist is required, the referral should be "hand-carried"—in other words, accomplished in person, with the two therapists overlapping in seeing the student and observing firsthand that the transfer is successful.

The exact prediction of suicide is extremely difficult, because suicide per se is a relatively rare event, and there are many more threats and attempts than suicides (Murphy, 1984); however, outright suicide is just a fragment of the huge phenomenon of morbidity. Thus, serious attention to signs of suicidal inclination is never wasted, even though a particular individual does not actually commit suicide and may not even be a "serious" suicide risk.

Psychotherapists who will be confronted with the challenge of intervening with suicidal college and university students need to know the literature on suicide, the ways in which it fits into the context of emergency phenomena, and the meanings of suicide threats and attempts in terms of mental disorder. The reader is referred to Linn (1985), Robins (1985), and Tucker (1975) for an understanding of emergency phenomena generally. Adolescent suicide is presented well in overview by Sudak, Ford, and Rushforth (1984). Considered together, the literature suggests that, although suicide and near-lethal suicide attempts are still not as frequent in adolescence or the college years as later in life, suicide and other lethal behaviors in youth may be especially volatile. Arieti and Bemporad (1978), in their excellent book *Severe and Mild Depression: The Psychotherapeutic Approach*, note that "the depressions of adolescents equal the adult form in severity, surpass them in self-destructiveness, and still betray a characteristic developmental stamp" (p. 198).

The psychodynamics and meanings of suicidal behavior need to be understood, and resolutions of underlying conflicts need to be achieved, in order to reduce both specific suicidal inclinations and general self-destructiveness. One must not treat the suicidal behavior or inclinations as if they are truly isolated phenomena. It should be understood that there are self-destructive inclinations in all forms of so-called psychopathology (Firestone & Seiden, 1987), that suicidal behavior is indirect as well as direct (Farberow, 1980), and that suicidal behavior represents "a more or less transient psychological constriction of affect and intellect" (Shneidman, 1984, p. 323). One of the essential tasks of the psychotherapist is to broaden the suicidal person's awareness of options to include more than the choice between unbearable pain and stopping that pain through self-inflicted death.

In expanding the suicidal student's view of life's possibilities, the therapist should not resort to hasty, merely expedient measures that "contain suicidal behavior" and make the student "manageable," but should consider psychotherapy as an opportunity to prevent college student suicide in a thorough way (Whitaker, 1986a). In this context, emergency room procedures, the containment aspect of hospitalization, and the use of psychiatric drugs can be seen as expedient and sometimes even necessary measures, but measures that can be constricting if not countered with the more liberating influence of psychotherapy. For example, hospital treatment that emphasizes surveillance may promote suicides, whereas hospitalization that emphasizes psychotherapy and a humane environment can make suicide quite unattractive (Deikman & Whitaker, 1979). In this light also, involuntary commitment to a hospital should be considered a psychologically costly resort as well as a complex legal procedure.

PSYCHOTHERAPY WITH SUICIDAL STUDENTS

It is a mistake to view a suicide threat or attempt as merely an unconstructive "manipulation." We are fortunate, actually, if there is a manipulative aspect; it should be viewed as a method (perhaps the only method currently within the student's ability) to ask for help. Similarly, it is a mistake to view the suicidal crisis as merely an expression of "dependency," which, like "manipulativeness," can be shorn (destructively) of any legitimacy if it is reacted to negatively. Quite often, the manipulativeness and dependency of students in crisis are expressions of a history of not being taken seriously enough through less desperate communications. Their normal dependency needs may not have been acknowledged and met. The challenge to the therapist, therefore, is to take seriously and respond affirmatively to the cry for help expressed in the "manipulation" and "dependency"—to legitimize and make constructive the student's dependency strivings. Essentially, the therapist needs to be therapeutic rather than judgmental.

In summary, the therapist needs to view the student in suicidal crisis as presenting a valid picture of the degree to which he or she is able, at the moment, to face and resolve conflict. The therapeutic challenge is to help the student confront the conflict more directly and effectively. To do this the therapist must provide support, understanding, and evident ability to tolerate the student's anxiety, rage, dependency, and manipulativeness, all of which are distinctly preferable to withdrawal.

The therapist must live with the fact that the student may respond antagonistically, perhaps by expressing rage. For example, a freshman at a large university was psychiatrically hospitalized following his climbing onto the roof of a fraternity house and talking to imaginary voices. The initial evaluation showed him to be variously suicidal, sullen, and withdrawn. On being introduced to his newly appointed psychotherapist, he first looked down at the floor, then looked at the therapist and said, "I feel like punching you right in the nose!", at which point the therapist, taken off guard, grinned at him. The student asked indignantly why the therapist would smile at such an expression of hostility. The therapist explained that there had been no time to think at that moment, but that he was glad that the student had looked right at him and told him how he felt rather than continue to look down and withdraw. It turned out that the student's father was a very shy and retiring man who could not face direct expression of strong feelings, and that the student was relieved that the therapist *could* do so.

Such rage as this young man expressed is generally the product of frustrated dependency needs and the fear of exposing these needs, in anticipation of rejection and further loss of self-esteem. In this case, the therapist fully accepted the student's dependency needs while also encouraging him to be highly assertive in constructive ways. Part of the psychotherapy consisted of actively encouraging the student to compete on a track team and to learn public speaking; the student confided to the therapist that having to address a group of people was his single greatest fear in life. This therapeutic combination of nurturant support and encouragement to confront his fears resulted eventually in his winning a track event and, on returning to his university, making the debating team. His suicidal and psychotic behavior receded quickly after only a couple of weeks, though resolution of underlying problems required another year of psychotherapy.

Many suicide threats and attempts are linked inextricably to severe, long-term depression, in which the frustration of dependency needs and the consequent rage have been transformed into an enormously effective system of rejecting help and rejecting anyone who would attempt to help. In such a case, would-be helpers are so held in contempt on the one hand, or so idolized on the other hand, that the suicidal person manages, as it were, to keep all helpers at a distance where they cannot be helpful. Concerning the second alternative, being placed on a "slippery pedestal" as the "perfect person" makes the therapist a vulnerable figure: Slippage is inevitable, and the therapist will be prodded where necessary to produce it. There is no security in this kind of distant therapist–client relationship, and therefore little influence to prevent suicide. A strong therapeutic relationship is often the single most crucial deterrent to actual suicide.

A severe depressive transformation is often accompanied by "splitting," a phenomenon most commonly associated with "borderline" personalities. Various surrounding people may be dichotomized into entirely bad or entirely good persons; therapists and all others who would be helpful may have to tolerate their resulting undeserved labels. One student's "totally wonderful" therapist may be another's "totally unhelpful" or even "malignant" therapist. One and the same therapist may be "wonderful," even for a long time, and then become "unhelpful" or "malignant" in accord with a change in the student's relationship with another person. For example, if the student experiences a rejection by a parent, friend, or lover of the same gender as the therapist, the student may not "forgive" the therapist. Such splitting, scapegoating, and volatility are based on deeply disturbed relationships with people in the student's early development.

Jill had an alcoholic father and aunt. Her mother died after an agonizing bout with cancer when Jill was 17, just before Jill went to college. She reacted to her mother's death with muting of emotional responsiveness, but without any more clearly severe symptoms. After a few months at college, however, she experienced gory fantasies of death and cut her wrist in an "experimental way to see how it would feel." After a few psychotherapy sessions with her male therapist, it became clear that there was great underlying rage and tension. The therapist was perceived as extremely nice and supportive, but not as someone who could get at the problem. The therapist referred Jill to another male therapist, who was also resented because he replaced the original therapist, who was a "real friend." Quite frank communications of suicidal intent and rage then emerged, and the student announced dates when the suicide might be consummated. Gradually, the second therapist was seen as having more power and insight and then was designated "perfect," while the first therapist and a helpful professor were labeled "weak," "ineffective," and "not truly caring." After the second therapist had weathered the student's intensely suicidal period, the actual suicide potential decreased and finally dissipated altogether. Then the student again befriended the recently "ineffective" first therapist and professor and became deprecating of her current therapist, apparently due to the stigma of having needed the current therapist and the painful comparison in her mind between this therapist and her alcoholic, rejecting father. While admittedly experiencing rage against her father, the student had to deprecate someone strong enough to tolerate it. Therapy ended at the student's volition, by which time there was no suicide threat or depression, though the need to split people into the protected and the deprecated had not been resolved.

In cases of severe depressive transformation, such as the one above, the therapist is challenged often and, in a way, complimented by the student's "choosing" to express an angry side that no one else has been fully permitted to hear or see. The extremely negative feelings, thoughts, and even actions (including suicide gestures) that are expressed convey a negative transference reaction to the therapist that can mark the creative beginning of psychotherapy or the abortive end. It may be creative in that, by becoming able to express anger, the student can begin to reverse the internalization of anger. It may be abortive in the sense that there is not enough rapport even to begin a psychotherapy relationship and/or the therapist cannot tolerate being treated with such hostility. In attempting to engage such hostile persons, the therapist sees firsthand how suicide dynamics may include an aspect of murderous impulses turned inward, as Sigmund Freud proposed. At the extreme, it may be difficult to evoke the compliment to the therapist whereby the severely depressed and suicidal person dares to express the anger outwardly. In cases of extreme depression, there even may be no viable alternative to daringly but skilfully evoking the murderous hostility, since alternative forms of "treatment" may actually serve to cover up rage and underlying frustrated dependency, and thereby to deepen the person's despair (Whitaker & Deikman, 1980).

Developing rapport with the suicidal student who has gone through a severe depressive transformation requires much more of the therapist than a "common sense" approach, because the transformation has led to a psychological construction that constricts affect and thought, and demands suicide as a solution. The student's logic of suicide (Caruso, 1987) must be understood and taken seriously, so that student and therapist can begin to share this crucial common ground and a common frame of reference. The student must feel understood and taken seriously in terms of his or her personal and subjective state of mind; otherwise, a would-be therapist may deepen the student's despair. Of course, an altogether alienating practice is to tell the severely depressed patient to cheer up, "because there is no reason to feel depressed." These messages, born of denial and insensitivity on the part of the well-wisher, give depressed persons a sinking feeling, since they show that there is indeed a wide gulf in understanding between themselves and other persons.

The effective therapist has a dual orientation. On the one hand, the therapist enters subjectively and empathically into the experiental world of the disturbed person and communicates this genuinely empathic understanding, so that the person is no longer subjectively isolated. The empathic listener shows the ability, willingness, and courage to join the person on the person's own ground. On the other hand, the therapist is also objective—that is, able to see the person and the person's situation from a distance that allows a greater understanding of the person's dilemma than he or she can obtain independently. It is this process of employing both empathic and objective viewpoints that helps the student to achieve a new perspective, that opens up options for continuing to live. By creating a path that begins with empathy and sensitivity and introduces greater objectivity, the dual orientation creates greater "psychological space" (Arieti, 1974) within which viable solutions can be sensed by the suicidal person as well as the therapist. This process of careful and usually gradual elucidation of perspective is not merely a cognitive undertaking, but a process that engages both the suicidal person and the therapist affectively; otherwise, therapy is a dry run that brings about no real change, because the basic premises of depressive transformations are highly emotional. There must develop an emotionally or affectively experienced resonance, vividly signaling the absurdity of the premises, for the severely depressed suicidal person to give up such premises decisively.

A mathematics graduate student came reluctantly into psychotherapy after a breakup with a young woman. Though the precipitant of his severe depression was obvious, the basis of his seemingly rock-hard assumption that he *should* kill himself was not clear at all. He was a person who placed great emphasis on logic both in his mathematical pursuits and in his personal life. Personally, he could see no reason why he should not kill himself. The therapist decided to enter into this student's own construction in order to understand his compulsion to kill himself. This approach immediately established a common ground, as the therapist showed genuine interest in understanding the logical basis for concluding that suicide was indicated. The question arose, then: "Indicated by what?" The student stated that he was worthless and that, being worthless, he was simply taking up space and getting in the way of others. When asked what made him worthless, he replied that although other people seemed worthwhile, he did not seem worthwhile (to himself). He did admit that he had been functioning as a worthwhile graduate student, so that his lack of worth was in his sense of himself personally. He assumed further that *he* must have done something to make himself personally worthless.

The therapist suggested that they carefully examine each period of the student's life to ascertain when he had made himself worthless and by what action he had done so. For the next few sessions, therapist and student systematically went back over the 24 years of his life, beginning with the most recent 2 years and working backward a couple of years at a time. The therapist asked the student to search his mind carefully over each segment of time for any deed that he had committed that could have made him worthless. As each segment was examined in detail, the student concluded that there was nothing he had done; he registered mild surprise at these findings, but was generally bland in affect until the very last "examination segment" during the fifth session. After the student concluded that he had done nothing in his infancy that would make him worthless, the therapist asked seriously whether, while in his mother's womb, he had done anything deserving of punishment; he replied in the negative. The therapist then asked him to consider very carefully whether he had done anything bad *prior to his conception*. He replied with a mild degree of indignation that he could not accept as even remotely reasonable the proposition that a person who had not yet been conceived could do anything bad. He then concluded, therefore, that he had never in his life done anything so bad as to make himself worthless and deserving of self-inflicted death. As he drew this seemingly airtight logical conclusion, he began suddenly to sob. He continued to sob in a fully expressive, nearly convulsive way for about 20 minutes, after which he said that he felt vastly relieved.

In this case, there was no further suicidal inclination, as shown by several more sessions and a follow-up a year later, when the student reflected on the great difference between his new and old orientations. Having had his own terms taken seriously, he had been able to arrive at his own conclusions.

ACUTE PSYCHOTIC BREAKDOWNS

Relatively sudden psychotic breakdowns occur on virtually every campus each year. Schizophrenic disorders, which in the United States are estimated to afflict about 1% of the general population, typically occur for the first time in clinically manifest form during late adolescence or early adulthood. Therefore, most campus mental health services will develop some experience with acutely schizophrenic students who need immediate help.

Since people of traditional college are relatively changeable, psychotherapists should be especially wary of assumptions that acutely psychotic students will not recover. The old but false adage, "Once a schizophrenic, always a schizophrenic," is especially invalid for this age group, particularly where there are skilled therapists available.

Though the almost universal response to people who are schizophrenic is to administer phenothiazines or "antipsychotic" drugs instead of offering psychotherapy, the drugs are of extremely limited long-term usefulness. Nor does hospitalization typically serve much purpose other than to place the person in what is, one hopes, a safe environment (Whitaker, in press). The social and psychological bases for acute schizophrenic breakdowns—like the bases for acute depressive breakdowns—must be addressed in order to maximize the person's ability to function productively, to lead a gratifying life, and to avoid chronic disablement.

The limitations imposed on college psychotherapists are, first of all, economic; chronically schizophrenic students generally need long-term psychotherapy. But many, if not most, students who are acutely schizophrenic may be prevented from becoming chronically so if the therapist is skilled, caring, and not easily daunted by the challenge of addressing someone who is not only terrified at times but can inspire fear and aversion in the therapist. Karon and Vandenbos (1981) have shown in their Michigan State University Psychotherapy Project that even severe and chronic schizophrenic persons respond favorably and in profound ways to skilled therapists. Even the minimal time and resources required for psychotherapeutic intervention in *acute* cases may be withheld, however, when the therapist is afraid of the student

(Karon, 1987). The following example illustrates what may be an internal struggle for the therapist.

Frank was a very bright but quite unstable freshman who came for his appointment on a cold November day dressed only in shirt and pants. His barefoot entrance, peculiar manner, and intense look of fear immediately caused a fear-inspired rush of adrenalin in the therapist. Frank disclosed a hospitalization a year earlier when he had had a schizophrenic breakdown, evidently featuring thought disorder, ideas of reference, and delusions that others were controlling his mind. He had been given phenothiazines but no psychotherapy to help him cope with a quite disturbed and disturbing family. This time, as he was feeling another breakdown coming on, he wanted psychotherapy and no phenothiazines.

The therapist began to realize that Frank's own terror and bizarre behavior were making him, the therapist, have a sense of panic at having to relate to Frank. This realization and previous experience with people in terror gave the therapist much-needed perspective. As the therapist relaxed, Frank tended to relax too. The therapist–student relationship became friendly and supportive, and clarified the therapy situation as safe and secure. During the remainder of the academic year, Frank managed to pass his courses and to avoid another breakdown, without phenothiazines, while seeing the therapist two or three times a month. He then took a year off from college, but wrote twice that year saying that he had had no further breakdowns.

There are situations when it is expedient to hospitalize a student who has been decompensating, especially when limited psychotherapy and social support on campus do not seem to be adequate and when there is imminent threat of life-threatening action. George, for example, was an exceptionally bright student who had been experimenting with LSD. The first time produced no apparent negative effects, but on the second occasion both psychotic and suicidal tendencies were stirred up, and he asked to be placed in a safe environment where neither he nor others could hurt him. Both friends and therapist assured him of their support, but he made it clear that he wanted to be hospitalized. A brief period in the hospital was effected, where he was administered phenothiazines and the immediate determinants of his breakdown were clarified. He was able to return to college with important realizations about the bases for his breakdown, including the realization that he was certainly too vulnerable to risk another LSD trip.

There are still other situations when students' needs for help, including psychotherapy, can be met only off campus; greater resources are required than most campus mental health sources possess. Even in those situations, it is important to pave the way for the student and provide encouragement, to make a meaningful learning experience out of the crisis or breakdown rather than a self-esteem-shattering experience.

SELF-ESTEEM AND THE MEANING OF CRISES

A central problem with self-esteem occurs in virtually all suicidal and other mental health crises. Typically, something has happened to precipitate a drastic drop in the person's sense of competence and/or lovability. Suicidal crises in particular tend to reflect extremely negative self-appraisals with varying degrees of acuteness and, usually, a chronic deficit of self-esteem that has made the student especially vulnerable. It is extremely important, therefore, to help in ways that enhance the student's self-esteem rather than to make him or her an object of impersonal treatment. In this light, merely "handling" or "managing" the crisis may be, by itself, actually harmful to the individual; the current rage to "target symptoms" may be especially likely to result in harmful or iatrogenic treatment, since the net effect is that the student feels mauled, controlled against his or her will, and personally attacked in ways that deny meaningfulness and creativity in crisis. Suicidal students have usually experienced especially great difficulty "getting through" to adults. Failure to get through to "expert" adults can result in an even greater degree of frustration, anger, and proclivity to violence of various kinds.

Psychotic breakdowns, including the schizophrenic types, also convey drastic losses of self-esteem. Psychosis itself is a kind of psychological dying or retreat from full engagement in life, which one can interpret in terms of regression to the destruction-oriented images that characterize psychotic mental "life."

The therapist's role in helping to raise self-esteem is difficult and complex but potentially profound. Simple attempts to try to convince students that they are competent and lovable seldom have favorable effects, and such attempts may backfire. What is typically needed are efforts showing a student that there is a persistent, highly reliable therapist who genuinely cares, who is active, and who is willing and able to help the student to address his or her deepest concerns. In contrast, an only superficially caring therapist who is eager to get rid of the student may accomplish that quite quickly, because the student will be all too prepared for rejection. Putting a rigid time limit on the frequency of sessions and the length of psychotherapy with a student in crisis will only serve as a "deadline" that may readily deepen the student's despair and increase the chance of suicide.

Eventually successful psychotherapeutic courses that resolve otherwise disastrously low self-esteem are marked by the student's increasing frankness and awareness of acceptance by the therapist. One student who had come close to what would have been a lethal suicide attempt said of his relationship with his therapist, "I realized that you would accept me no matter what!" Such realizations are essential to preventing further breakdowns and to developing the often long-term psychotherapy process that is needed.

Whereas high self-esteem is life-promoting, low self-esteem is death-promoting. Drunken and careless driving, debilitating and death-enhancing drugs, and violent acts against others are not perpetrated by individuals who have truly high self-esteem. Persons who experience high self-esteem have a generous and caring attitude toward themselves and others. Thus, successful long-term outcomes for students who have been in suicidal and other severe crises are characterized by a certain stable assurance that they will treat themselves and others well. In essence, they have developed consistent ability to maintain both self-respect and self-love.

REFERENCES

Amada, G. (1986). Dealing with the disruptive college student: Some theoretical and practical considerations. *Journal of American College Health, 34,* 221–225.

Arieti, S. (1974). *Interpretation of schizophrenia.* New York: Basic Books.

Arieti, S., & Bemporad, J. (1978). *Severe and mild depression: The psychotherapeutic approach.* New York: Basic Books.

Boswinkel, J. (1986). The college resident assistant (RA) and the fine art of referral for psychotherapy. *Journal of College Student Psychotherapy, 1,* 53–62.

Burns, W. K., & Sloane, D. C. (Eds.). (1987). Students, alcohol and college health [Special issue]. *Journal of American College Health, 36.*

Caruso, A. (1987). The logic of suicide. *Journal of College Student Psychotherapy, 1,* 63–69.

Centers for Disease Control. (1985, April). *Suicide Surveillance, 1970–1980.* Atlanta: Author.

Centers for Disease Control. (1986, November). *Youth suicide in the United States, 1970–1980.* Atlanta: Author.

Dasheff, S. S. (1984). Active suicide intervention by a campus mental health service: Operation and rationale. *Journal of American College Health, 33,* 118–122.

Deikman, A., & Whitaker, L. C. (1979). Humanizing a psychiatric ward: Changing from drugs to psychotherapy. *Psychotherapy: Theory, Research, and Practice, 16,* 204–214.

Dickstein, L. (1987). Social change and dependency in university men: The white knight complex unresolved. *Journal of College Student Psychotherapy, 1,* 31–41.

Farberow, N. L. (Ed.). (1980). *The many faces of suicide: Indirect self-destructive behavior.* New York: McGraw-Hill.

Firestone, R. W., & Seiden, R. H. (1987). Microsuicide and suicidal threats of everyday life. *Psychotherapy: Theory, Research, and Practice, 24*, 31–39.

Hersh, J. B., & Lathan, C. (1985). The mental health walk-in clinic: The University of Massachusetts experience. *Journal of American College Health, 34*, 15–17.

Johnson, N. J., Whitaker, L. C., & Porter, G. (1980). The development and efficacy of a university mental health service walk-in service. *Journal of the American College Health Association, 28*, 269–271.

Karon, B. P. (1987, May 28). *Avoidance of the acutely disturbed college student and the fear of understanding schizophrenia.* David Dorosin Memorial Lecture, presented at the annual meeting of the American College Health Association, Chicago.

Karon, B. P., & Vandenbos, G. R. (1981). *Psychotherapy of schizophrenia: The treatment of choice.* New York: Jason Aronson.

Kathol, R. G., & Henn, R. A. (1983). Tricyclics—the most common agent in potential lethal overdoses. *Journal of Nervous and Mental Disease, 171*, 250–252.

Linn, L. (1985). Other psychiatric emergencies. In H. I. Kaplan & B. J. Sadock (Eds.), *Comprehensive textbook of psychiatry IV* (pp. 1315–1330). Baltimore: Williams & Wilkins.

Love, R. L. (1983). A walk-in clinic in a university mental health service: Some preliminary findings. *Journal of American College Health, 31*, 224–225.

Murphy, G. E. (1984). The prediction of suicide: Why is it so difficult? *American Journal of Psychotherapy, 38*, 341–349.

Nicholi, A. M. (1985). Characteristics of college students who use psychoactive drugs for nonmedical reasons. *Journal of American College Health, 33*, 189–192.

Offer, D., & Spiro, R. P. (1987). The disturbed adolescent goes to college. *Journal of American College Health, 35*, 209–214.

Pavela, G. (1985). *The dismissal of students with mental disorders.* Asheville, NC: College Administration.

Perlmutter, R. A., Schwartz, A. J., & Reifler, C. B. (1984). The college student psychiatric emergency: A descriptive study. *Journal of American College Health, 32*, 191–196.

Rivinus, T. M. (Ed.). (1988). *Alcohol and other substance abuse in college students.* New York: Haworth Press.

Robins, E. (1985). Suicide. In H. I. Kaplan & B. J. Sadock (Eds.). *Comprehensive textbook of psychiatry IV* (pp. 1311–1315). Baltimore: Williams & Wilkins.

Rockwell, W. J. K. (1983). Initial communications with the parents of emotionally disturbed university students. *Journal of American College Health, 32*, 104–109.

Ross, N. (1969). Suicide among college students. *American Journal of Psychiatry, 126*, 106–111.

Schwartz, A. J., & Reifler, C. B. (1980). Suicide among American college and university students from 1970–71 through 1975–76. *Journal of the American College Health Association, 28*, 205–210.

Schwartz, A. J., & Reifler, C. B. (1984). Quantitative aspects of college mental health: Usage rates, prevalence and incidence, suicide. *Psychiatric Annals, 14*, 681–688.

Schwartz, A. J., & Reifler, C. B. (1988). College student suicide in the United States: Incidence data and prospects for demonstrating the efficacy of preventative programs. *Journal of American College Health, 37* (2), 52–59.

Selzer, M. L. (1980). The accident process and drunken driving as indirect self-destructive activity. In N. L. Farberow (Ed.), *The many faces of suicide: Indirect self-destructive behavior* (pp. 284–299). New York: McGraw-Hill.

Shneidman, E. S. (1984). Aphorisms of suicide and some implications for psychotherapy. *American Journal of Psychotherapy, 38,* 319–328.

Thomas Speer, Administrator v. State of Connecticut, 4 Conn. App. 535 (1985).

Sudak, H. S., Ford, A. B., & Rushforth, N. B. (1984). Adolescent suicide: An overview. *American Journal of Psychotherapy, 38,* 350–363.

Tabachnik, N. (1973). Creative suicidal crises. *Archives of General Psychiatry, 29,* 258–263.

Tarasoff v. Regents of the University of California, 555 P. 2d. 334 Cal. (1976).

Tucker, G. J. (1975). Psychiatric emergencies: Evaluation and management. In D. X. Freedman & J. E. Dyrud (Eds.), *American handbook of psychiatry* (pp. 569–592). New York: Basic Books.

Wagener, J. M., Sanders, R. S., & Thompson, G. E. (1983). Reacting to the uncooperative, severely disturbed student: A survey of health center policies. *Journal of American College Health, 31,* 196–199.

Whitaker, L. C. (1986a). Psychotherapy as opportunity to prevent college student suicide. *Journal of College Student Psychotherapy, 1,* 71–88.

Whitaker, L. C. (Ed.). (1986b). Special symposium papers: Voices and boundaries in college mental health [Special issue]. *Journal of College Student Psychotherapy, 1,* 1–2.

Whitaker, L. C. (1987). Macho and morbidity: The emotional need vs. fear dilemma in men. *Journal of College Student Psychotherapy, 1,* 33–47.

Whitaker, L. C. (ed.). (1988). *Parental concerns in college student mental health.* New York: Haworth Press.

Whitaker, L. C. (in press) *Assessment of schizophrenic disorders: Sense and nonsense.* New York: Plenum.

Whitaker, L. C., & Deikman, A. (1980). Psychotherapy of severe depression. *Psychotherapy: Theory, Research, and Practice, 17,* 85–93.

Widen, H. A. (1987). The risk of AIDS and the defense of disavowal: Dilemmas for the college psychotherapist. *Journal of American College Health, 35,* 268–273.

4

Developmental Opportunities

GARY MARGOLIS

> For age is opportunity no less
> Than youth itself, though in another dress
> And as the evening twilight fades away,
> The sky is filled with stars, invisible by day.
>
> —HENRY WADSWORTH LONGFELLOW,
> "Morituri Salutanus"

> Whenever treatment directly neglects the experience as
> such and hastens to reduce or overcome it, something is
> being done against the soul. For experience is the soul's
> one and only nourishment.
>
> —JAMES HILLMAN,
> *Suicide and the Soul* (1964, p. 23)

When I think of the developmental issues of college students—our late adolescents, our adolescing adults—I imagine their development multidimensionally. First, I imagine it in time: We talk with these young men and women during this particular segment in their life-and-death cycles. This time is framed on one side by their families, peers, former teachers, mentors, and dreams, and on the other side by employers, more permanent intimate relationships, and experiences of deeper meaning and creativity. Second, I imagine their development in space: We speak with our student clients in the security of our offices—the office of our position as well as our private rooms—within the boxes of our buildings and the landscapes of our campuses. Each has varying degrees of geographical and emotional distance from our students' homes. And, third, I imagine their development in spirit: In doing therapy with students, we are communicating with their conscious selves and with their psyches, their souls—the part of them that dreams, imagines, and divines.

I think of development as a series of events and tasks college students need to encounter and master in order to engage increasingly complex adult roles—a development forward and up. I also envision students developing downward, realizing within their intellectual, social, sexual, and imaginary selves the quality of their depths: They can rise into ecstasy and plunge into depression, sometimes within the same day, the same hour. Often I experience my office as a photographer's darkroom, illuminated by the small sun of a protective, tinted bulb in which students, in my presence, are developing themselves, lifting the images of who they were, are, and wish to become up through the treated waters of therapeutic reflection and talking.

I have written before (Margolis, 1976, 1978, 1980, 1981) that I understand the developmental issues of students to be a pattern of somewhat predictable crises. I use the word "crisis" in the Chinese sense, as a dangerous or lucky opportunity for change. Because resolving a crisis often implies, to our Western minds, succeeding or failing, and because we tend to be so crisis-oriented and thus need "crisis intervention," I want to replace that concept with Harry Stack Sullivan's phrase "developmental opportunities" (Sullivan, 1953). There are necessary and predictable developmental opportunities for college students, by which they strengthen their personalities and enrich their souls. This process increases the likelihood of their being able, as James Hillman (1964) has written, to translate the events of their lives into experience.

In this chapter, I identify these opportunities and some therapeutic responses to them within the context of short-term or brief therapy—not only because that is what I primarily do with college students, but also because it seems to be philosophically and financially necessary on many campuses today. In addition, college counseling often takes place outside of college counseling centers and traditional clinical roles. Deans, chaplains, nurses, coaches, and faculty members find themselves in their own darkrooms with their own developing trays. They, too, need to have a picture of the developmental opportunities of college students; they need to have a sense, technically and conceptually, of what clinicians do, so that they can appropriately use therapeutic methods in their settings.

Although I speak of these issues sequentially, as if they occur in a line, these psychological tasks and markers curve, wiggle, and circle back on themselves. Completion or mastery of them can be complete or partial.

When students ask, "Why do I need to be feeling this pain and dealing with that problem?" we can, after empathizing with them, acknowledge the wisdom of psychological development. We can note that although each difficulty in their lives exists in its own moment, it also anticipates an event, a time in the future, which will require what they are coping with now as a precedent. The compression of developmental opportunities during the college years replays and anticipates many of life's most meaningful dynamics—separating, individuating, intimating (the ability to love others and oneself), working, and creating a psychological self.

FRESHMEN

> I am growing again, I have not stopped—
> I can see my falling age
> freshly, it is new to me, it takes hold
> collecting my whole mind.
>
> —ROBERT PACK, "Narcissus"

Context

Is there a more tender developmental moment, save graduation, than that of 18-year-olds saying goodbye to their parents, setting up their dormitory rooms, meeting their roommates and hallmates, buying their stacks of textbooks, and going to their first college classes? Is there an event that evokes as much anxiety and excitement as this moment that *is* and *represents* the separation process—the moving away from parents, siblings, pets, friends, neighborhood, high school, church, temple, and everything that students experience as the familiar and (even with all of their ambivalence) the secure? First-year students begin to let go of and exchange major anchors of their lives—their childhoods, their early and middle adolescences—for only a fantasy of what they would like to be: that is, graduated adults. They do this, often for the first time, in a context of almost unlimited freedom, where they are allowed to decide most aspects of their lives for themselves (i.e., food, clothes, sleeping, partying, studying, praying), without much immediate accountability and within their homogeneous first-year peer group. Freshmen risk testing their previous competencies—intellectual, social, and physical—in the new college environment, where initially they do not receive as much feedback as they need or are accustomed to, and where the abilities of other students mirror or go beyond their own.

Doing this without the immediate responses of their parents, they have freedom about which they are both terrified and enthusiastic. Each of these opportunities—to begin separating, to gain competence, and to manage freedom—is also experienced at a moment when students may choose to continue their given religious practice or reject their attachment to it. Freshmen explore their spiritual commitment and questions, even if indirectly, through other rituals and through the unconscious (dreams, writing, music). Spirituality and religious practice are theirs, too, to relinquish and to find.

Presentations and Clinical Responses

It does not take much clinical sophistication to recognize freshmen in pain, in psychological crisis. First-year students who seek therapy on their own, or who are referred by deans, faculty, health staff, or parents, often are *visibly* agitated, depressed, or straining to mask panic and confusion. We tend to call their evident anxiety and grief "homesickness" or "adolescent adjustment reaction" and not to identify their response as the mourning it is. This mourning, as I have said to groups of first-year students, is like barbecued chicken wings; it comes with three sauces—mild, hot, and volcanic. Although students have experienced external losses before, they probably have not mourned the losses of personal identity and family attachment to this extent; they have not felt themselves dying. Freshmen also describe a variety of somatic responses to these changes—headaches, appetite loss, sleeping too much or too little—because that is what they experience, and because their bodies sometimes are the doors through which they can legitimately seek help or express their feelings.

What typifies freshmen in turmoil, however, is their difficulty in coping, in applying strategies that have worked for them in the past, or in inventing new ones. Lacking coping strategies for their grief, they instead try to resolve or anesthetize it by wanting to withdraw from school or friends, blaming others (e.g., parents, high school counselors), studying obsessively and perfectionistically, numbing their feelings with food, using alcohol and/or other drugs, engaging in sexual activity, or thinking and acting suicidally. They want relief from their own grief, and also from the projected pain and reorganization their families are undergoing without their daily presence. I am thinking primarily of students who go away to college, those who move away from their homes and families. I am also speaking primarily of generic psychological responses to these developmental changes rather than psychopathological responses.

What can we do clinically with students experiencing this first developmental opportunity? How can we be with them?

First, it is important for us as clinicians to recognize that freshmen may be using professional psychological services for the first time; they may have misconceptions about us, based on their experience with high school guidance or pastoral counselors or their fantasies about what adult "shrinks" do. Part of our initial work is clarifying for students who we are and what they can expect—that is, teaching them how to use this relationship. For example, a therapist might say, "I would like to tell you about what you can expect from me and our therapy relationship. As we begin, now is a good time, too, to ask me any questions you might have about this new experience." Given that structure and feedback are often what freshmen need, I think it is useful for the clinician to establish the parameters for therapy, so that deeper affective and cognitive chaos can be safely expressed.

Second, it is useful for the therapist to intuit and recognize a student's primary mechanism for managing developmental or situational stress. Is the student attempting to cope by feeling or by thinking, intellectualizing? Consequently, how can the therapist nurture and teach the less dominant coping skill? I think feelers need to think more, and thinkers need to feel. How can therapists also help students turn their thinking and feeling into appropriate action? A therapist might observe of his or her client, "I notice you are telling me a lot about how you emotionally experience your situation. What do you also *think* about your girlfriend wanting to see other men? Is there anything you want to discuss or do now or over time in response to this?"

Third, given an understanding of this developmental opportunity, clinicians can empathize with students' mourning, their multiple feelings of sadness, anger, and excitement, by using and giving them the language of death and grief. An appropriate therapeutic reflection and interpretation might be this: "I hear the sadness and anxiety in your voice as you are telling me what it's been like for you these first weeks of college. Do you feel as if a part of you has died and that you are grieving and saying goodbye to some things?" With these words, they can identify and speak about the experience of this transition, which, like any mourning, can last in one form or another for weeks and months.

Fourth, freshmen may be uneasy at the thought that parents, faculty, and other freshmen are all watching and evaluating their performance. Therapists can help freshmen form a more realistic picture and timetable for how and when developmental skills are acquired and mastered. Newborns are expected to eat, sleep, and eliminate, and only later to smile and make sounds we can understand. Freshmen, too, learn to survive in their new environment before they learn to relax and sing. Describing this sequence to them—in effect, giving them a psychological road map—can help some freshmen lower their anxiety.

Fifth, in addition to fostering a relationship in which students can express themselves, therapists can concretely identify coping strategies that their freshmen clients have used in the past to survive and to enrich their growth. They can resourcefully imagine, model, and teach new skills that can be helpful during a student's first year at college. In subsequent therapy sessions, a review as to which behaviors and attitudes seem to help will coincide with meeting freshmen's developmental needs for external feedback. Helping students manage their immediate predicaments does not preclude attending to the deeper conscious and unconscious transformational currents.

Finally, therapists need to attend to the unresolved issues a freshman's initial presentation may represent—for example, dysfunctional families and marriages, unresolved losses and separations (e.g., deaths, rejections, illnesses, injuries, starting and/or changing schools), multigenerational deprivations, victimizations, and other unexpressed traumas. For example, a therapist working with a first-year student's classroom anxiety may explore previous times in the student's life when losses or moves affected that person's school performance or comfort: "Sometimes starting a major new enterprise like college brings up feelings of other times when we experienced loss or were in a transition that felt as if it were out of our control. Does this ring any emotional bells and stir up memories for you?" Some students may request or need a long-term healing relationship for discussion and resolution of these events; others ride them through or take them to another time, another place, another therapist.

In therapists' relationships to freshmen, they can compassionately create an atmosphere in which students can experience and reveal their dependencies, their inadequacies, at the same time that they begin to find their competence, their ability to direct their own lives.

SOPHOMORES

So much of adolescence is an ill-defined dying,
An intolerable waiting,
A longing for another place and time,
Another condition.

—THEODORE ROETHKE, "Meditations of an Old Woman"

Context

I have never liked the term "slump" that is used to characterize the developmental opportunities of second-year students. "Sophomore identity crisis" comes closer to this experience. Although "slump" implies its counterpart, "rise," I think it trivializes the necessary psychological process that these students undergo. It also tends to portray sophomores' painful feelings as just "a phase they will grow through," a position we sometimes take when we are avoiding contact or deeper understanding.

I once heard freshmen referred to as "adrenalin junkies." If they are the recipients of college's best endorphins—the highs of leaving home and beginning to be competent at the tasks of adult life—then sophomores are the ones who typically feel down, often in what they call the "pits." "Pit" is the right word for their struggle, with its unique depression. Part of what causes their plunge is obviously based on their *not* beginning for the first time. Returning to college for their second year, some feel overwhelmed by the 3-year landscape of routine they see stretched in front of them. Excitement gives way to boredom; challenges are not as thoroughly built into their role, as they were during freshman year.

In many schools, the squads of first-year students living in homogeneous dormitories for freshmen only give way to integrated housing for upperclassmen. Sophomores must live with *their* choice of roommates, without the excuse of having the college choose for them; they also live in groups that do not as readily (for better and for worse) identify with the group experience, as freshmen do, as a way of surviving their transition. Boot camp is over. It is more difficult for them to cope with their feelings and existential predicaments when they do not hear their peers talking about similar experiences, when it seems that no one else is feeling what they are and to quite such an extent.

Colleges and universities also often ask sophomores to declare their majors, symbolically a request that they again engage time—that is, their future. "Declare" is the right term for this process; the institution wants students to focus their academic interest and, by association, their vocational choice, and to make that choice public. This, in effect, requires from students an attachment and commitment to ideas, interests, and a group of faculty members at a time when they may well be continuing to separate from the original ideas and society of their families. Choosing a major can help resolve ambivalence for some students, but prematurely forecloses exploration for others. The degree to which students have the psychological and behavioral skills to renegotiate unsatisfactory decisions may be one indicator of the strength of their developing selves.

Less visible, however, is the existential turmoil that sophomores engage, or rather that engages them. Having demonstrated their capabilities to survive, and, in most instances, having succeeded academically and socially in college, second-year students begin their inevitable search for meaning. No longer do they only ask themselves, "How do I make it?", but now, more profoundly, "Why should I be studying and doing this here?" and by extension, "Why am I living?" Their psychological development has enlarged to the degree that they can begin tolerating some of life's most enriching and painful dilemmas: complex questions and feelings that have few easy or immediate resolutions. As they search for meaning and ways to *create* meaning, they are in sight of land, yet drifting in their own small boats, waiting for wind and current. Late adolescents in college generally do not have the luxury of acting out their psychological whirlpools in the style of teenagers. Without as many answers to resolve the frustration these questions raise, sophomores turn inward and downward. It is not as if they have not asked these questions before; the developmental opportunity is that they ask them at this moment, as they are disengaging from home and have the terrific and terrifying freedom of more choice, more personal responsibility. At this existential level, they continue the experience of dying that was begun freshman year, so they can continue to live with greater self-determination.

Presentations and Clinical Responses

Sophomores who experience the angst of this developmental opportunity can look the way they feel: sad or despondent, irritated or enraged, apathetic or withdrawn, fatigued, confused, and despairing. They evidence depression, including, at times, the organic signs of disturbed sleep and appetite; they may also think suicidally, as a way of managing their immediate and anticipated pain, and may again defensively blame the outside (faculty, governments, parents, God) in order to protect themselves and maintain their vulnerable ego-selves. The level of inadequacy they feel often parallels this psychological configuration; that is, they feel inadequate at managing these feelings or using coping mechanisms that could help resolve this struggle. Perhaps this inadequacy is the wisdom of their souls, which know that any fast cure is not in their best long-term interests. In addition, this may be the first time in their relatively "successful" lives that they have felt these depths and have been so self-consciously aware of their own experience. Not infrequently, previous, semifunctional coping responses may emerge. Over- or undereating, food purging, excessive drinking and/or drug using, compulsive sexual activity—all these are behaviors that people use to manage stress and chaos, but addictive behaviors that create their own distracting and potentially destructive worlds. Sophomores honestly ask the paradoxical question, "Why am I feeling so depressed, so stuck, when things have been going so well, when finally I am gaining my independence?"

How can clinicians sit with sophomores? What can they say? Therapists must be prepared for the expression of deep feelings of ambivalence and ambiguity and/or the necessary anxiety brought about by trying to give meaning to one's life. Again, therapists should identify the feelings of their sophomore clients, particularly because the intensity of these feelings may not have been felt or may not have been permissible in the past. Both sides of seemingly contradictory feelings and thoughts (e.g., "I like my courses but hate being in school now") should be acknowledged; this acknowledgment helps the clients to experience and tolerate ambivalence and paradox.

Second, therapists can support any direct or indirect philosophical statements students make that ask "Why?" Doing so lends structure: it encourages and legitimizes students' need to ask and explore large questions, to experience and survive existential pain. Of course, all concerns about suicide, violence, or destruction of property need to be addressed first—not only so that appropriate protection can be provided, but also so that other issues can be discussed in an atmosphere of safety and reduced tension.

Third, although students may wish for an immediate solution (e.g., dropping a course, switching roommates, leaving college) to resolve their confusing feelings and questions, clinicians should resist early resolutions. This will demonstrate both counselors' and clients' ability to experience, tolerate, and learn from these feelings and questions. Of course, such decisions may later be appropriate, but more as a choice than a reaction. Whereas therapists may need to offer feedback and gentle direction in working with freshmen's separation issues, with sophomores therapists may find that their own existential experience— their uncertainties and questions—consciously or unconsciously speak to students' dilemmas. For example, a therapist could briefly talk about a moment in his or her own college career when significant mixed feelings were felt: "I know my experience isn't yours, but I want to share a dilemma I faced in college when I was trying to decide whether or not I should or could stop out of college for a year. I had many conflicting feelings that I couldn't quickly resolve." It does not seem to hinder the young to *know* that someone else has been where they are, even though they too have the developmental opportunity to make their own decisions, to make meaning of their own confusions.

Finally, it is useful to help sophomores understand the necessary wisdom of the developmental process. Therapists can explain that questions of meaning will continue to plague and please them throughout their self-examined lives; now, at 19 and 20, they have a chance to deepen their dialogue with their inner selves.

JUNIORS

> We exist in those who,
> by letting us love them,
> teach us our own
> faithfulness. . . .
>
> —GALWAY KINNELL

Context

Freud identified satisfying love and work as two of life's most important experiences and goals. Add Jung's (1938) engagement with psyche—soul and spirit—and we have the three-cornered developmental opportunity that, although it also affects students at other points, particularly applies to third-year students.

With graduation from college in sight and with their process of separation from their families more behind them, juniors seem readier to risk a variety of commitments and to entertain the *idea* of commitment. Although in the past they have had temporary jobs, serious and frivolous intimacies, and sometimes a given relationship with God, now they are asked by society, hormones, and themselves to become attached again—this time (one hopes) from a position of greater autonomy, self-awareness, and self-esteem. Having begun the process of leaving home and strengthening their personalities and deepening their souls, they now have the developmental platform from which to dive into deeper emotional waters. They can risk saying, "I love you"; they can acknowledge to themselves and to other persons that they feel sexual; they can use their imagined vocational selves at job interviews or continued training and education; often they can acknowledge their need for God or something larger outside themselves. They can allow themselves to think and feel more independently, to risk rejection *and* confirmation, and, as graduation lurks within the coming year, to take more personal responsibility. Although intimacy, spirituality, and vocational choice can be issues for students during any of their 4 years, they seem particularly pertinent to discuss here in the context of the junior year. This is the time when students have coped with separation and depression sufficiently to allow themselves further individuation through making decisions and commitments.

Presentations and Clinical Responses

Intimacy Issues

A junior's response to what I call "intimacy stress" can be terrific—terrifically frightening and/or terrifically exciting. As usual, if the student does not have experience with or permission for these feelings, they can be covered up, distorted, or disowned by the widest variety of defenses (e.g., depression, avoidance, substance abuse, psychosis). The stress of becoming close has five particular sources.

First, students can feel anxious as they become interested in others, as they let their desire and need for intimacy emerge. A student is both excited and unsettled when he or she focuses interest on a specific person who has a name, lives in the same dormitory, and has a similar class schedule. Our adolescing, adult juniors leave safe land when they acknowledge their wish for and pursue ongoing, intimate relationships.

Second, in order to engage such relationships, they have to end, in reality and fantasy, any previous relationships. They have to relinquish whatever protection and link to home and childhood the previous persons were serving, which means, in effect, that they experience more loss, more grieving.

Third, many young adults transfer the struggle for autonomy with their parents onto their new relationships. They want to connect with their partners, but at the same time they need and require their independence. This dynamic often stimulates conflict in college-age people, some of whom have few conflict-resolving skills. Students in the midst of this conflict can focus on their feelings of jealousy and their guilt for feeling jealous; they feel angry when they think they are not enough for their intimates and sad when they fantasize the loss of those persons. Jealousy is often the covering emotional experience for the underlying dependence–independence struggle.

Fourth, intimacy for students also involves feeling and acting sexual. No matter how much previous sexual experience a student has had or fantasizing he or she has done, exploring their sexuality in a more committed relationship stimulates a range of anxiety-laden issues. These include bringing sexual feelings into awareness; experimenting with, exploring, and/or consolidating sexual orientation (homo-, bi-, or heterosexuality); developing relational trust so that pleasuring can occur; and creating a more complete sexual picture of one's self. Exacerbating these dynamics are the usual stresses of college life (completing assignments, exams, extracurricular activities, etc.) and the issues of students' individual personal histories. Therapists can therefore expect to hear students talk about (1) problems of sexual comfort and performance, a behavioral value confusion ("How do I want to behave sexually with my partner?"); (2) issues of responsibility regarding sexually transmitted diseases and birth control; and (3) concerns of privacy and publicity ("Whom do I want to know about my sexual activity, and to what degree do I want to behave sexually beyond my partner?")

Finally, college therapists can expect to see students who are in various stages of ending intimate relationships, breaking up. Other than the loss of a family member or sexual abuse, I can think of no other event that so significantly traumatizes our late adolescents. This experience is extremely painful no matter when it occurs during the 4 years; it can be particularly difficult for students whose postgraduate plans have been based on being in particular intimate relationships. All the emotional elements of grieving—sadness, anger, numbness—are evident when students deal with the loss of another and, to a greater or lesser degree, with a concomitant loss of self. At this age, much of students' social, emotional, and intellectual lives revolve around their partners; when their relationships are lost, they, in effect, are lost too. Therapists should not be surprised at how desperate and suicidal these rejected lovers can feel and should explore any suicidal feeling or thought, even if a student does not initially or directly discuss this issue. Again, experiencing, surviving, and living beyond the loss of a relationship can be one of the most important pieces of individuation a young person can encounter.

Although there are many interventions to help students deal with intimacy stress and specific techniques for sexual performance problems, I suggest that therapists primarily focus on how clients create emotional distance and closeness and on clients' communication skills. It is useful for students to receive feedback (using the therapy relationship as a model) as to how they create intimacy, and it is helpful to explore their experiences of intimacy in the past, specifically those concerning their parents and siblings. How students regulate their levels of closeness is, I believe, symbolically indicative of deeper psychological processes. Their ability to tolerate and embolden their intimacy can simultaneously effect greater attachment to their deeper selves and enhance the capability to let go of any particular version of themselves. Therapists can observe, attend to, and question students about how they feel at various points in therapy relationships; the point is to help students understand which coping mechanisms are functional and which new attitudes or responses may be desirable to deepen their relationships. Thus the therapy relationship is used not only to exemplify students' relationships with authority figures, but more generally to illustrate the way students stay away from or become closer to other persons. With a sensitivity to appropriateness, therapists can be as concrete as possible in disclosing their own experiences to model different ways of thinking, acting, and feeling. A therapist might say to a client, "Given that you are wanting to feel more personal authority, I want to share with you that in our relationship you wait for me to initiate the direction of our conversation. When I was feeling anxious with myself or thinking myself inadequate in regard to my thesis advisor, I waited too. I'd like to invite you to experiment with taking the initiative with me and see how that feels."

Communication skills are an essential aspect of any intimate relationship. Students seeking therapy to discuss intimacy stress may for the first time have the chance to look at how they express themselves to others. Do they recognize and express their feelings? Do they know and ask for what they need? Are they willing to and capable of listening to their boyfriends or girlfriends? Do they know their personal and cultural histories well enough to see what they are mimicking or acting out in their present relationships? Obviously, these are skills that are acquired over a lifetime, and yet college students, often juniors, can begin to acquire them in the context of individual or couples therapy or in relationship therapy (a term sometimes more palatable to students). For example, a therapist can reduce the projecting and blaming of a couple with self-esteem issues by asking each partner to relate his or her own experience from an "I" point of view (e.g., "I feel ... " and "I am thinking ... ").

Vocational Issues

A second major theme is that of vocational dilemmas—the developmental opportunity to form a picture of and start practicing a working self. Although most campuses provide career and placement counselors, college therapists can also expect to talk with their clients, often juniors, about vocational issues, which are related to the psychological issues of separation, individuation, and soul-making.

In our society, the question "What do you want to be when you grow up?" basically means "What work do you want to do?" Students bring this search to their psychotherapists because unconsciously they need to separate being from doing; they need to distinguish who they are from how they earn a living, as if one's living needed to be "earned." This is a discussion primarily about differentiating who one is from what working group or task one wants to belong to. Therapists can aid students in making this differentiation. This task is similar to helping students (particularly North American students) know that they, as persons, are not equivalent to their examination and essay scores. On the other hand, it is true that these identities—vocational and self—do overlap; discussing personal identity issues can bring self-awareness and choice to vocational explorations and decisions.

Also, juniors and other students often feel ambivalent or discouraged about a premature vocational or educational choice—college major, program, or thesis. At this point, many simply do not know what work they want to do or what their real skills and interests are. And yet parents, school, peers, and employers all seem to be saying, "Decide now!" The therapist's task, I believe, is to help students tolerate, at least for a while, their specifically vocational and existential anxiety, and to help them ward off external pressures from others, so that their true vocational selves have a chance to gradually emerge. Students first need to cope with themselves before other people and realities invoke their inevitable requirements. How many of us have needed this preliminary experience of drifting? How many of us "went through something like this in college" before we survived and grew during life's subsequent difficulties?

In addition, therapists often talk with students who want to make a vocational decision that strenuously conflicts with their parents' or others' (peers or faculty members) expectations. Choosing a course other than the family business or a generally approved occupation, or deciding not to live out the unfulfilled dreams of one's parents or teachers, requires independent thinking and action by students. Therapists must be cautious to leave both the feeling experience and any decisions to students, no matter how much students may try to give away their responsibility or growth to their therapists. Parents may try to involve themselves in the counseling process, either to support this independence or to undercut their children's autonomy—to attempt, for whatever family or marital reason, to maintain the status quo. At this point, therapists' independent, ethical, and clinical behavior is essential for their clients. For example, if a client has apparently acceded to his or her parents' demands to move back home after college without thinking through the decision, the therapist might ask, "What are the conflicts this decision raises for you? What kind of internal and external support might you need to make a growth-enhancing decision for yourself?"

Finally, developing a vocational self and choosing a first job also involve another significant, psychological dynamic: coping and compromising with reality, in the face of one's dreams and wishes. Again, this is one of life's continual dilemmas, with which upperclass students and their therapists deal concretely through discussions of vocational choice; preferences for career, residence, and salary may not fit what is available or what is offered. I encourage therapists to use the therapeutic relationship as a way of bringing this issue to life, by asking their clients near the therapeutic midpoint to share what they had hoped for from therapy, and asking them what their actual experience has been. These questions give them the opportunity to explore the necessary tension between wish and reality.

Spiritual issues

A third major theme concerns spirit and soul—the developmental opportunity to retrieve and create a relationship with the self and God. Each developmental phase over the college cycle involves students determining for themselves their connection (or disconnection) to their unconscious (i.e., soul, imagination) and to God (higher power, mystery, cosmos). Students talk about their comfort and discomfort with their given religious background, their peers' spiritual affiliation or lack of one, and their own confusion in both attitude and practice. But if God is and represents the sublime, upperclass men and women in particular often need to explore the heights. They want to define, based on their understanding and their needs, either a relationship or no relationship to God and denominational practice. Or they want to give themselves space and time in which to continue their exploration, before they choose a particular representation and experience of God.

Discussion of religiosity and spirituality is not the exclusive domain of college chaplains. In the process of separating and individuating, students need to have this part of themselves acknowledged by their therapists. I think it is appropriate for therapists to ask at least opening questions in regard to students' religious histories, current beliefs, and practices. Even if students do not choose to respond in depth, asking these questions validates and stimulates these issues. Students may discuss encounters with religious prejudice on campus, conflicts with parents or others over religious choice or practice, and spiritual experiences (through prayer, sexuality, contemplation, drug use, or hallucination). They need to talk about these topics for present management of feelings and for deeper understanding and contemplation.

As for the unconscious (soul and imagination), it appears that some of the developmental opportunities I have discussed—that is, initiating separation, coping with disillusionment and abandonment, risking interpersonal and sexual intimacy, and creating self-esteem—first need to be engaged in order for the materials and experiences of the unconscious to be apprehended and incorporated. Not uncommonly, this process may coincide for upperclass students with discussion of these subjects in academic courses (psychology, the arts, religion, anthropology, literature, philosophy, and, more recently, science), as well as in the courses' laboratory or studio components (experiments with extrasensory perception, writing poems, sculpting, chemistry, dancing). Some students, whether developmentally ready or not, will directly or indirectly reveal their unconscious in therapy. Their bodies will speak with and for them. Their stories will be touched with metaphor. And, simultaneously, they will want to talk about interesting or unsettling dreams, unusual emotional experiences, strange coincidences, memories, and premonitions. They will bring their poems, journals, drawings, letters, and performances to therapy, and, more subtly, their clothes, the messages on their sweatshirts, their choice of colors, costume, and jewelry. A therapist who notices and attends to these expressions is acknowledging a student's inner life, a bridge between the student's rational and irrational selves, and the self's relationship to archetypal images and universal human experience. For example, a therapist seeing a client's T-shirt printed with the phrase "Born Free" and a family of lions could open the session by inviting the student's responses to those words, those animals. The shirt design could be interpreted as statements about the self or the student's relationship to things, images, and patterns outside of the self, or perhaps as a statement about the student's developing autonomy.

Even in short-term therapy, the unconscious, the soul, or the imagination needs to be acknowledged and honored. Religious experience from one perspective explores the heights and God; in revealing the unconscious, students also encounter the depths—the gods, goddesses, and demons. They begin to experience the relationships between their roles and themselves, between their personalities and their spirits. Despite various levels of training and comfort in this area, college therapists should validate these parts of their clients' experience, so that these parts are not split off from clients' total sense of themselves. One student talked about her anxiety in dating a man who practiced a religion different from her own. She used to worry about disapproval from others for dating this man as a way to explore with her therapist feelings that she had disowned, and ultimately to confirm and broaden her spiritual self. In this instance, a therapist could ask, "What aspects of your partner's religion are you attracted to and/or afraid of? Can your experience of differences help you consolidate your sense of self or broaden your spirituality?" Young people, in particular, want to have these parts recognized by their adult confidants. They want their therapists, like Hermes, to guide them through the shadows; to help give voice, names, and shelter to their spirits; and to help them integrate these perceptions and experiences into meaning.

SENIORS

> . . . and I step once more
> Through a hoop of tears and walk on, holding this
> Buoy of flowers in front of my beauty,
> Wishing myself the good voyage.
>
> —W. S. MERWIN, "Departure's Girlfriend"

Context

Students ending their undergraduate cycle again face the developmental opportunity of completion and separation, of continuing their movement toward autonomy and *chosen* dependencies/interdependencies; consequently, they deepen their sense of life and death. Graduation is education's ritualization of these goodbyes, of this transition. In order to graduate, seniors must have fulfilled academic requirements; they also must have begun, to varying degrees, exploring psychological processes necessary for further adult living. Each of the developmental opportunities engaged during the college years—separation/individuation, depression, intimacy, self- and soul-making, and completion—becomes a block on which further psychological competencies are built. Seniors have the structure of graduation—its ceremony—to demarcate their developmental accumulations. At the same time, when their schoolwork is completed and while they wait for graduation itself, they are truly lost in their transition. In an in-between state, they are left to contemplate their psychological selves, their reaction to what they have done and what they have created. About to leave and let go, to say goodbye, they are once again metaphorically dying, as they move on to the next phase of their lives.

Presentation and Clinical Responses

Seniors may bring a variety of problems and obstacles to college therapists, many of which relate to the dynamic process of ending this developmental sequence and moving on to the next. An example is apathy toward and "inability" to complete final academic papers; another is leaving seemingly small responsibilities unfinished, such as returning library books or paying campus parking fines. Some seniors become mired in final projects as they struggle with unresolved authority issues *vis-à-vis* their faculty advisors. Others begin imagining how the post-college world will be different from their present place and relationships.

For many students, participating in the graduation ceremony means gathering their families—families that may be blended or divorced, or that may include chemically dependent members. And often for seniors, there is the conflict between spending time with families and with college friends. In the months and weeks preceding graduation, seniors sometimes do not take time to acknowledge their deeper feelings of excitement, fear, sadness, and anger as they are going through this moment, this developmental opportunity. Great feeling becomes ritualized and anesthetized in massive partying. I think it is the primary task of therapists to help seniors emotionally complete college, to help them recognize and name their feelings, to express feelings to meaningful others, and to reflect on their intellectual and psychological changes. This process, as in any other developmental "accounting," means that they can acknowledge their regrets and unfulfilled dreams—that is, their human limitations. College therapists can expect that working through these feelings may evoke previous instances of loss and transition. Clients have a chance to gather and restore pieces of the past, while moving toward the future.

It is important, too, for therapists to recognize that some seniors are *not* developmentally ready to graduate; however difficult that may be for parents and students themselves, these seniors need to postpone this event until they can master the necessary feelings and tasks of this psychological time. Continued, in-depth therapy is recommended.

As graduation nears, it is also common for both old and new clients to discuss, for the first time, significant historic issues of pain, victimization, or guilt. As this period in their lives is closing and the availability of free therapy is ending, some seniors broach these topics before they leave, often as a way of saying goodbye to that piece of their past and to solicit encouragement from their therapists to seek further therapy.

Not the least of these changes is the process of separation and goodbyes between college therapists and their clients. Graduation for a senior often means terminating therapy, ending this specific relationship, and thus experiencing another kind of death. As this may have been the student's first therapeutic contact, as therapeutic work may have been done at a variety of times during the 4 years, and as the therapist is often a significant other or "transitional object" for the student, it is important for the therapist to use graduation to effect closure, to deeply say goodbye. Closure is also important for college therapists themselves, who, by the nature of their educational setting and use of short-term therapy, work with large numbers of people. They too need to let go, to say goodbye to their seniors for the sake of those relationships, and to make emotional room for their coming freshmen clients and for their own ongoing lives.

CASE STUDY

If there is one example that particularly illustrates the developmental opportunities of late adolescence and the college years, it is our own. Probably, by now, readers have been remembering and imagining clients they have seen or anticipate seeing. They may have been thinking of their own young adult journeys, with their logjams and fast currents. In the service of our clients and ourselves, I encourage us all to think of our college experiences, of that developmental time, as specifically as possible in relation to the dynamics I have discussed. Which issues were ours and which were not? What sequence did they follow? Which emotional tasks were completed? Which ones are still in process and deepening? What did we manage on our own? What conscious and unconscious help did we receive, and from whom, from what? What did these people and spirits say, do, or not do? What meanings did we attribute to them? How did we survive and turn our survival into growth, a deepening of our imaginations?

INTERVENINGS

I would like to suggest a few generic questions that therapists can use in considering the larger developmental issues that often underlie the specific dilemmas and turmoils of college students. Perhaps, too, they are questions on which to meditate.

1. How do you feel being away from home and your family?
2. How is it for you having a roommate who isn't your brother or sister?
3. How do you manage your anxiety in these new situations?
4. How is your eating, drinking, and/or using drugs affecting how you feel, think, and act?
5. What personal qualities or interpersonal skills would you like to gain?
6. What pain have you brought with you?
7. What do you most fear? What do you despair of?
8. What losses and deaths have you experienced?
9. Are you thinking suicidally?
10. Whom else would you like to know your struggles?
11. Whom do you love?
12. Whom do you feel sexy toward?
13. How do you experience your differences from other students (e.g., racial, religious, cultural)?

14. What are your beliefs about yourself, others, and the world that foster your status quo? What beliefs foster your growth and deepening?
15. How do you experience the differences between who you want to be and what others want of you?
16. What do you dream, imagine, and make with your hands, your voice, your instruments?
17. Do you dance, walk, run, or swim?
18. What internal voices do you talk with?
19. Who are your guiding spirits? Your demons?
20. What poems and stories are meaningful to you?
21. What things have you left unsaid to significant people in your life?
22. What is your experience of God?
23. What do you need from me?
24. To what and to whom are you saying hello and goodbye?

OTHER CONSIDERATIONS

In this discussion, I have remembered students with whom I have talked, psychological models I have been taught, books I have read, and dreams I have dreamt, in order to generate this concept of the developmental opportunities of college students. Although I have described this sequence as if I were thinking of one student, I do not believe that any general formulation can exactly fit a particular personality or the unique experiences and developmental process of any specific group, whether defined by gender, race, culture, religion, or sexual orientation. The same qualification applies to cases of unique physical or intellectual ability or disability. Therapists must take these circumstances into their clinical awareness by understanding how they both stimulate and interact with clients' immediate dilemmas, and simultaneously with the developmental moment surrounding their problems. At the same time, if therapists pay attention *psychologically*, they listen to and encourage students' souls, the imagination that speaks above and below any particular moment, any particular personality.

It is also important for college therapists to respect the psychological protection some students need in order to defend against premature, developmental change. Leaving biochemistry temporarily aside, I am thinking of students who experience psychosis or consistently alter their reality with alcohol or other psychoactive drugs. These methods may be the best and only means some students have of demonstrating where they are and what they need, in order to eventually continue their growing.

Finally, therapists' own developmental position and the degree to which they are aware of it, through self-exploration, therapy, or supervision, affects their perception of their student clients' developmental opportunities. How individuated therapists are, how much depression they have worked through, how they create platonic and sexual intimacy, what access they have to their souls and imaginations, and how they join and separate from others—all are important dynamics that impede or facilitate developmental change in their clients.

In discussing psychotherapy with college students, I have imagined the photographer's darkroom, in whose muted darkness and solitude images and representations are allowed to emerge. No matter how available, competent, and well-regarded therapists may be on campus, it is still an act of courage and grace when these late adolescents ask for help and enter into therapy relationships, when they allow us the opportunity to work with them and be together in this moment of their lives.

REFERENCES

Hillman, J. (1964). *Suicide and the soul* (p. 23). Dallas: Spring.

Jung, C. G. (1938). *Psychology and religion*. New Haven, CT: Yale University Press.

Margolis, G. (1976). Unslumping our sophomores: Some clinical observations and strategies. *Journal of the American College Health Association, 25,* 133–136.

Margolis, G. (1978). Becoming close: Intimate relations among college students. *Journal of the American College Health Association, 27,* 153–156.

Margolis, G. (1980). Learning to leave: Problems of graduating—clinical observations and strategies. *Journal of the American College Health Association, 28,* 336–338.

Margolis, G. (1981). Moving away: Perspectives on counseling anxious freshmen. *Adolescence, 16,* 633–640.

Sullivan, H. S. (1953). *The interpersonal theory of psychiatry*. New York: Norton.

5

Family Problems

JOANNE D. MEDALIE
W. J. KENNETH ROCKWELL

Family problems are among the most prevalent issues dealt with in college counseling. These problems most often involve contemporary conflicts—disruptions and/or crises both within the family and between the student and salient family members. Common problems causing acute crises are the serious illness or death of a parent or sibling, or a parental separation or divorce. In addition to the threat (actual or potential) that such losses pose to the student's emotional stability, they frequently impose many "reality" demands that generate conflicts and additional stress.

Family problems are often students' primary reason for seeking therapy. (In a survey taken at Duke University, 33% of therapy clients, in the judgment of their therapist, fell into this category.) But even when family problems are not a presenting complaint or a precipitating event, they tend to lie beneath the surface of other presenting complaints, both academic and social, and frequently become the focus of treatment. Although family problems, broadly defined, are likely to be uncovered in any open-ended psychotherapy, we limit our discussion here to those problems that are, in the therapist's judgment, the obvious source of the student's distress or symptomatic behavior.

Early parental loss (i.e., death, divorce, or an emotional loss) is the one major family problem that is not strictly ongoing yet contributes to current stress. Though largely an "internal" psychological issue as distinct from a current relational problem, an early loss frequently presents an acute problem during the college years. This is because children frequently do not mourn (Wolfenstein, 1966). An unmourned dead or lost parent casts a shadow over the child until the loss can be acknowledged, confronted, and worked through. The accomplishment of mourning may be possible only after the student reaches college and must come to grips with being alone.

The prevalence of family problems in college students is a function of two factors. One is the nature of the family in the contemporary cohort of students. The families of these students reflect the changes that have occurred since the early 1960s as a result of women's liberation, the changing sexual division of labor, and particularly the very high incidence of divorce. Parental divorce during a student's childhood may lead, for example, to conflicts during the college years about which parent will provide financial support for college, and may stir up old feelings of rage and depression associated with a total or partial abandonment by a parent (usually a father). Divorces that occur when students leave home for college create a sense of instability that impedes students' adjustment at school. In general, college students today are more likely than in the past to have experienced a major disruption in their family structure and relationships. An informal study by Medalie of 112 cases of randomly assigned undergraduate students at her counseling service found that 27% of students were from divorced families and 12% came from families in which there had been a parental death (an unusually high figure). Thus, two students in five did not come from traditionally intact nuclear families.

The other major reason for the prevalence of family problems in this population is the developmental status of college students, who are in the process of separating and establishing themselves as autonomous adults. They are therefore particularly vulnerable to disruptions and conflicts within and between themselves and their "home base." Threats to the stability of families or to students' support network back home may disrupt the separation process, with destructive consequences for the students' adaptation to college.

THEORETICAL PERSPECTIVES

The Developmental Framework

In addressing the therapeutic needs of college students, we employ a developmental, object-relational approach. Before a diagnosis of psychopathology is made, we consider the student's developmental status—the degree to which he or she is addressing age-appropriate developmental tasks. How far along is the student in developing as a differentiated person who takes responsibility for values and decisions? To what degree has the student been able to define interests and goals, to establish close ties with peers, and to begin to experience a mutually caring relationship with a loved "other"? The accomplishment of such tasks is assessed in relation to the student's place in the "college life cycle." Hence, a freshman who has undifferentiated interests, goals, and relationships would be regarded quite differently from a senior who remains diffuse and undifferentiated (Medalie, 1981).

Clearly, the psychosocial assessment of the student's developmental progress has diagnostic implications that bear on choice of treatment. The preferred defenses and adaptive style, the degree to which anxiety is contained and productively channeled, and hence the impulse–defense balance must all be taken into account in assessing the appropriate therapeutic approach. The degree to which the student is capable of taking emotional distance, living with ambivalence and ambiguity, and benefiting from insight are also critical. In general, the more immature or developmentally arrested student will benefit from support and a direct cognitive–behavioral approach, whereas a psychologically minded student with higher-level defenses can profit from gaining insight into the less conscious feelings and fantasies associated with the problem. In the latter case, a nondirective though appropriately supportive approach to therapy is often indicated.

The developmental framework also helps us to understand the roles students play, and the modes of adaptation and defense they employ, in coping with family conflict. Their "input" into the family problem will reflect their autonomy conflicts, sexual needs and inhibitions, and fears of abandonment and loss. An important therapeutic function with family problems is to help students to identify and ventilate feelings about these underlying developmental concerns.

The Systems Framework

The systems approach developed in the family therapy literature (e.g., Minuchin, 1974) provides a useful lens for viewing family problems presented by college students. Although family therapy per se is rarely practiced in a college setting, its perspective is nonetheless useful (Fulmer & Medalie, 1987). It alerts the therapist to possibly unseen pressures, demands, and events within the family that may be generating the student's current distress.

This approach focuses on the family system rather than on individual intrapsychic problems. It treats symptoms and problematic behavior patterns as products of distortion in the family system, rather than simply as manifestations of one member's unconscious infantile or developmental conflicts. It conceptualizes family problems along a continuum from "enmeshed" relationships, in which boundaries between family members are blurred and individual growth and separation are prevented, to "disengaged" families, which provide insufficient structure and support. Overinvolved families on the one side and distant families on the other are less extreme versions of this polarity. This approach allows us to focus on the developmental requirements of the several generations that make up a family and to keep in mind the family life cycle when addressing particular problems within a family (Carter & McGoldrick, 1980). It also alerts us to the resistance of the family (including the student himself or herself) to changes in the dysfunctional student. Any threat to the family homeostasis will tend to be met with opposition.

Many of the family problems presented by college students involve changes in the family system brought about by the student's developmental progress—for example, the student's leaving home for college, impending graduation, or commitment to a boyfriend or girlfriend. An explanation of how the family system is disrupted by the student's individual changes may give the student a handle to cope with family pressures.

It is important to stress that using the family system to frame the student's conflict should not preclude exploring internalized conflicts. Mourning a lost parent is a case in point. A systems framework alerts us to inquire about how the loss was dealt with in the family and how needs previously filled by the lost parent were filled, or ignored, after the loss. However, the student's sense of abandonment, identification with the lost parent, and/or the denial about the loss must be explored from a psychodynamic perspective.

Similarly, an overt conflict between a student and parents over their frequency of contact can be profitably addressed from both perspectives. The systems perspective alerts us to the possibility of parents' "empty nest" issues, which move them to resist the student's efforts to leave home. This perspective also suggests that the student, while outwardly protesting, may actually want to maintain homeostasis in the family by assuring parents that they are still needed. On the other hand, the psychodynamic perspective raises the possibility that the struggle is largely a product of the student's efforts to externalize an inner conflict about separation—an externalization with which the parents may have colluded.

GENERAL TREATMENT STRATEGY

Time-Limited versus Long-Term Treatment

The treatment of family problems, like other problems of college students, is circumscribed by the available service and structure of a college counseling center. It is also limited by students' readiness and ability to address family problems. The most readily treated family problems are acute crises and transient developmental conflicts. By their very nature, these problems are time-limited and are amenable to treatment within the time frame and structure of most student counseling centers. For example, a student in her junior year wishes to take a summer job in a city far from home; her parents object, and tension between them grows. The therapist explores with the student the family issue surrounding this conflict, learning that she is an adored only child of high-functioning but overinvolved parents who nevertheless have generally supported her moves toward autonomy. Once it is clear to the therapist that the parents will adapt to her decision, the treatment task is to focus on the woman's internal conflict. The decision must be implemented in a few months. The time frame and treatment agenda are thus set.

Another student has just learned that his mother is about to have surgery for breast cancer. A hard-working premedical student, he is unable to concentrate in preparation for his organic chemistry midterm next week. He feels guilty about his desire to push aside concern for his mother in order to focus on his studying, although she supports his goal unambivalently. The therapist can help him to sort out his feelings so that he can both respond to his mother's needs and continue his own functioning. The task requires only a few therapy sessions, and perhaps a future follow-up.

In contrast to these examples, chronic family problems that reflect a severely enmeshed family system or that have become embedded in the student's personality structure frequently require longer courses of individual therapy or perhaps family therapy. If feasible, the work may be performed at the college mental health facilities. If not, the treatment goal is referral (Fulmer & Medalie, 1987; Medalie, 1987).

Identification and Framing

An early task with any college student's therapy is to assess to what degree and how family problems are implicated in the presenting problem. This is done by inquiring about the student's present and past family situation. The inquiry must include information about losses, disruptions, illnesses, or other traumas; about the parents' relationship with each other, as well as their general adaptation with regard to work and the world; and about the student's relationship with each parent and sibling.

In cases where the family problem is not part of the presenting complaint, students may resist the therapist's efforts to explore unresolved family issues. This is often the case with students who have adopted counterdependent defenses against their yearnings for parenting, or who have used denial in dealing with the loss of a parent; they are not developmentally prepared to cope with unfinished family business. As their peer-centered conflicts or work inhibitions are addressed, however, these students may become ready to explore family problems. They may realize that troubling patterns in contemporary relationships parallel problematic interactions in the family.

A critical judgment must often be made as to whether to probe and vigorously pursue hints of family problems. Some students need to resist connecting their complaints with family issues in order to see themselves as independent. For them, it may be wise to honor this wish as a means of supporting their thrust toward autonomy. In such instances, the therapist can only suggest that there seem to be unresolved issues that the student might find useful to pursue at some future point.

The Therapeutic Stance

The stance of the therapist toward family problems is complicated because of students' developmental status. On the one hand, students may look for support against family members with whom they are angry. Sometimes the anger is justified and it would benefit them to be able to ventilate it. At the same time, a student may become guilt-ridden and fearful if the therapist seems to attack the offending family members, and may react with resistance and even withdrawal from therapy. Thus, the therapist may want to reassure the student that the aim of treatment is to gain understanding, not assign blame, and that the end result may be better relationships for all.

Yet a strictly neutral stance on the part of the therapist is not always indicated. The separating late adolescent may need validation of a perception that parents are behaving inappropriately or irrationally. Sometimes students with psychotic or borderline parents have never been given adequate information about their parents' mental status or support for distancing themselves from irrational or destructive demands. The college therapist can offer a perspective on the parents' behavior that facilitates the deidealization needed to foster separation/individuation. In short, the therapist should identify parents' problems and psychodynamics nonjudgmentally while at the same time legitimizing students' negative feelings about these problems. Recognition of parents' limits and conflicts may free up students' internalized resources and enable them to separate from relationships with disturbed parents.

On the other hand, particularly in cases of clearly enmeshed families, students may be acutely aware of parents' vulnerability and inappropriateness, but may be unable to disengage from the "system" because of fears of precipitating further deterioration in their parents. Here the therapist's stance might be characterized as "in the best interest of the child." The therapist must help students to recognize and come to terms with their own age-appropriate developmental needs and with the reciprocal role of parents at this stage in the family life cycle. The therapist should explain that college students need to invest their social energies in forging ties with their own generation so that they can grow into competent adulthood, while parents need to come to terms with the "empty nest" by finding new outlets for their attachment and generative needs. The therapist may point out that a child's ability to grow into competent adulthood is ultimately in the best interest of parents. The therapist may also need to question a student's perception of parents' vulnerability or inflexibility, confronting what may be the student's own need to maintain the status quo. Feelings of being special and safe, based on a sense of power over sick or inadequate parents, may inhibit the separation process.

The family problems of students may "pull" strong countertransference feelings from therapists. Particularly common are competitive feelings with inadequate or destructive parents and unconscious needs to "rescue" students. These feelings must be carefully monitored so as not to threaten students' loyalty to their families. However inadequate parents may seem, students fear losing them. Walking the thin line between empathy and overinvolvement is a special challenge in working with young people at the late adolescent life stage.

Treatment Options

Family problems, insofar as they are in part "reality" problems, call for a flexible approach to treatment. For example, a cognitive–behavioral approach may be combined with insight–oriented techniques. Thus the therapist might at one point identify the underlying issues in the family problem and plan with the student how to act in appropriate ways to cope with it, and at another point focus on the student's fantasies and feelings that underlie resistance to solving the problem. As the counseling proceeds, the therapist must continue to evaluate the degree of leverage for change in the family system in order to orient the treatment toward a realistic goal. The degree to which a family is enmeshed or disengaged and therefore resistant to change may only become apparent over time.

In addition to the understanding, insight, support, advice, and/or treatment recommendation and referral that college therapists ordinarily provide within the context of short-term treatment, therapists may use the additional option of long-term treatment. Particularly for students from disengaged families, in which there are too little support and inadequate models for making developmentally progressive steps, college therapists may provide a reparative experience to partially make up for what has been missing. (Short-term work provides somewhat of a reparative experience, too, but obviously to a lesser extent.) Students who benefit from this option may have insufficient inner resources to develop supportive relationships with teachers and others who might play mentor roles or act as role models. They frequently seek to fulfill their needs for parenting from their college peers, putting excessive burdens on these relationships. Subsequent rejections, losses, and disappointments with peers bring such students to the counseling service. In these cases, therapists can sometimes effectively function as "pinch hitters" for disengaged parents by providing, in Winnicott's (1953) terms, a "holding environment" for students. A therapist who acts as a "transitional object" has intimate knowledge of the student and is available as needed during the student's college career for support, insight, or advice. With sufficient "refueling," a student may eventually be able to reach out for additional reparative inputs from other parental substitutes in the college community.

TYPES OF FAMILY PROBLEMS

Several types of family problems may be identified among college students. These are (1) autonomy struggles in conflicted family systems, (2) problems stemming from loss, (3) problems in separating from enmeshed family systems, and (4) attachment problems associated with disengaged families.

We focus here on the role these family problems play in students' presenting problems or conflicts. Since no psychological problem is unidimensional, the cases we discuss are not "pure" and to some extent overlap the categories.

Autonomy Struggles in Conflicted Family Systems

Students' internal conflicts about becoming independent are likely to have special intensity and meaning when their families are divided and hence insecure. Students then may be afraid to become autonomous and disrupt the family further; expressing dependency needs may represent an unconscious wish to distract warring parents from their battles in order to unite them. Autonomy struggles most frequently manifest themselves in crises centered around academic performance—the most obvious avenue to autonomy and independence at this life stage. The college therapist's task is to frame the issue, explore its ramifications in the family system, assess the reality constraints with the student, and address the student's own conflicted wishes and needs. Below are two examples of autonomy conflicts and therapeutic interventions.

Struggle Expressed as Inhibition

Anne, an 18-year-old freshman, came to the counseling service tearfully, asking to see a counselor right away. She felt unable to complete her first term paper in college and feared that this meant she would be unable to succeed at the school. This was an unlikely prospect, since she was quite obviously a very bright young woman who had previously been an exceptional student. She associated her current academic block to an experience the previous year, when she was having acute conflicts with her parents about her wish to go to college away from home. Then, too, she had had problems completing a paper.

On inquiry, she revealed that she was the youngest of several children in her family and the last to leave home. Her decision to go away to school appeared to have activated an "empty nest" crisis in her parents' conflict-ridden marriage, in which there had been frequent brief separations and threats of divorce. There had even been a suggestion that the parents might divorce when Anne left home. The parents could unite, however, on where Anne should go to college. They pressured her to apply to a prestigious college near home. Anne overtly complied, but managed to sabotage the application by failing to send crucial data to the college her parents chose. This left her with no other good alternative but to go to her first-choice school, which was away from home. She did so, albeit with much acrimony and misgivings from her parents.

The therapist explored Anne's recent role as focus of conflict in her parents' marriage, and her ambivalent feelings about taking a decisive step to detach herself from them by leaving home. Anne was able to understand her problem with the paper as a symptom of her fear of succeeding in her new college world, and of her unconscious wish to return to the threatened "nest" that might come apart once her parents no longer had her to fight over. This very bright, labile, still adolescent girl was consciously quite prepared for the possible dissolution of her parents' marriage and could use the therapist's interpretations to good advantage. She returned for a second session a few days later, reporting that she had completed the paper and received positive feedback from her teacher. She wanted no further counseling for the moment, but suggested that she would return if needed.

Anne had already partially resolved her autonomy sturggle by coming away to college in the face of strong opposition from her parents. However, the presence of the therapist as a transitional parental substitute supplied a boost at a crucial point. Since her intellectual gifts were critical for her autonomous development, support for overcoming the academic block was essential to forestall a regression. The therapist supported her during a temporary regression when she could not turn to her parents for "refueling," for fear of confirming their dire forecasts. Such brief interventions, with the therapist's promise of being "on call," are often appropriate for freshmen who may need to touch base with a parental substitute but want to avoid becoming dependent, with its threat of further regression.

Struggle Expressed as Resistance

Whereas Anne's focal conflict involved an unconscious inhibition in her performance, Joe's autonomy struggle manifested itself in a crisis of will. Also a freshman, Joe came to counseling because of loss of motivation to do his schoolwork. He justified himself by complaining about the quality of his teachers, and showed surprisingly little guilt about skipping classes and neglecting assignments. This was quite out of character with his performance in high school, where he had been a conscientious, very capable student. Joe's stance now was to sabotage any fruitful outcome. His absence from class and refusal to work made it clear that he had no intention of finishing the year, yet he resisted the next best course of withdrawing from school before he failed. He preferred the passive–aggressive strategy of playing the helpless victim who is asked to leave after failing.

It was quite apparent that Joe's resistance to his studies reflected an autonomy struggle with his father, an alumnus of the college, who had pressured Joe to go there. Joe had preferred to join some of his high school friends at a less prestigious college much closer to home. The father had refused to pay for that school, leaving Joe feeling trapped and enraged. Joe was not ready to risk the loss of his father's financial support by asserting his own choice of college. Rather, he chose the strategy of failure, thus frustrating his ambitious father while escaping the responsibility for his aggression by labeling himself psychologically impaired. He sought counseling to verify his impairment.

Joe's helpless anger was greatly intensifed by the family drama that had transpired in the 3 years prior to his freshman year. His seemingly

stable, well-functioning middle American family had erupted in separation and divorce, precipitated by his father's romance with and subsequent marriage to the mother's best friend. Subsequently, Joe had
been forced into a joint custody arrangement that had disrupted his
social life. He empathized with his mother and greatly resented his
father's authoritarian control. Given the collapse of his stable world at
age 15, it is no wonder that he did not wish to separate from his high
school peer group or to comply with his father's demand that Joe identify with him by attending his alma mater.

Interpretations of his motives for resisting academic work were
ineffective in turning Joe's passivity into activity. Joe was not interested
in using counseling in a constructive way; he was determined to resist
counseling too. The therapist could only point out his passive aims and
the obvious anger that was animating him. The counseling concluded
after five visits, with the recommendation that after Joe left school he
should address the conflict with a family therapist whom he had previously found helpful.

Joe's case illustrates the impact of family breakups on adolescents'
capacity to achieve autonomy and separation. College students often
cannot leave home until they have worked through anger at parents
that family conflicts and disruptions have instilled.

Problems Stemming from Loss

Parental divorce, death, and disabling illness constitute significant losses
for college students. Though these losses may not necessarily be mentioned in the complaint brought to the college therapist, in most cases
they are implicated in the presenting problem, especially when the problem concerns current relationships. When the parental loss is recent, the
task of mourning is clear-cut and can often be accomplished within the
context of a college counseling center. For example, Mary, a very competent sophomore with counterdependent defenses, came to the service 4
months after her father's death from cancer, feeling unsure of herself and
unaccountably detached from her boyfriend. These were unfamiliar and
frightening feelings for her. She had dealt with her father's fatal illness
by playing the caretaker of both parents, and after his death had continued to divert her own grief by focusing on her mother's loss. She generally reacted to sad feelings by fleeing from them. While encouraging her
to talk about her father and their relationship, her therapist also had to
respect her defenses, and therefore did not insist that she focus exclusively on her massive trauma and loss. In this way, Mary was helped to
grieve at a pace that she could manage.

Usually, the college therapist encounters students whose losses have taken place prior to the college years. These losses are apt to manifest themselves in chronic depressive positions and conflicted identities. In addition to the death or physical absence of a parent, the temporary emotional withdrawal of a physically present parent because of depression must also be treated as a loss that requires mourning. These often unacknowledged losses may significantly increase a student's fears and sense of aloneness during current periods of separation, and they complicate the student's developmental task of separating from the rest of the family. It is of note that students with significant past losses frequently turn up for counseling during their sophomore year, a time when they are generally faced with the experience of feeling alone.

Mourning earlier losses may or may not be a feasible task within the college setting. Success depends upon the degree to which past losses have been activated in students' current lives; the degree to which students have conflicting feelings toward the lost parent; the degree of identification with the lost parent; and the degree to which students are psychologically minded and have some capacity for making meaningful attachments. A frequent complicating feature is pseudoindependence, whereby students as children projected themselves into an adult stance and unconsciously adopted the philosophy of "I will not want what I cannot have." One issue in therapy with these students is finding ways by which they are able to obtain and accept emotional supplies, because they are resistive to feeling dependent.

Successful Mourning for a Lost Parent

The case of Donna, a 19-year-old sophomore whose mother died of breast cancer when she was 14, illustrates a significant mourning experience achieved within a college therapy setting. Like most such experiences, it was activated both by her life stage and by triggers in the current family situation. She sought counseling because she had been feeling very depressed, even having some suicidal ideation. She was angry at her all-male suitemates, at her father, and even at her best girlfriends. The impetus for the depression was her father's remarriage several months earlier, coupled with the sale of her childhood home. To make matters worse, her father and his new wife had moved into a new apartment in which there was no permanent room for Donna. Her older sister was far away in graduate school, and Donna felt quite alone and unsupported. She felt particularly estranged from her "insensitive" suitemates—a feeling partly displaced from her younger brother, who did have a permanent room in her father's new home.

Donna was a bright, psychologically minded girl who could quite readily make the connection between her anger at current family events and the impact of the death of her mother. With support, she was ready to explore the feelings about her past that had previously been unavailable to her. It became obvious that her loyalty to her mother had kept her at arm's length from the new stepmother and fueled her anger at her father and brother. She reviewed her early life and family relationships prior to her mother's illness and death, allowing both parents to emerge in her narrative as real people, warts and all. At the same time, she developed an intense, ambivalent maternal transference to the therapist, bringing dream material that bespoke her fears of becoming too dependent and thus exposing herself to further loss.

After doing some useful mourning during the fall term, Donna failed to return to therapy immediately after the Christmas break. An intense transference dream brought her back in the middle of the spring term. By now she had greatly improved her relationship with her father and stepmother. The theme of leaving home was now addressed with regard to the therapist as she anticipated spending her junior year abroad. She needed both support for leaving, which was a developmentally appropriate step, and reassurance that if necessary she could return in the future for "refueling."

The combination of her feelings of aloneness in her all-male suite, the absence of her freshman-year supports, and the fresh wound of the loss of her home all contributed to Donna's readiness to express grief for her mother. The therapist's tuning in to this material facilitated the mourning process, which took place within a few months.

Unexpressed Mourning for a Lost Parent

Unlike Donna, many students with parental losses are not readily able to do grief work. This is especially true of students with parents who have died by suicide, usually preceded by serious mental illness. The guilt at having not prevented the suicide and the sense of helpless rage it has engendered result in isolation of affect and other defenses that make such students inaccessible to brief therapy. These students seek counseling when current relationships are disappointing, but usually leave treatment when it is clear that it will inevitably involve facing the painful loss. A college therapist can do little here except to communicate the importance of a student's facing feelings associated with his or her deceased parent in order to free up the capacity for future attachments.

With students who are highly defended against painful early losses, the main therapeutic ally is time. Repeated disappointing relationships revealing a pattern of self-defeating behavior may bring home what a therapist's mere words and predictions will not. Whereas sophomores may experience and disregard some depression, seniors usually begin to worry about their prospects for adult life when current relationships fail. Such was the case with Allen, a 20-year-old senior, whose defenses probably would have made therapy futile earlier in his college career. Allen, who had a very sophisticated, psychologically minded veneer, sought treatment for "anhedonia." His inability to be more responsive led to the loss of a girlfriend he greatly valued. In addition, he was unable to make a career decision, and he was preoccupied with death. He revealed a chronic depressive position that seemed clearly associated with the death of his father when he was 13. His father's accidental death had followed a downhill course of alcoholism and was clearly a conflicted issue for his son, who was just entering adolescence. Allen especially regretted not having attended his father's funeral. His own career conflicts were quite parallel to the conflicts he knew his father had experienced, and they indicated the strength of his identification. A further current event that perhaps finally prompted Allen to break out of his self-defeating, frozen grief was the threatened loss of his mother, with whom he had always been especially close, to a new man in her life. Although Allen would not have profited from brief therapy, his position as a senior with career choices to make and his capacity for productive use of his intellect made him a suitable candidate now for intensive psychoanalytic therapy. This treatment might penetrate his obsessional defenses, bringing him closer to his feelings. A referral was arranged.

Problems in Separating from Enmeshed Family Systems

Students who come from enmeshed family systems present some of the most intractable problems encountered in college counseling. Rarely can these problems be truly resolved within the limited time frame available, even when students are relatively well motivated to work on them. Not infrequently, the enmeshment is regarded as a problem by therapists, but not by students themselves. One kind of enmeshment appears in same-sex parent–child relationships, in which a parent over-identifies with and attempts to live through the child to such an extent that boundaries between them are blurred. Another form is present in caretaker parent–child relationships, in which there are role reversals and blurred generational boundaries. The degree to which students are part of an enmeshed family system may only become apparent over the course of what initially appear to be ordinary separation problems.

In each of the following cases, as with most cases of enmeshment, both elements—parental overidentification and blurred generational boundaries—were present.

Ellen came to the counseling service as a senior, with serious separation problems stemming from her enmeshed tie with her mother. She
had accumulated an outstanding college record and was apparently
headed for a high-powered graduate program abroad after graduation.
Her presenting complaint was an obsessive fear of being pregnant,
despite assurances that she was not. This anxiety was fueled by her
impulsive sexuality and was given some reality basis in her amenor-
rhea, which was soon diagnosed as a symptom of an ovarian disorder.
The unconscious wish underlying her fear of pregnancy was to resolve
her separation crisis, since clearly a pregnancy would interfere with
her career plans.

Ellen was the older of two daughters born too soon in her parents'
marriage to permit the parents to comfortably establish themselves. The
mother was very disappointed in her husband's modest schoolteacher
career and had continually urged Ellen to look for a man with better
prospects and higher social status than her father. Ellen's mother had
a conflicted relationship with her own disapproving mother. In turn,
Ellen's mother behaved with intense ambivalence toward Ellen, often
directing uncontrollable fits of anger at her for not living up to the
mother's expectations and for not being attentive enough. Ellen would
become enraged at her mother, but continued to be caught up in trying to be the idealized woman her mother would have liked to have
been herself.

Ellen was seen for the better part of the academic year to facilitate
her senior transition. Although she eventually decided to go to the
graduate school and thus physically separate herself from her family,
the enmeshment with her mother was far from resolved. She continued
to feel the pull toward attaching herself to a promising "yuppie" mate,
thereby remaining close to her mother. Despite the repeated opportunities Ellen had in therapy to observe, dissect, and anticipate the
dynamics of the mother–daughter relationship, its conflict-addicted
quality did not significantly abate, nor were firm boundaries established.
Her therapist facilitated only one phase of the separation process, and
hoped that a door had been opened for future work.

A second case illustrates the possibilities for therapeutic change in
cases of enmeshment. Dan, a 22-year-old senior, encountered severe
examination anxiety as he neared the end of his college career. This
unaccountable anxiety had led him to drop critical courses and decide
to take a leave of absence from school. Previously academically successful although socially inhibited, he had transferred from a smaller,
supportive college to a highly competitive one. His current inhibition
seemed to point in the direction of his relationship with his father.

Dan was the younger son of well-educated parents. His father, who worked at a level lower than his abilities and training would warrant, was mainly interested in his two sons. Dan's academically successful brother found it necessary to move far away to escape the father's over-involvement with him. Dan, on the other hand, was regressing to greater dependency on his father, constantly seeking his advice and support concerning his academic trouble. As this relationship was explored, Dan revealed that he regarded his father, who had had an unhappy childhood, as quite psychologically vulnerable; his father would be very threatened if Dan were to become more independent and separate after graduating from college. Thus, "choking" on examinations allowed Dan to stay attached; he could gratify his father's need to support him only by failing. Over a two-session consultation, Dan showed considerable interest in confronting the dynamics of his situation and readily accepted a referral.

It is worth noting that truly enmeshed students are most likely to turn up at counseling centers when a separation decision is imminent. Hence, Ellen and Dan were both seniors, on the verge of making important adult career commitments. Symptoms that might undermine their graduation or career success (failing to complete papers, dropping courses, or becoming pregnant) brought them to counseling. They accepted their enmeshment as a given, seeking help only for their troublesome immediate symptoms. Such symptoms in heretofore high-achieving seniors often signal enmeshment problems with overinvolved parents.

Attachment Problems Associated with Disengaged Families

Students from disengaged families suffer from a lack of psychological inputs, which in turn limits their capacity to make use of many resources within the college. Disengagement is a matter of kind and degree; it rarely means that there has been a total lack of available parenting over a prolonged period. Few students have been without at least one caring parent through their preadolescent years. Disengagement may consist of emotional distance from at least one parent in an intact family or, in divorced families, a frequently absent father and an affectively withdrawn or self-absorbed mother. It may refer to lack of attunement and emotional support or to a failure of structure and control. Depending upon which parent is more disengaged and the chronicity of the disengagement, students present with varying symptoms and character pathology. They may express diffuse feelings of dissatisfaction, indifferent achievement, and extreme sensitivity to rejection. Unlike students from enmeshed families, they are apt to lack deep interests and have rather shallow attachments. They often have low self-esteem, especially regarding their sexual selves.

Disengaged parenting cannot be easily repaired. The task of college therapy in most cases is to identify the disengagement and the feelings associated with it, and to help the student find a reparative relationship that might at least partially replace what has been missed. Like students with enmeshed parents, students who have been insufficiently nourished or supported are often candidates for referral to long-term supportive therapy. However, their difficulty in making emotional commitments may deter them from going beyond seeking a "quick fix" from the college therapist.

Most often in counseling, disengagement in young women involves the father–daughter relationship. In some of these cases, the disengagement of fathers is a result of the marital instability so common to parents who were young adults in the 1960s. In others, fathers began to disengage emotionally because of extreme discomfort with their adolescent daughters' sexuality.

Amy, a 20-year-old sophomore, came to therapy because of difficulty in giving up a boyfriend who had seduced and abandoned her in a very brief but intense relationship. The hurt was so great that she had moved her dorm room in order to avoid him, but she continued to date him intermittently even though he also dated other girls. She wanted help with her masochistic prolongation of this relationship.

A feisty, ambitious girl, Amy was the second of four closely spaced children. Her conservative parents had a somewhat skewed relationship in which the mother was dominant. Amy considered herself the rebel in the family, by far the most academically ambitious, and generally quite self-sufficient. Although she got some support for her intellectual achievement from her father, a teacher, she complained of his lack of emotional availability and his passivity. Indeed, she attributed her poor self-esteem with men to his lack of attention. She was able to verbalize her yearning for a close, supportive, attentive relationship with a man, and she became aware of the appeal of this younger boyfriend who had so admired her. Her depression lifted after a few sessions, and by the last one she had broken off entirely with her rejecting lover and had begun what appeared to be a more satisfying relationship with a graduate student.

Amy was a more emotionally and intellectually differentiated young woman than many children of disengaged parents. She was masochistically vulnerable, but not narcissistically fixated. Her father's lack of support for her feminine self made her vulnerable to a relationship with an immature partner that re-enacted aspects of her parents' skewed relationship. But her ability to rebound and use insight productively indicated a basis of early "good enough" mothering that made it possible for her to take nourishment from the therapy. The brief therapy of seven sessions was sufficient to point her to a reparative relationship in the person of her mature new boyfriend.

In some cases where students are unusually socially constricted, a college therapist may provide the reparative relationship, rather than being simply a facilitator. In the case of Alex, for example, the college therapist acted as a substitute parent by providing some intimacy and guidance that this developmentally arrested young man had missed. Alex was referred to counseling by a dean during his junior year. Although he spent almost all of his time on his academic work, he had done poorly and was thinking of withdrawing from college before his finals. In addition, he was extremely unhappy about having no girl-friend; he was in fact quite socially isolated because of his low self-esteem. He was from a mixed racial background, and was self-conscious about his physical appearance as well.

The only child of parents who divorced when he was about 6, Alex spent a lonely childhood in which his main satisfactions were school achievements. His father had disappeared from his life, and his mother, an upwardly mobile nurse, moved with Alex to a setting away from familiar family and friends. Although she was a responsible, stable par-ent, she was quite emotionally withdrawn and embittered. She had not been tuned in to her son's loneliness or to his insecurity about his masculinity. As counseling proceeded, it became apparent that Alex had little memory of and no real knowledge about his father, and that he felt inhibited in asking his embittered mother about the past; this had left a huge gap in his sense of identity.

Although not psychologically minded and quite passive, Alex finally responded to the therapist's repeated inquiries about his past by acknowledging his curiosity about his father and exploring his fanta-sies about him. In addition to addressing his feelings about his iden-tity and his insecurity as a male, his counselor addressed his academic problems by supporting a change of major and use of tutoring. The therapy was especially important to him because it allowed him to speak about the previously unspeakable, to share his intimate thoughts and feelings with a parental substitute, and to break out of his loneliness. He continued to see the counselor periodically until graduation. With-out this support, it is unlikely that he could have sustained himself in college.

Especially for students from relatively deprived, often minority-group backgrounds, the availability of ego-strengthening reparative rela-tionships within the college itself is important. For many of these stu-dents, school has provided essential organization, and teachers have been important mentors. Such students often make an "institutional transference" to the counseling service, allowing it to function as a kind of substitute parent. The college therapist can supply psychological structure and understanding that may enable them to utilize their college experience productively.

WORKING WITH FAMILY MEMBERS

Direct contact with parents and other family members is a relatively infrequent but important activity of most counseling center therapists. Contacts are most frequently made by telephone at times of crisis, such as when a student is hospitalized or is suicidal. These calls are sometimes initiated by the therapist, especially if there is a question about the student's fitness to remain in school. Family members may also contact therapists to establish whether a student is in treatment, to lend support, to give information, or to check on progress during treatment. Occasionally a contact is deliberately disruptive of treatment, testing the tact of the therapist.

It is well to consider that all contact between parents and the therapist occurs under conditions of stress for the family, and often during a crisis. As a stranger, the therapist has no standing except as it inheres in the occupation; unless the family has knowledge or positive experience with mental health practitioners, fear and skepticism of the therapist are common. The burden is on the therapist to reduce the family's stress level without treating the members as if they are patients, a status implying loss of control. A further impediment to work with families is the tendency for all people to dislike the bearer of bad news—a primitive and "unacceptable" reaction that may bewilder family members and therapist alike.

The therapist must be careful not to threaten or challenge whatever sense of control over their child parents may feel, and to bolster parents' sense of control over their own feelings. To accomplish these goals, the therapist must quickly establish an alliance with the family members in a joint effort to help their child.

Confidentiality

Contact between the therapist and family members is often useful in a crisis, for it gives the therapist an opportunity to independently evaluate the family context with which the student must cope. Therapists should not use the issue of confidentiality to avoid contact with parents. When crucial decisions must be made about treatment plans or withdrawal from school, students more often than not welcome contact between their therapist and their families, which validates their distress and need for help. When a student has already authorized the therapist to speak with parents, confidentiality is not the problem, but what to communicate may be problematic. The therapist and student can sometimes work out beforehand the most useful approach and level of information to convey to the parents.

Sometimes the therapist can anticipate that a parent will call and can ask the student for authorization to communicate. If family members call before authorization is given, the therapist can give a brief explanation of confidentiality and express a general willingness to speak with family members, while neither affirming nor denying that the particular student has been seen. Family members should be encouraged to give as much information as possible to which the therapist can respond without violating confidentiality. Family members can often provide missing data about a student and sometimes about themselves that will clarify the situation. Based on the discussion, the therapist can make specific recommendations such as whether a family member should arrive at once on the scene, whom else they might contact, and whether there is a need for the student to authorize further communication. Time spent with concerned parents may prevent further escalation of the crisis situation and/or facilitate a quick resolution.

Family Consultations

Parents who have denied their children's problems, overidealized their children, or detached themselves prematurely from the parenting role may contribute to students' reluctance to enlist family support in a crisis. When a student is unable to inform the parents about his or her problems or feels that the parents will not accept this news, a joint consultation involving therapist, student, and parents is often useful. Parents who feel helpless in the face of their child's reluctance to talk with them also may seek out the therapist to facilitate communications between them and their child.

The therapist has a delicate role in a family consultation. The goal of such consultations usually involves acknowledging the problem and developing treatment recommendations for the student. The therapist has the task of confronting mutually reinforcing denials between parents and child, firmly emphasizing the realistic consequences of failure to follow through on treatment recommendations, and yet offering some hope to both student and parents that the crisis can be resolved. Although the identified patient is the student, a family consultation may elicit acknowledgment from one or both parents of family problems that have contributed to the student's crisis. The therapist must deflect blame and mutual recrimination, and focus on practical means of addressing the current situation. It is usually inadvisable to suggest treatment for parents unless they solicit such advice, for such a recommendation may be experienced as blame.

Given that college students are in the process of separation and need reinforcement in the direction of becoming more autonomous, family therapy is usually not the treatment of choice, even when family problems are a prominent aspect of a student's difficulties. However, in cases of severe enmeshment, this recommendation may be most acceptable to both students and parents, since it initially promises that therapy will not threaten their relationship with each other. In such situations, a future family therapist can work toward developing the psychological context from which students can finally leave home.

REFERENCES

Carter, E., & McGoldrick, M. (1980). The family life cycle and family therapy: An overview. In E. Carter & M. McGoldrick (Eds.), *The family life cycle: A framework for family therapy.* New York: Gardner Press.

Fulmer, R. H., & Medalie, M. D. (1987). Treating the male college student from a family systems perspective. In J. C. Coleman (Ed.), *Working with troubled adolescents: A handbook* (pp. 31–45). New York: Academic Press.

Medalie, J. D. (1981). The college years as a mini-life cycle: Developmental tasks and adaptive options. *Journal of the American College Health Association, 30,* 75–79.

Medalie, J. D. (1987). Psychotherapy referral as a therapeutic goal of college counseling. *Journal of College Student Psychotherapy, 1,* 83–103.

Minuchin, S. (1974). *Families and family therapy.* Cambridge, MA: Harvard University Press.

Winnicott, D. W. (1953). Transitional objects and transitional phenomena. *International Journal of Psycho-Analysis, 34,* 89–97.

Wolfenstein, M. (1966). How is mourning possible? *Psychoanalytic Study of the Child, 21,* 93–123.

6

Relationships

MARVIN H. GELLER

In a fundamental way, this entire book is about relationships. When I was first asked whether I was interested in writing a chapter on "relationship issues" for this edited volume, I felt the topic to be so broad that I feared I would get lost in trying to coherently present work that would be useful to potential readers. After thought and discussion, the focus was narrowed to heterosexual relationships from a clinical and pragmatic perspective. The editors would like a chapter presenting the typical problems that students bring to university counseling or mental health centers, and examples of how one might think about and work with the students and the relationship concerns that they bring. Although this perspective clearly narrows the focus, it nevertheless is a topic that is as complex as life itself. Life is about relationships.

In order to orient the reader to what follows, let me state that my theoretical perspective is psychoanalytic, and in particular I am interested in an object-relations perspective. The fundamental questions about relationships explored from an object-relations point of view can be stated as follows: How do our significant early relationships become internalized and affect our subsequent view of the world and other people? How do early relationships affect our choice of partners, our ability to be satisfied with our partners, and the satisfaction and love we are able to experience in our heterosexual relationships?

How do we understand and work with the young woman who seeks help because she continues to select the wrong partner? Or the young woman who is chronically dissatisfied with her boyfriends, always criticizing them, while at the same time feeling dependent upon them? What do we explore with the young man who seeks counsel because his girlfriend of 3 years is offering an ultimatum: Either make a formal engagement or end the relationship? What should we focus on with the young man who is constantly on the lookout for the "right" woman, but is never able to find her? Shall we offer support to the young man unable to overcome his depression about the breakup of a relationship, or shall we explore more deeply what has been lost and what might be underlying his sadness? What about the female freshman who becomes involved with a male classmate the first week of school and is devastated later when he wants to break it off?

All of these are relatively familiar issues to those of us working in university or college counseling or mental health centers. How we think about these issues and how we intervene psychotherapeutically depend upon our theoretical perspective as well as the length of time available for treatment. Those of us who use short-term approaches within university mental health settings utilize different interventions and have different expectations than therapists who work on a more long-term basis, usually outside of the university setting.

The tension contained within this chapter relates to my commitment to psychoanalytic object-relations theory on the one hand, and the necessity on the other to translate this perspective into relatively short-term interventions within the context of a university counseling service. The goal of therapy from a psychoanalytic point of view would be an increase in ego strength and an enlargement of ego boundaries. We can think of this enlargement of ego as an increase in the ability to know more about unconscious needs and motives, as well as the ability to tolerate and deal more effectively with those aspects of the unconscious that have been brought into awareness; this allows the individual to behave more frequently in his or her own best interest. Most typically this process occurs within the context of long-term treatment (either psychoanalysis proper or psychoanalytically oriented psychotherapy), the transference relationship with the therapist being a key element in the expansion and strengthening of ego boundaries. The two key elements are (1) making the unconscious conscious through emotionally laden insight; and (2) effecting growth and change in psychic structure because of the reparative aspects of the relationship with the psychotherapist.

The challenge within the context of a college mental health center is to adapt this model to a short-term approach—to help develop genuine insights that can start a process of change and offer the individual a method for exploring his or her problems. If the process works well, the student becomes aware that something new and valid has been added to his or her sense of self and that psychotherapy is a useful tool in the search for self-knowledge. Some students are ready for self-search and self-evaluation. Others are seeking concrete solutions to complex problems, and some are seeking soothing in the form of immediate relief from their pain. Although in-depth work can be more personally enriching for therapist and student, immediate relief or concrete solutions can be valid ends in themselves. Although I am committed to the psychoanalytic perspective on the world, there is room for a wide variety of approaches within the context of a university counseling center. This chapter focuses exclusively on a short-term psychoanalytic approach.

SOME THEORETICAL BACKGROUND

It is universally accepted within the psychoanalytic framework that the ability to love and form meaningful interpersonal relationships has its roots in early parent–child interactions. The infant's ability to form a sense of self separate from the mother, a self that begins to develop coherence and esteem, is determined by the complex subtleties of their interpersonal experience. The "good enough" mother (Winnicott, 1965) is one who can provide a holding environment in which the infant can flourish both physically and psychologically. Mahler (1981) has sensitized us to the tasks of early childhood and the effect of the resolution of those tasks on later development. We know that if a young child is to eventually gain a relatively healthy sense of self, he or she must be able gradually to leave the mother's side and eventually move into the world beyond the home. This process of separation and individuation is a complex phenomenon and is achieved through the process of internalization. In the day-to-day interactions with the significant people in its environment, the young child begins to develop an inner world of experiences that shapes his or her self-perception, as well as how he or she feels and relates to others. The child fortunate enough to have parents who are reliable, caring, and dependable is more likely to develop a healthy sense of self-esteem and trust in the world than is the child reared in an anxious and insecure environment with parents whose needs take precedence over the needs of the developing youngster. The recent contributions of Kohut (1977), like the previous contributions of Erikson (1963) and a host of other psychoanalytic writers, have placed strong emphasis on the lifelong role of early relationships in development, and, specifically, their influence in determining a person's sense of self-worth. It is this sense of self-esteem and the yearning to fulfill long-standing desires that will be the cornerstone of my observations about the vicissitudes of relationships and the problems encountered in their pursuit.

It is a truism among mental health professionals working within a college environment that the tasks of late adolescence, especially during college years, center around the issues of separation from family; the consolidation of gender identity; the formation of a career goal; and the ability to eventually form intimate, meaningful, and committed relationships. What was in early childhood a need to move from the symbolic attachment to mother into an individuated toddler becomes, in adolescence, the shedding of family dependencies and the loosening of infantile ties, in order to become an adult member of society. These ties and attachments, whether negative or positive, are extremely powerful. The critical issue for the adolescent is how to shift from these powerful emotional ties of love and hate with parents to investments in peers and adults outside the family. Going off to college can be seen as a major step in the adolescent's move toward separation from family and home. For those young people who have been doing reasonably well at developing self-esteem and autonomy, college and extrafamilial relationships may be exciting challenges that can be mastered without encountering serious psychological problems. For those students who have not been so successful in establishing psychological autonomy and healthy self-esteem, the path through college may be filled with many pitfalls and difficulties.

Another important aspect of theory is contributed by the object-relations focus. Arlow (1986), in his book chapter on object concept and object choice, draws our attention to the distinction between interpersonal relations and object relations. Simply put, the "object" in object-relations theory does not refer to the person or thing in the outside world, but rather to the "mental representation" that one holds about that person or thing outside of one's self. In working with students who bring relationship problems, it can be useful for clinicians to keep this distinction in mind. How an actual person is seen, experienced, desired, or related to by students is profoundly affected by their "inner objects." These objects have been formed through a lifetime of experience with the important people in their world, especially in relationships with early parenting figures. From this perspective, the focus of therapy is on how object relations affect interpersonal relationships.

Horner (1986) focuses upon the centrality of early mother–infant relationships as the foundation for one's capacity to love. If a basic attachment exists, then the child's ability to love develops normally. Parents who have the ability to empathize with and respond to their children's needs, rather than impose their own, are more likely to foster autonomous individuals with a strong sense of self-esteem who will be free themselves to express genuine love and concern for others. Relationship difficulties, as well as other problems, are more likely to arise when childhood experiences lead to what Winnicott (1965) has called the "false self." The false self is a self that reacts and responds rather than initiates; it is the child who has had to hide his or her uniqueness in order to feel secure. His or her special qualities have not been accepted or admired—this child has been told directly or subtly what is required in order to be loved. In this climate, autonomy, healthy self-esteem, and a genuine capacity to care about and love others cannot flourish.

Horner draws a parallel between being and loving. The individual who has had the fortunes of good parenting is able to *be* the genuine and real person he or she is, and also has the capacity to accept and genuinely love others; the person whose "real self" has been forced into hiding will not have the same capacity to love genuinely. This person is likely to need others, perform for others, fight others, or comply with others, but rarely will genuinely love. Others are needed as regulators for self-esteem, but are feared for the same reasons that they are needed. In order for these individuals to genuinely love and establish enduring and mutually satisfying intimate relationships, significant transformations in their sense of self must occur.

THE COLLEGE COUNSELING CENTER

I now turn more directly to the issues and problems involved in working psychotherapeutically with students who bring relationship issues to a college counseling or mental health center.

The college years have been regarded as a transitional period between adolescence and young adulthood. Levinson, Darrow, Klein, Levinson, and McKee (1978) designate this period as "the early adult transition." It is a time during which individuals can test new roles, discover new interests, and explore relationships without making long-term commitments. In her paper on the college years as a mini-life cycle, Medalie (1981) suggests that college psychotherapists are "apt to regard student problems as coming in part from the anxiety generated by their transitional developmental status in which one or more psychosocial tasks are not being adequately confronted" (p. 75). One of these tasks is the forming of intimate social and sexual relationships. Although forming intimate relationships can be viewed as a typical life cycle task essential for the process of separating from one's family of origin, it is important to distinguish, when possible, between the inevitable anxieties that are part of a mutable developmental process and those concerns that flow from more entrenched and long-standing character issues.

Although the solutions to developmental tasks are affected by the context in which they occur, in this case the college environment, it is my belief that one's developmental history is always a major factor to be considered, especially when matters go awry. As Erikson (1963) has pointed out, the successful mastery of one stage of development significantly increases the probability of coping successfully with the next. Those students who enter college with a sturdy sense of self obviously will negotiate the tasks of this stage of life more effectively and with more satisfaction than those students whose early experiences have been harmful to their self-esteem.

The challenge for psychoanalytic clinicians working in a college counseling center is to effectively utilize their theoretical orientation within the context of a short-term treatment model. An object-relations framework appears to be more at home in a long-term therapy setting, where the individual's internal life can eventually unfold in the transference relationship. The demands of a college setting make it more difficult to settle in psychotherapeutically; the setting does not allow the work to unfold gradually. In a short-term framework, the therapist has to develop a working hypothesis rapidly, focus actively upon a given problem, and be more active in uncovering covert issues before having an opportunity to work with defensive structures. Nevertheless, an object-relations perspective can inform the process of treatment even in a college mental health center.

OPENING ISSUES

Langs (1976) has written extensively about the structure of the work frame and its impact upon the conduct and outcome of psychotherapy. Organizations typically provide a general work frame that sets parameters within and around which individuals may formulate their own styles. In college psychotherapy, a key dimension of the work frame is length of treatment. In my own work with students, which is generally once per week for each student, I typically do not set specific time limits but usually have a short-term perspective in mind. A student coming to the counseling center is therefore entering into a somewhat ambiguous situation. On the one hand I am trying to provide an open-ended work frame, but on the other I am establishing an uncertainty about the length of treatment, which can create covert tensions in our work. When these tensions surface, I attempt to use them therapeutically. With more severely disturbed students, this approach is contraindicated; with them one needs to be explicit about length of treatment, and usually a long-term relationship (and perhaps a referral) is necessary.

My therapeutic work with students bringing relationship problems does not vary from my work with students in general. The first interview with each student is diagnostic. I am trying to understand the student's problem, decide what approach to take (e.g., expressive or supportive), evaluate the student's motivation, and discern the student's conscious and unconscious expectations of counseling. I will, if possible, attempt trial interventions to assess the student's openness to his or her own psychological processes.

A sophomore, Rachael, came to the counseling center wanting help with her depression. Her boyfriend had recently left her, and after 3 weeks she found her depression still interfering with her academic work. A friend suggested she try the counseling center. After telling me her story, she fell silent, looking as if she wanted me to do something. Feeling somewhat uncertain, I asked her what she hoped we would work on. She said, "What! I told you I have been depressed for 3 weeks; it's interfering with my work." She again fell silent. I said, "I guess you had expected it would have lifted by now; perhaps it means that you still have feelings that you haven't explored." "Look," she said, "I told you I am depressed and my friend suggested I come here for help! Can you help me get rid of my depression now?" "I can help you," I responded, "but it will take time. Being depressed after being rejected is not an unusual thing. [I was consciously trying to normalize her experience.] It doesn't always go away when you want it to." I told her I thought it would be helpful to talk more about her feelings toward her boyfriend, and perhaps it would help alleviate her depression and provide her with some insights. I did not deal directly with her dependency or her anger at me, except to acknowledge that she might be disappointed. I did suggest that she was angry at her boyfriend but had not been able to express it. My hypothesis may not have been correct, but I was trying to see whether she was open to joining me in work. Despite my efforts to engage her, she obviously felt that what I had to offer was not what she needed. She was in pain that was interfering with her life, and she wanted someone to remove it. I offered her the opportunity to return, suggesting that she might find it useful. I had the perhaps fanciful notion that her disappointment and anger toward me could lead her to decide to help herself; this could be the catalyst to resolving her depression. However, she never came back.

In contrast, Janet, a senior, came to the counseling center to talk about the problems she was having with her boyfriend. She let me know early on that this was not the first boyfriend with whom she had had trouble. Although she was focusing upon her criticism of him, I felt part of her knew that her own issues were at work. She liked John, but found herself feeling very critical and annoyed with his "rational thinking." She attacked him for not having feelings and for being so "damn logical—when we tie-dye shirts he puts the dye on with a ruler." Though I did not doubt her description of him, I did wonder out loud what it was about his rational thinking that made her so angry with him. She wasn't clear. "We aren't on the same wavelength." I asked her whether she felt that he did not value her emotional side. She agreed that he did not. As the hour progressed, there were hints that she felt uncertain about her intellectual capacities, especially her ability to be a clear and rational thinker. I felt her emphasis on the value of feeling was masking some of her self-critical attitudes toward her logical side. I decided to present a working hypothesis to see how open she was to exploring her own internal dynamics. I said, "I wonder if some of the anger you feel toward John's rational thinking is fueled by envy you feel for his abilities." She did not reject what I said, and I felt she was open for exploration. She spent the rest of the hour talking about her previous boyfriend, for whom she still had positive feelings; she had left him because she was critical of his substance abuse. She was telling me indirectly that she felt dependent upon men, but was aware after a short time that their shortcomings disappointed her. I suggested that we work together for a while. She agreed, and we began a course of therapy that lasted 3 months.

These two vignettes highlight the differences in how students bring themselves to the counseling center. The flow of the initial hour provides information on how prepared a student is to work on his or her inner dynamics. For many students, such as Rachael, any attempt to interpret dynamics or inner conflicts would probably be disastrous. Feeling helpless, they simply want someone to alleviate their depression. If the therapist is able to respond to initially resistant students' felt need, they may eventually be able to look inward. Many counseling contacts fail within the first hour because the therapist moves too rapidly or is unable to find a way to an empathic connection.

Hanfmann (1978), in discussing cases of "striking progress," asks, "[W]hat kind of client is most likely to move vigorously in counseling?" (p. 127). From Hanfmann's experience, the students who make "striking progress" do not expect to solve their problems in one or two sessions. Their readiness to commit themselves to the work involved in counseling is either present from the start or emerges in the first session. This readiness also correlates with a kind of perception or ability to move from external issues to internal reactions. Trouble in a relationship or a depressed mood or difficulty studying, Hanfmann says, "is almost from the start ready to be viewed as psychological in the sense of having some roots not in the external events but in his or her own feelings, attitudes and resulting ways of dealing with problems" (pp. 127–128). These students do not focus for long on what to do about this or that particular problem, but rather on their own inner processes, feelings, and reactions. When this occurs with a student, a great deal can be learned in a brief period of time. My assumption is that these students, despite having problems, have a "good enough" sense of self-esteem that permits them to look inward, not in a self-blaming fashion, but in a genuine search for self-knowledge.

COURSE OF THERAPY

In order to discuss clinical material more systematically, I present relationship problems under several clinical headings—narcissistic issues, dependency conflicts, and commitment concerns. People rarely fit neatly into any single category, and similarly, many relationship concerns cut across categories. Nevertheless, it may be useful to categorize the nature of a student's problem in order to explore a specific internal issue more fully.

Narcissistic Concerns

From a psychoanalytic perspective, "primary narcissism" refers to the circumstances of the first months of life when the child cannot distinguish between self and other; we assume that the child feels at one with the world around him or her. Those young adults with a primary narcissistic disturbance have a fragile sense of self and, when psychically threatened, can experience intense anxiety, fearing their sense of self may crumble. Students with primary or very early ego disturbances are not good candidates for short-term insight-oriented therapy. They are more likely to need a constant and long-lasting relationship that allows them to develop a sense of trust and constancy about their inner selves. In interpersonal relationships, they find it difficult to differentiate between their own selves and others. There is always a risk that they will fall into that undefined primal state where the world around them exists only as a function of themselves. Students with early narcissistic disturbances need a great deal of support; they are in desperate need of relationships, yet they fear intimacy. They tend to monopolize the attention of the persons they are involved with, who eventually withdraw because of the overwhelming demands. These students often evoke concern for their well-being in a number of people on the campus.

"Secondary narcissism" can best be described as a turning away from others because of disappointments, and toward the self (self-love) in reaction to an alien or frustrating environment. Young adults who have secondary narcissistic concerns are usually easily wounded. Although they frequently position themselves in relationships so as to avoid injury, they are generally insecure and, despite outward appearances, have low self-esteem. Trying not to need others, they are exceedingly dependent upon others for their self-esteem. These students are not typically threatened by the fear of a disintegrating ego, as are the primary narcissists, but are vulnerable to severe breakdowns in their sense of self-worth. In my experience, some of these students with narcissistic conflicts can benefit from relatively short-term insight-oriented psychotherapy, although it is not possible to work through major transformations within a short period of time.

As an example of secondary narcissism, Ralph, a senior who had been seen previously at our service for an entire academic year, was referred to me by his previous therapist, who had left the service. In our first session, I felt his sense of entitlement expressed in his taking for granted my willingness to work with him for the entire year. His girlfriend had broken up with him, and he was upset because he did not understand what had gone wrong. I decided to see him with a time-limited agreement of 12 sessions. Setting a time limit was atypical for me; I knew it was connected to the countertransference feelings evoked in me by his sense of entitlement. However, I convinced myself that it could be useful for him if the time limit helped us focus on his sense of entitlement and illuminate some of his underlying narcissistic conflicts. My opportunity arose in the first hour, when I explained to Ralph that I would work with him for the set period of time. He reacted with anger and said I was not taking him seriously. I held my position, trying to explore his sense of injury. I told him that his anger came because he did not get what he wanted, not because he believed that short-term work would not be of value. Although it was difficult for me to hold my position because of the countertransferential aspect of my decision, I felt the decision was an appropriate one. The hour was difficult, but ended with his agreeing to see me for 12 sessions. We selected an ending date.

Our subsequent work focused on Ralph's relationships with his former girlfriend, his mother, and me. His girlfriend had accused him of being self-involved, which he did not really understand. He felt he cared for and loved her, although as we talked in greater detail it became clear to both of us that he really needed her to bolster his sense of esteem. In our fourth session, I opened a window because it was warm in my office; he reacted critically, feeling I was not giving him my full attention. At this point, we had enough of an alliance that he was able to explore his reaction to my opening the window. He realized how easily he was injured and how he wanted others to make him feel needed, loved, and special, while at the same time denying that he needed anything from others. Any behavior indicating that he was not special aroused a sense of injury and anger.

We spent time talking about Ralph's mother, who he felt was never there for him in any genuine way. He felt her approval was contingent upon his being what she needed him to be, rather than on what he genuinely needed from her. In our eighth hour, he reported an event that had had a major impact upon him. He had been doing errands and suddenly felt depressed. After giving it some thought, he recognized it had occurred while he was at the bank. He said he had been "taken care of" by a woman teller whom he was trying to chat with; "she was unresponsive and did not even give me a smile." He had no sense at the moment that it had any impact upon him; only later was he able to feel the injury he had experienced. Ralph explored his need to talk with and get her to respond to him. What he thought initially to be a simple gesture of friendliness on his side blossomed into the recognition that he needed everyone to mirror back to him that he was a valued person. This was an important event; he was able to feel the depth of his need for others' responsiveness to him and his lack of regard for their feelings.

When our 12th session ended, he genuinely thanked me; I felt we had done a piece of good work. A year later he wrote and asked whether I would write a letter on his behalf; he was hoping to be selected as a psychoanalytic control case. It was clear that the work we had done was the beginning of a self-exploration of his object world and how it influenced his interpersonal relationships.

My experience with Ralph affirmed my belief that it is possible to help students discover important aspects of their character structure in a brief period of time. Clearly, our work together did not lead to any major transformation in Ralph's character structure, but it opened up his view, shifted his perspective, and enabled him to find a connection between his inner and outer worlds. This shift in perspective created hope; he was now able to see that he was struggling with internal dilemmas and might be able to change. That this shift occurred was confirmed, I believe, by his decision to enter psychoanalysis.

Another case that illustrates the problems inherent in working with more complex narcissistic concerns within the framework of a university counseling center is that of Donald, a junior majoring in English literature, whom I am still seeing. He came to the counseling center to "explore moods and problems." In our first session he managed to tell me a great deal about himself, including some very painful sexual traumas he had experienced within his family. He wanted to explore two issues: The first had to do with "strange feelings that were hard to describe"; the other was about his relationships with women. Although currently in love with a girl who was spending the year in Sweden, he was dating other girls. He had been in love twice before, ending the relationships when he felt disappointment with the women.

During our first session, Donald described his impulsive visit with a former girlfriend—someone with whom he had not had a satisfying relationship—while on a school vacation. Calling her at home, he was told she was out and the family was unsure of when she would return. "I didn't know why I wanted to see her," he said, "but decided to make the 3-hour trip, knowing she might not be at home." He called when he arrived in her hometown and was again told she was not at home. "While waiting for her on a hillside near her house, I began to experience those strange internal sensations that I had experienced many times before. I always thought of them as fostering my creative potential. Now I find they are interfering with my life, and I would like them to stop." They sounded to me like dissociative experiences. When his former girlfriend arrived home, he was aware that she felt as uncomfortable and confused by his visit as he was himself. I too was struck with the driven quality of his visit, a visit that had little to do with the reality of their relationship. His anxiety and dissociative-like states also raised questions in my mind about his ego stability, particularly when Donald unselfconsciously told me about painful and deeply disturbing childhood and adolescent sexual experiences.

At the end of our first interview, I knew I was working with a student who would probably need more extensive psychotherapy than I could comfortably provide within the context of the counseling center. I did not raise this issue because I felt it would only serve to discourage him. Clearly, he had significant problems, and he was becoming increasingly concerned about his "strange feelings" and finding it harder to rationalize their creative aspects. I found myself wondering if his defenses were beginning to give way and whether I should offer support rather than exploration. I invited him to come and talk with me again.

In our following two sessions, Donald began to talk in greater detail about his relationships with women. He told me of a recent experience with a young woman he had met at a party whom he really did not like because she seemed self-centered and overly taken with her physical appearance. Two weeks later he invited her to a formal dance; this was the first time he had contacted her, and she was "excited." At the party he was cold and distant, but did not know why. In fact, he was not even sure why he had invited her. They ended up in bed, as he "knew they would." After having sex he wanted her to leave, but since he felt it would be too hurtful to her, he decided to stay with her for a few hours. Nevertheless, he was filled with angry and critical feelings, especially about what he felt to be her self-inflated attitude. At one point she asked him what he thought of her. He said, "If I told you that you were beautiful, would I sound too much like your echo?" He told me she wasn't smart enough to get it. He felt caught between two feelings, being aware of the cruelty of his comment and yet feeling it was a wonderfully creative moment; the clever aspect of his comment filled him with a sense of esteem and specialness. He managed to take her home at 5 A.M., and while walking back to his room he began feeling "like a monster."

Despite the clear narcissistic issues in Donald's relationships, I felt there was a possibility of working with him about these aspects of his character, because of the remorse and regret he felt. I took his feeling cruel as a positive sign, an indication that he could be empathic with the other person, or at least guilty about the way he treated others. I did nothing more than tell him that I thought her self-centeredness, as he perceived it, seemed to arouse in him a wish to knock her down. I also wondered whether in some subtle way her self-centeredness aroused in him the thought that she felt superior to him, which made him want to hurt her. He listened, reflecting on what I said. I was trying to move away from focusing exclusively on his guilt and attempting to see whether he could think about what this woman had aroused in him that might lead him to treat her the way he did. I was attempting to move inward to his own object world. At the end of this session, it was clear that I was working with a student for whom issues of ego integrity and self-esteem were paramount. Future sessions corroborated this.

In a later session, Donald told me that his previous girlfriend was beautiful and intelligent. In fact, he was aware that all of the girls he was attracted to were beautiful and intelligent. His previous girlfriend admired him, made him feel special, took him to California, helped him pick out new clothes, and in general enhanced his self-esteem. She had taken pictures of him after they had spent time in the California sunshine; he thought he "looked fantastic." He told me this without a trace of self-consciousness. After a while he lost interest in her, feeling she was not the right woman for him, but he was puzzled by his loss of interest. I talked with him about how important women were to him; he depended upon them to bolster his self-esteem and sense of specialness. I said I thought he tended to idealize some of the women he became involved with, and that if they were special, then their interest in him made him special. I also suggested that he lost interest in them when they turned out to be real rather than ideal people. Donald was able to hear and work with what I said.

After having seen this student for a short period of time, I have been able to formulate the core psychological issue for our work together. My goal is to help him deepen his understanding about his feelings of insecurity and how they affect his relationships with women. I hope he can come to see how he unconsciously assigns to other people the task of enhancing his self-esteem. I am operating on the hypothesis that Donald's difficulties in relationships can best be understood from an object-relations perspective. I will try to keep the focus on his use of women as narcissistic self-objects who are a means of bolstering his precarious sense of self-esteem and fending off an inner sense of emptiness. Donald knows something is wrong because of his concern about "moods and mysteries." Though I am not certain I can help in a short period of time, I will try to help him enlarge his ego-sphere enough so that now and in the future he will have a better sense of the conflicts that need to be more fully explored.

Given the characterological issues Donald is dealing with, it is reasonable to ask whether supportive psychotherapy (which involves a reduced emphasis on the interpretations of defenses and unconscious conflicts in favor of ego-supportive interventions) might not be more appropriate in our short-term work. It has been my experience, however, that it is possible to do useful, relatively short-term work centered on characterological problems in cases of secondary narcissism. With such students, I always end our work letting them know that I am available in the future if they feel the need to return. I have seen a number of students like Donald who, in a few months, make some progress, end therapy, and continue with their lives knowing that I am available if the need arises. Often these students return 6 months or a year later, ready to work again.

In general, I have found it possible to work profitably with students whose narcissistic concerns have led them to seek help because of problematic or unsatisfactory interpersonal relationships. With most of these students, however, my work has been longer than average. It is important for the therapist to insure that this longer commitment, which may last 5 or 6 months, will not become a burden and lead to counter-transference problems (e.g., feeling resentful toward the student). Under any circumstances, ending with students in this group can be difficult because of the potentially strong, although frequently denied, dependency attachment to the therapist. The unwanted termination can be experienced as an injury and, at an unconscious level, as a re-enactment of an earlier parental rejection. Therefore, it is sometimes useful to let narcissistic students know at the outset that the therapy cannot be open-ended, as I did with Ralph, and the therapist must pay attention to issues of injury and anger at termination even if the student seems to be agreeable. It has been my experience that many of these students are fearful of directly expressing their real feelings and are likely to comply with whatever the therapist suggests.

Dependency Concerns

In relationship issues that focus primarily on dependency concerns, the themes of caring for, being cared for, and being protected are central. With a college population, it is important to distinguish students whose dependency concerns are transitory from students whose dependency problems are more deeply entrenched in early child–parent relationships. The former are typically in the process of separating from home and need an intimate relationship as a transitional experience; once settled into college life, they function quite well. Students with more deeply entrenched dependency problems also suffer from the process of separating from home, but are less able to adjust because of complex unresolved pre-oedipal issues. These students are less autonomous and depend excessively upon others for their internal stability. They often feel the problems in relationships are their partners. Frequently, their underlying wish in therapy is to learn how to get and keep the object of their desire. Though it is often difficult to differentiate between these two groups, it is important, if possible, to determine how early the developmental conflict is and therefore how entrenched the problem is. Students with transitory concerns about separation are more likely to benefit from a short-term intervention that is supportive and also applies object-relations insights. Students with entrenched dependency problems usually need a long-term therapeutic relationship.

Catherine first came to the counseling center in her sophomore year because she had been upset for some time about her relationship with her boyfriend, Mark. She wanted a more intense and committed involvement than he seemed to want. Catherine's mother had died when she was 11 years old. Since then, she had been cared for by her very dependable maternal grandmother and her somewhat unreliable and immature but loving father. After her mother's death, her father was unable to provide a stable and secure place for her or her sister. He was very involved in his own life and frequently left Catherine to fend for herself, though he did supply money. In therapy, her presenting concerns about her boyfriend moved to the background as she began focusing upon her anger at her father. In my efforts to find out what had brought her for therapy "now," I learned that her father had taken a job in the Middle East and would be leaving the country within the month. She felt frightened and insecure about his being so far away, and angry that he was not and never had been as reliable and dependable as she wished he would be. I made a connection between her feelings about her boyfriend and her feelings about her father. The focus remained on her feelings about her father, and within a short period of time she was feeling better. I was busy and suggested that we end for now. She was angry with me, but I felt it was a sign of her strength that she could express it directly. I felt we had established a positive enough relationship so that, despite her anger, she would return to see me if the need arose.

From a technical point of view, uncovering the immediate factors that bring a student to therapy is an important first step. Especially when the relationship problem is long-standing, the question of "Why now?" is critical, and the current context for the problem should be explored. In Catherine's case, the precipitating factor for her seeking counseling was her father's imminent departure.

Catherine returned for our second series of sessions about a year later. Her concerns again were about her boyfriend, from whom she still wanted more than he was apparently able or willing to give. He was now a graduating senior, and she wanted to know what would happen to their relationship after he graduated. But he was noncommittal, which made her angry. This time our work turned toward her desire to know "for certain" that the other person would not leave her. Her feelings about her mother's death came to the surface for the first time in our work. Her mother had been a loving and available person who always was "there" for her; her death had been a terrible blow. However, Catherine was also able to express anger at what she had experienced (despite rationally knowing otherwise) as an abandonment by her mother. The connections between her feelings about the loss of her mother and her wishes to have her boyfriend provide certainty became apparent to her. These insights also freed her to look more realistically at her own needs as well as at her boyfriend's conflicts. I felt that her ability to see her boyfriend as a person with conflicts and unresolved issues of his own that limited his ability to meet her needs was an important move forward. It provided her with alternatives; she could either accept his current limitations or leave if the relationship remained unfulfilling.

As a general point, it is important to help students who present relationship issues recognize that both partners bring their inner conflicts and unresolved issues into the relationship. I encourage students to think of relationship problems as the mixture of a "two-person" psychology, so as to increase their awareness that relationships, in order to survive, require work on the part of both people.

Despite Catherine's dependency needs and her wishes to find

someone who would provide her with the sense of certainty she yearned for, I did not feel that she had serious separation issues. Working with Catherine allowed me to experience her underlying strength and solid self-esteem. She was able to be alone, had traveled through Europe on her own, and in general coped quite well with her world. I assumed because of her ego strength that the first 11 years of her life were filled with good parenting experiences. She was easily able to establish a working alliance with me, could work with the interpretations I offered, yet did not need me in her life in a continuous fashion—all factors that were central to her ability to profit from short-term therapy.

In contrast, Virginia, a first-year graduate student, came to the counseling center because of "depression and problems with her boyfriends." In our first session, she told me she was suffering because she was currently involved with two men—Tom, her boyfriend of 6 years, who lived in a distant city, and Bill, with whom she had become involved since starting graduate school. Although she presented with relationship conflicts, she wanted me to help her "get rid" of her depression because it was interfering with her studies. Virginia's self-presentation had a quality that aroused a sense of helplessness in me. I took my countertransference reaction to be a response to her helplessness and her wish to have someone soothe her, take away her pain, and make certain that no harm (in this instance, academic problems) would come to her. Her self-presentation was in marked contrast to that of Catherine, who despite her sadness and depression conveyed an inner sense of strength and autonomy. It is clinically useful to attend to the feelings that students arouse in us, particularly during the initial interview. Exploring these feelings can help formulate a picture of the students' conflicts, strengths, and desires in relation to us. They can also help us understand the students' "self-representations" (the mental representations of self that have evolved in interaction with significant others), as well as the reactions the students arouse in other people.

Virginia was the only child of divorced parents. Her mother had remarried when Virginia was 6 years old. She was never fond of her stepfather, feeling uncomfortable with his "excessive closeness" on the one hand and his "authoritarian" manner on the other. Her mother was totally captivated by her husband, idealized him, and depended on him. Virginia felt abandoned by her mother, whose own needs for safety and security made it impossible for her to attend to the serious problems her daughter was having with her husband. At age 16, Virginia confronted her mother with some painful facts about her stepfather; she hoped her mother would feel compelled to take some action.

Her mother, however, was unable to act on her behalf, which Virginia experienced as the "final betrayal." She was forcibly struck with how needy and dependent her mother was, and realized that she would never get from her what she needed.

Virginia had met Tom when she was a high school senior. He was 6 years older than she, and became both her lover and good parent. She dated him exclusively through college and felt that through his guidance she had become the person she was today. However, she was beginning to feel she could not separate her ideas from his. Although he had provided a presence that was needed, she increasingly felt she had to find herself. What she told Tom, and genuinely believed herself, was that she needed to separate from him in order to grow. She also felt that he would accept this plan without abandoning her. What she could not talk about was her involvement with Bill, which she feared might cause Tom to end their relationship. Thus, although she felt she needed to separate from Tom, she could not tolerate the idea of losing him. It was as if Tom were the good parent she needed, but now she had to test her own wings while knowing that he would be there if she wanted to return. Virginia was understandably confused by her conflicting motives. In some moments of distress, she would express the desire to be on her own. Whenever she felt upset or was having trouble with academics, however, she would immediately turn to Bill for comfort and soothing. She was continuously caught between her wish for self-reliance, her need for comfort from Bill, and her fear of losing Tom; any position she took felt as if it threatened her other needs.

The dilemma in working with a student like Virginia in a university counseling service is that a short-term perspective may be insufficient. Virginia's struggles with dependency and separation were embedded in early mother–child difficulties, and therefore long-term therapy, where important transference and countertransference conflicts could be worked through, would have been more conducive to significant emotional change in her. It is, of course, possible with a short-term focus to interpret early dynamics, thereby helping students to know more about their inner life, acquire some sense of internal changes that need to occur, and achieve an understanding of how the unresolved issues of their formative years led to their current difficulties. In other words, short-term work can lead to expansion of their egos. However, interpretations offered in short-term work are often rejected, and insights gained are often only intellectual. Therefore, in the short run it is best with people like Virginia to (1) point out their strengths, (2) reward their efforts at self-sufficiency, and (3) encourage and help them to find methods of self-soothing. Doing so helps encourage the growth of independence and toleration of anxiety.

In the past 4 or 5 years, we have seen an increasing number of students from family backgrounds that failed to provide the security necessary for a reasonable degree of autonomy, self-sufficiency, and self-esteem. Although many of these students managed to function adequately before college, the greater self-reliance required during college years has made it harder for them to cope emotionally. We are seeing more students who come to us needing a form of psychotherapy that contains a substantial amount of good parenting. Many of these students move in and out of relationships because their need for support is so intense that they drive their partners away. For many of these students, the driving force in relationships is not love and mutuality, but their inability to function on their own. These students typically can only profit minimally from short-term therapy, because they need the presence of a steady and reliable figure for an extended period of time. It has been my experience that many of these students are also helped by forming alliances with other adults in the university community who make themselves available on a more spontaneous basis.

Commitment Concerns

The issue of commitment is a central theme in the realm of interpersonal relationships. Commitment involves not only the ability to make a positive choice, but the ability to close off other possibilities. Commitment also involves the maturity to accept one's own and others' limitations, through the giving up of a fantasied omnipotence in which all things are possible and one is able to be all things to all people. Therapists will also come across students who on the surface appear to have no trouble at all making commitments but who actually may be making defensive choices. Defensive choices may be especially prevalent among younger students, who seek intimacy with one person in order to avoid the anxiety and complexity involved in social relationships.

It has been my experience that women, more often than men, feel prepared to enter into an ongoing committed relationship. More women express concern about their boyfriends' inability to make a commitment than vice versa. Gilligan (1982) points out that women are more relationship-oriented than men; the male focus is typically on doing rather than being, on achieving and accomplishing rather than relating. Similarly, it is my impression that college-age men are anxious about their autonomy and independence, and that beneath their growing self-sufficiency is the fear of being drawn, through a relationship with a woman, into passivity. Rochlin (1980) speaks about the young boy's unconscious pull toward femininity, based upon his early attachment to his mother, which from the boy's perspective makes masculinity "a precariously held, endlessly tested, unstable condition. There are not only special difficulties in becoming masculine but also in maintaining it throughout life" (p. 91). It is my impression that the comparable fear for women, of losing their femininity, is less often a threatening issue.

In working with students who present commitment concerns, it is important to try to separate the healthy developmental aspects of exploring or "playing the field" from exploration based on fears of involvement and commitment. Though typically we think of the college years as a time to experiment with new relationships—an opportunity to learn about oneself before making a long-term commitment—a pattern of frequent or brief explorations may reflect deep, unresolved personality conflicts, perhaps fear of loss of self and autonomy. Similarly important is differentiating the adaptive, growth-oriented aspects of committing oneself to intimate relationships from the defensive aspects of clinging to relationships out of a fear of experiencing oneself as alone or separate.

Karen came to the counseling center in her junior year because her boyfriend, Dennis, had encouraged her to work on the difficulty she was having in committing herself to their relationship. She felt comfortable with Dennis and felt he was a good person, but increasingly found herself desiring a new relationship; this was not the first time she had experienced this difficulty. Karen was often energized by attractive people who were not necessarily or obviously available; Dennis had initially been one of those people. As he became more interested in her and more deeply committed to the relationship, she found herself dissatisfied and unhappy. The repetitiveness of this pattern made her feel that the problem was primarily hers. At the time I saw Karen she was also attracted to Bill, a young man whom she had been unable to win over despite repeated efforts.

Karen was the youngest and only female child in a family of four children; her next oldest sibling was 6 years her senior. Her parents had divorced when she was 10 years old, and her father, a successful businessman, was relatively unavailable during her childhood, leaving her almost exclusively involved with her mother and a housekeeper. As a young child, she would "perform" in an effort to capture the attention of the adults around her. After her parents' divorce and her brothers' departures her attention turned almost exclusively toward her mother. She suffered because of the envious and competitive feelings she experienced toward the men her mother was interested in.

In our work together, her pressing needs to win people over, to seduce them away from others, and to feel the power of her own attractiveness emerged as central themes. As relationships became more settled and the "seduction" was over, she not only lost interest, but lost her own energy. It seemed that her sense of well-being and vitality depended on the excitement of winning someone to her; her desire to have a career as a singer was a derivative of this need. She reacted to the short-term focus of our work by trying to make herself an "interesting patient," hoping I would therefore want to continue seeing her. Her attraction to women, especially women involved and committed to men, also emerged as a theme in our sessions. Her conscious wish was to have them become more interested in her than they were in their boyfriends. The longer we worked on the issue of commitment to a given relationship, the more we discovered the complexity of her situation. She was clearly gaining in insight, but the strengths of her desires did not diminish in a short period of time. It was clear that we had brought a deeper focus to the problems she encountered in her relationships, but I knew, and she came to understand, that the working through of these issues would take a longer period of time than we had. Our work ended when she decided to take a year abroad.

Fred, a second-year graduate student who was engaged to be married, came to the counseling center because as the marriage date drew closer, his sense of commitment began to diminish. Fred had had two previous committed and long-standing relationships with women, and I therefore assumed that there might be some specific concern about his current relationship and, most probably, some conflict about marriage. He also had been in psychotherapy as an undergraduate and had found it helpful. I told Fred I thought there might be some specific issues involved in his conflict that we might try to uncover. He agreed to work with me on a short-term basis until the end of the semester.

What emerged in our work was Fred's complicated relationship with his "feminist" mother, whom he had always had an intense desire to please. His father had died when he was 4 years old and his mother had not remarried until he was 12. Since she often talked with him about the plight of women, in his desire to please her he took up her cause and her point of view—he was an enlightened young man. In our sessions, he began to realize that despite his efforts to please his mother, she had a wish to have a daughter. It was this emerging insight that became the bridge to his current feelings of ambivalence toward his fiancee, Ellen.

Fred's mother was very fond of Ellen; at times he felt she was more interested in Ellen than she was in him. He wondered whether his task was to marry a woman in order to bring a daughter to his mother. He was able to experience his anger and deep sense of hurt toward his mother because, despite having done his best to please her, she apparently felt he was not enough. He was able to link his ambivalence about his upcoming marriage with his fear of losing his mother's attention. He also uncovered his desire to deprive his mother of what he felt she wanted—a daughter. Our work ended shortly after he had these insights. Although he gladly would have continued therapy, he ended feeling that he knew what he was struggling with. I felt that he would marry Ellen, because he had made a very appropriate choice and they were both committed to the relationship.

CONCLUSION

Although relationship issues are certainly broader and more complex than I have been able to demonstrate in this chapter, my effort has been to emphasize the connection between an individual's inner life and his or her interpersonal relationships. It is my experience that it is possible, within the context of a university counseling or mental health center, to provide students with an opportunity to learn about their internal conflicts and how these unrecognized concerns affect the quality of their lives. Though short-term psychotherapy limits the depth to which one may be able to explore the inner life, it can provide enough insight to enable individuals to struggle more effectively with relationship problems.

My view of the therapeutic process has at its base an educational perspective. Students may come seeking help with the unconscious wish for perfection or with the overt desire to inure themselves to the pain of rejection or abandonment. It is our task to help them find the connections between such inner themes and the complexities of their interpersonal relationships. We must also help them recognize that relationships require work and that perfection is impossible.

REFERENCES

Arlow, J. A. (1986). Object concept and object choice. In P. Buckley (Ed.), *Essential papers on object relations* (pp. 127–146). New York: New York University Press.
Erikson, E. H. (1963). *Childhood and society*. New York: Norton.
Gilligan, C. (1982). *In a different voice*. Cambridge, MA: Harvard University Press.
Hanfmann, E. (1978). *Effective therapy for college students*. San Francisco: Jossey-Bass.
Horner, A. J. (1986). *Being and loving*. Northvale, NJ: Jason Aronson.
Kohut, H. (1977). *The restoration of the self*. New York: International Universities Press.
Langs, R. (1976). *The bipersonal field*. New York: Jason Aronson.

Levinson, D., Darrow, C. N., Klein, E. B., Levinson, M. H., & McKee, B. (1978). *The seasons of a man's life*. New York: Knopf.

Mahler, M. S. (1981). *On human symbiosis and the vicissitudes of individuation*. New York: International Universities Press.

Medalie, J. (1981). The college years as a mini-life cycle: Developmental tasks and adaptive options. *Journal of the American College Health Association, 30*, 75–79.

Rochlin, G. (1980). *The masculine dilemma*. Boston: Little, Brown.

Winnicott, D. W. (1965). *The maturational process and the facilitating environment*. New York: International Universities Press.

7

Depression

PAUL A. WALTERS, JR.

Mental health professionals in a college or university have a constant in their clinical work. Each day they are likely to be confronted by troubled, self-preoccupied, lonely, vulnerable, ashamed, and apologetic young students who diligently attempt to ascribe their misery to outside forces such as troubles with intimates, family, instructors, or whatever. During their recitation, however, they seem uncomfortably aware that this face of things—outside forces—does not adequately depict or explain the depressive feelings they are experiencing. Indeed, they often express bewilderment as to why they, amidst so much challenge and opportunity, should feel depressed. This chapter attempts to explain some of the underlying reasons why they are troubled.

Depression is by far the most ubiquitous symptom among this young adult age group and has been so for at least two decades. Beck and Young (1978) have noted that 78% of college students will show depressive symptoms in any given year, and of these 46% will seek some form of professional help. In all likelihood this is an overstatement for most campuses, but it does call attention to a pressing issue for students in higher education.

A number of years ago, I (Walters, 1970) observed that the primary responsibility of a clinician in treating depression in adolescents and young adults is to distinguish among depression as an illness, depression as a character problem, and depression as a developmental reaction. In the ensuing years, much has been learned about the first two kinds of depression, but less about the third kind. This differentiation among three types of depression is still critical to assessment and treatment, however.

Although I classify depression as a reaction to developmental issues as one of three categories of depression, *every* case of depression in the college population is affected by these developmental issues. In the broadest terms, these issues involve (1) changes in the equilibrium between the capacity for autonomy and the availability for attachment, and (2) overreliance on external standards of success at the expense of ideals. Difficulties in these areas are often signaled by fluctuations in self-esteem. In addition, all three categories of depression are usually associated with recent stressful events. Therapeutically, the difference among the three types of depression is that these developmental themes and stressful events can be directly addressed in therapy with the third type—depression as a developmental reaction—whereas with the first two types the basic illness or character problem must be addressed first, or at least concurrently with the developmental issues and stressful events.

To illustrate the differences among the three types of depression, three representative clinical vignettes selected from a 3-year sample are presented. Names and certain biographical details have been changed to insure confidentiality, but in general the genetic histories and presenting complaints are depicted accurately. Though all three students happened to be graduate students, the characteristics they illustrate apply to undergraduates as well.

ILLUSTRATIVE CASES

Depression as an Illness

Depression as an illness is characterized by the presence of vegetative or somatic symptoms such as anhedonia, somatic heaviness, early morning awakening, impaired cognition, loss of sexual drive, constipation, and loss of weight. According to an old psychiatric saw, at some point during the development of the illness, such symptoms take on a life of their own that is unrelated to outside stress. This type of depression is also usually accompanied by a family history of depression and perhaps by early loss and neglect, and it tends not to respond to a strictly psychotherapeutic intervention.

Ralph, a 24-year-old graduate student, showed clear vegetative signs of depression. He originally called for an appointment because of a deepening inability to concentrate, insomnia and early morning awakening, loss of sexual drive, and a slight loss of weight over a 6-week period. He cited as significant recent events difficulties with a girlfriend, the death of a close relative by suicide, and doubts about his career. He also felt that he had been becoming more isolated over the past 2 years. Lack of a social network made him vulnerable to the difficulties in the relationship with his girlfriend and ultimately contributed to their separating. His early life had been disrupted by the death of his chronically depressed father, after which the family atmosphere became distant. His adolescence was without obvious turmoil, and there was no history of mood swings.

After the initial interview, the symptoms of depression deepened, and the patient became unable to work. Because the symptoms were clearly those of a major unipolar depression, the patient was started on an antidepressant medication (imipramine) while clinical interviews were continued. He gradually improved over a 2-month period, and was able to resume his relationship with his girlfriend and re-establish some recently neglected peer relationships.

In a formulation of this case, several factors stand out. First, there were clear-cut vegetative symptoms (weight loss, early morning awakening, slowed cognition, and loss of libido), which along with the family history of depression indicated the presence of a depressive illness. His genetic potential for the development of illness was augmented by the childhood history of distant relationships among family members and the feeling that he had been abandoned by his father at an early age. Finally, there was a gradually increasing pattern of isolation and difficulty with intimates. Thus, genetic vulnerability (the illness factor) combined with current loss of connectedness (a developmental issue and a current stressor) to bring on his depression.

Depression as an Expression of Character Problems

The second type of depression is hard both to evaluate and to treat. Cases in this category comprise a spectrum of diagnoses, from dysthymic reaction (in which there is chronicity for 1 to 2 years) to the personality disorders (where symptoms of depression may extend back into childhood and early adolescence). The defining features of this category are early onset and chronicity. These persons also typically respond slowly to psychotherapeutic interventions, and they frequently come from troubled families, in which depression, alcoholism, and unstable marriages may be found. Narcissistic problems, involving low self-esteem and grandiosity, are commonly part of the clinical picture. (We must remember, however, that low self-esteem is a barometer of all kinds of depression.) Although these patients may have one or two somatic complaints, they do not have the full array of vegetative signs found in depression as an illness.

Helen, a 26-year-old graduate student, requested a consultation after hearing a lecture on depression. She complained of difficulties that had begun in the distant past and become more obvious in early adolescence. Prominent among these were difficulties in relationships, particularly with men; intermittent periods of moderate depression; constant feelings of low self-esteem and guilt; and pessimism about the future. Her mother had died when she was quite young, and her father, who was alcoholic, had then married a woman with whom Helen had an exceedingly difficult relationship. She described the family atmosphere as filled with turmoil, disagreement, and anxiety about the future. Because of her high intelligence she won admittance to a highly competitive private school, which furnished her with a stable environment during adolescence. Under these circumstances she became outwardly stable, and remained so. Inwardly, however, she had been for a long time filled with the self-doubt and periodic feelings of depression that continued to the present. She now viewed therapy as essential to help her to continue a close relationship that would balance her commitment to a career.

In this case, the absence of vegetative symptoms argued against depression as an illness, while the onset of depressive affect in early adolescence—coupled with repeated loss and family alcoholism and turmoil—indicated depression as a character problem. Her condition would not have responded psychopharmacologically, but called for psychotherapy with limited goals.

Depression as a Reaction to Developmental Issues

In the third category, the syndrome of vegetative symptoms does not appear, and the onset of depression is relatively recent. The depression is brought on by a recent stressful event that upsets the balance between autonomy and connectedness. Furthermore, early responsiveness is shown to psychotherapy, with a relatively quick recovery to a sense of optimism and sense of control.

Clyde, a 24-year-old visiting graduate student from another university, was referred by a colleague for evaluation of difficulties with his wife, from whom he was geographically separated because of the demands of their careers. He revealed that he was very sensitive to his wife's absences. He had been unfaithful to her on three occasions: when she had left temporarily while he was under academic stress; when she spent a year away while he was beginning his graduate studies; and, finally, when she refused because of a conflict with her work priorities to accompany him during his current temporary relocation. During each of these occasions he was resentful and depressed, but was unable to acknowledge his feelings and to admit the depth of his need for her. His wife perceived him as a highly intelligent, ambitious, self-reliant man who satisfied his needs through work, comradeship with peers, and a good relationship with her. In contrast to her view, the patient felt needy and always felt the pressure to be perfect and self-sufficient. Peer relationships brought him no pleasure, and therefore his relationship with his wife was his most important and only intimate one; he counted on her for fulfillment of his emotional needs.

This complex pattern of superior external adaptation accompanied by internal self-doubt had begun in early adolescence, when he recognized that most of his relationships were competitive in nature and did not fulfill his wishes for intimacy and acceptance. He had been an accomplished athlete and a student leader for much of his career, but he recognized that success made him feel distant from his peers. In addition, he felt that he had related to his parents and siblings through his success; he had never been accepted for what he was, only for what he did.

Clyde was seen in therapy for a number of months, which helped him get in touch with his resentment, admit his needs for intimacy to his wife, and broaden his circle of relationships. It also helped him to see success as a choice rather than a necessity.

Clyde's case would not be categorized as an illness because of the absence of vegetative symptoms. It would also not be categorized as a character problem because his depression, though rooted in early adolescent issues, was not chronic. Furthermore, he had come from an intact family in which his parents had been available as respected role models; early childhood trauma did not contribute to the etiology of his depression. Rather, the cause was to be found in the poverty of his social network; in his difficulty with the adolescent developmental task of integrating autonomy with the need for connectedness; and also in his difficulty in modifying, in Kohut's (1977) terms, his ego ideal from one driven by ambition to one that was also led by ideals.

Discussion

These cases are illustrative both for their differences and their similarities. The chief differences among the categories are the presence of vegetative symptoms and often a family history of depression or early loss and neglect in depression as an illness; chronicity and often at least some form of family disturbance, but few or no vegetative symptoms, in depression as a character problem; and the absence of these symptoms coupled with a relatively quick responsiveness to psychotherapy in depression as a developmental reaction.

One important similarity to note is that there is little to distinguish these categories in regard to depth of depression or degree of impairment. Students who have "merely" a developmental reaction can be just as depressed as those in the other two categories. Furthermore, all three of the students described above showed growth during adolescence, all left home readily enough, and all showed a history of accomplishment. Therefore, a thorough anamnesis and a careful clinical evaluation are necessary to differentiate among the three types of depression.

All of these students also showed the effects of recent stresses and shared important concerns centered around developmental themes. Autonomy was achieved at the expense of relationships, causing concern about isolation. They were concerned about the quality of their relationships with the family, and expressed difficulty in establishing friendships or intimate relationships with peers. They all felt that their self-esteem was disproportionately based on accomplishment; they now found it hard to maintain self-esteem without the affirmation and validation that relationships and inner ideals bring.

These developmental themes involving the balances between autonomy and connectedness, and between outer accomplishments and inner ideals, are critical to the etiology of depression in the college student population. This perspective differs, however, from traditional models for the etiology of depression in this age group, which in my opinion overemphasize the influence of loss as the central cause of depression. Indisputably, the loss of the primary caregiver in early childhood creates a vulnerability that may lead to disturbance, but this loss is not sufficient to explain all depression in adolescence. Of equal importance are late adolescent developmental issues and also lack of family cohesiveness, a family history of depression (or at least family psychopathology), and recent stressful life events. Thus O'Neil and Mingie (1988) point out in a study of university students that recent stressful life events, lack of social support, and a family history of psychiatric illness are more important in the etiology of depressive symptoms than past traumatic events such as the loss of a nurturing person.

Recent theorists have attempted to redress this imbalance by broadening the concept of early attachment deficits to include faulty, ongoing parent–child interactions that interfere with separation/individuation and the maintenance of self-esteem. Most of these theories, however, describe depression as an expression of chronic character problems rather than as a reaction to current crises in development. It is of questionable value to apply data gained from models of illness and character problems as an explanation of normal development. As Masterson (1968) explained, illness and character problems among adolescents are distinct from problems related to developmental issues. What is necessary is a model that can cover the spectrum of depressive disorders in adolescence and furnish the clinician with treatment guidelines for each disorder.

GUIDELINES FOR TREATMENT

Practically speaking, there are three goals of therapy with all three categories of depression: reduction of symptoms, creation of a more positive assessment of life, and establishment of a balance between autonomy and connectedness and between external and internal sources of approval. The following clinical material offers guidelines for reaching these goals for each category of depression. Because every case of depression is unique, these are guidelines rather than prescriptions.

Depression as an Illness

Monica was a recently graduated senior whose therapist requested a consultation because her depressive symptoms had deepened. This change occurred following the breakup of a serious recent relationship. A clinical evaluation revealed psychological symptoms of agitation, anxiety, and depression, and bodily symptoms of weight loss, early morning awakening, loss of libido, somatic feelings of heaviness and constriction, and frequent episodes of tearfulness. Preoccupation about the futility of life was present, but there were no suicidal plans. Careful questioning about family history revealed depressive illness in a maternal uncle.

Because of the presence of somatic symptoms and a family history of depressive illness, the patient was evaluated as suffering from depression as an illness. In cases like hers, antidepressant medication is indicated.

A discussion of the choice of antidepressant is beyond the scope of this chapter. The decision is best left up to the experience of the therapist or consultant. In my opinion, the manner in which the drug is presented is as important as the choice of drug. A full discussion about the drugs available should take place, and the final decision should include the student's input. In addition, the student should be advised about side effects, including long-term ones such as weight gain. Finally, the drug should be introduced slowly, since most young people are more intolerant of side effects than of depressive symptoms. These collaborative steps reinforce a sense of autonomy and thus support compliance.

Since Monica was initially hesitant about medication, it was clearly important in her case that the antidepressant be introduced slowly and increased gradually to therapeutic levels. Over the ensuing weeks, she gradually improved and regained optimism about the future. With her sense of self-confidence restored, the primary importance of the breakup began to recede. In its place, concerns emerged about making the transition to postgraduate life—adjusting to a job, living on her own, and finding a new social group.

These concerns prompted Monica to discuss how her wishes were pre-empted by goals set by her family. These discussions concerning issues of autonomy and identity enabled her to assume more ownership of her wishes and capabilities. Her growing self-confidence augmented her self-esteem and helped her to make a more positive assessment of the future. Thus, when the depressive symptoms ameliorated, the therapist could better evaluate Monica's developmental issues and focus on her insufficient closure in the area of autonomy. Although Monica might need to explore difficulties with intimacy in the future, for now the major developmental themes involved autonomy and ideals. By establishing her own priorities, she was able to resume her life with renewed confidence.

The important lesson from this vignette is that the possibility of illness must be carefully evaluated by looking for the signs of vegetative symptoms and a family history of depression. Once the illness is recognized and then treated through use of antidepressant medication, depressive symptoms will be ameliorated, and the treatment can address the other two goals of creating a more positive assessment of life and establishing a balance between autonomy and connectedness.

Depression as an Expression of Character Problems

The case of Stephanie, a 21-year-old junior, illustrates some of the difficulties that may occur in evaluating and treating character problems. Her presenting symptoms were loss of interest in her academic work, hypersomnia and weight gain, and difficulty with a current intimate relationship. She saw this relationship as the crucial problem that explained all her current difficulties, whereas the therapist initially formulated her symptoms in the wider context of developmental issues centered around intimacy. However, the patient did not improve, and meanwhile developed an attachment to the therapist. At this point a more careful history was taken, which revealed prolonged periods of depressive feelings, periodic weight gain, tendencies toward isolation, few close friendships, and a rather pronounced lack of empathy. For much of her life she had felt like a sham, and for this reason she was shy and retiring, fearing that people would find her shallow. Although she had had many romantic relationships, she felt pessimistic about achieving genuine mutual commitment. Most important, her pessimistic feelings had been present throughout her adolescence, and had not been ameliorated by her romantic relationships. In addition, she had little insight into her lack of commitment to an ideal or a career, and how this fact might be related to negative feelings about herself. Such long-standing symptoms and slowness to benefit from psychotherapy indicated the characterological basis of her depression.

In these cases where chronicity is a defining feature, it is often appropriate to focus on clients' views about themselves. These depressed persons usually have cognitive biases against the self, which result in low self-esteem and pessimism about or devaluation of the future. They are most cognitively efficient when processing negative information; they tend to focus on evidence that supports their negative views, rather than on evidence or specific actions they could take that might contradict them. Such negative views often interfere with educational progress, leading to procrastination, low work output, and lack of commitment to a career path.

To aid these patients to break free from their negative beliefs and behavioral impasses, cognitive approaches offer an appropriate therapeutic strategy. Childress and Burns (1981) advocate techniques to pinpoint silent negative assumptions about the self and to substitute a more reasonable and self-enhancing belief system. Trautman and Rotheram-Borus (1988) emphasize that in the initial stage of therapy, the two most important steps are to identify social resources and to help the patient to view them positively. The patient is then encouraged to focus on a list of both problems and strengths, which helps the student see that current problems are less overwhelming than they have seemed, while there are strengths the student has overlooked that may be helpful in relieving the current impasse.

The therapist used this form of cognitive therapy with Stephanie, focusing on her doubts and negative assumptions and her overlooked strengths. As a result, her self-esteem improved, and she became more optimistic about the future and more socially outgoing. This approach was also helpful with Helen, the student in the first vignette, who was able to see how attention to her difficulties in relationships had obscured her more positive academic and career accomplishments. Focusing on these strengths enabled her to feel more positive and to improve her self-esteem, which in turn helped her broaden her social network and lessen her needs for an intense but distracting relationship. With this more optimistic view, she decided to postpone her quest for intimacy until she felt more established in her career and her outside life. Connectedness in the new scheme of things became a choice rather than a need, and so she was able to reorder her priorities in a more positive and less biased way.

Cognitive approaches work well with the college population, since they are problem-focused, present-oriented, and time-limited. They fit both the developmental themes of adolescence and the goals of most college mental health centers. Cognitive therapy is particularly efficacious when educational progress is at issue, which is often the case with chronic, characterological depression.

Depression as a Reaction to Developmental Stress

Most depressed students have this third type of depression. Though cognitive therapy may help them, they need at least to supplement this approach with a therapy that emphasizes developmental issues. For example, Ellie, a 20-year-old senior, sought counseling because of her concerns about a depressed roommate. As she told her story, it became clear to her that her susceptibility to her roommate's issues stemmed from her own feelings about a current relationship. She now realized that she only felt completely worthwhile in a close relationship in which she could subsume her wishes to those of another. Her self-esteem was rarely based on her own achievements, but depended on praise from someone close to her, preferably a man. Her concern about the opinion of others stood in the way of establishment of true autonomy and the internalization of self-esteem. After some work on this issue, including exploration of its source in family relationships, she focused more on extending her social network beyond intimate relationships. She was able to develop a close friendship with a female peer, which she found to be genuinely supportive. In this broadened network of friends and intimates, she was able to re-establish goals of her own without having to seek approval first.

Therapy with this young woman illustrates the importance of evaluating development in understanding a precipitating event. She had had close and apparently rewarding relationships with a number of men, and seemingly had achieved a capacity for intimacy. Upon closer examination, however, her intimacy often masked her doubts about competence and autonomy. Her development featured an imbalance in which connectedness was emphasized at the expense of autonomy and independent achievement. This asymmetry surfaced clinically in her fragility of self-esteem and depressive affect. Therapy helped her focus on finding ideals and goals that belonged to her.

Cases like this, in which depression primarily stems from developmental issues, are in my opinion more related to events in the present than to traumas of the past. At issue are the ways in which stressful life events bear on developmental issues—particularly the balance between autonomy and connectedness, and the resulting implications for self-esteem. For example, stressful events such as financial difficulties, poor academic performance, or disciplinary problems often threaten students' sense of autonomy and in turn may impair self-esteem. Problems in living arrangements often stress a perhaps tenuous social network, leading to fears of isolation and loneliness. The death of a parent jeopardizes a sense of connectedness. The breakup of an important relationship cancels an important source of validation and affirmation. A healthy response to any of these crises is to repair the balance between autonomy and connectedness, and so to restore self-esteem, by finding additional work or increased involvement in a social network. Some students, however, react to the stressful event by developing depressive symptoms.

What form of therapy is recommended for these cases? Klerman and Weissman's (1982) interpersonal therapy is one obviously appropriate choice. These therapists state that depression, regardless of severity, genetic vulnerability, or personality traits, occurs in an interpersonal context. Clarifying and renegotiating the social context is then crucial to recovery and the prevention of future episodes. As useful as this approach is, however, it fails to emphasize autonomy along with connectedness. Any of the contemporary forms of short-term therapy may be helpful for these students, provided the approach takes into account the balance between autonomy and connectedness, and focuses on self-esteem and the here-and-now.

FINAL THOUGHTS: DEPRESSION AND THE CONTEMPORARY COLLEGE STUDENT

In working with college students, I am impressed that most of them have achieved, if not full psychological autonomy, at least a measure of independence. Generally, they have departed the family of origin and established the early foundations for a career. Their personalities have been integrated into reasonably functioning entities on most external measures, allowing them, for example, to negotiate the educational system. All of these accomplishments contribute to a sense of identity and the ability to make a conscious choice, in Arnstein's (1984) terms, and live with it.

For some periods in history, this would have been the proper goal of education. However, Kett (1977) has made the observation that adolescence is a changing and cyclical phenomenon from a historical point of view. Autonomy, or "self-reliance" (to use a quainter term), may be more important when there is a frontier to be settled or farms to leave for cities. But as society has become more industrial and technological and more dependent on specialized knowledge, education has been prolonged, and thus now it is essential for children and parents to maintain a longer relationship. Similarly, the skills of autonomy necessary in the first two-thirds of the 20th century, when large corporations were founded, world wars were fought, and means were created to enter space, may not be sufficient for the final third of the century. The skills necessary today include learning to lead through cooperation; managing dual-career marriages; relating with diverse, multinational networks of people; and dealing with repeated changes of community. Under the present circumstances, connectedness is of as much importance as autonomy.

As the psychosocial milieu changes, so does the epidemiology of depression. Goldin and Gershon (1988), using data from several epidemiological studies, make the observation (which is supported by clinical data from the college population) that starting around 1940, successive cohorts defined by decade of birth have had significantly higher rates of depression. Along these lines, Offer, Ostrova, and Howard (1981) conclude that adolescents in the late 1970s and early 1980s, compared to adolescents in the early 1960s, have a more negative social image, are more lonely, and think worse of themselves. In other words, depression may be on the rise.

Yet depressive symptoms among this age group are nothing new. What has perhaps changed more than incidence are the *causes* of depressive symptoms, the developmental etiology. For the alienated and idealistic students of the 1960s it was a difficult task to reconcile the ideal world and self with the real world and self. The disparity between ideal and real, according to Nicoli (1967), led to depression. In contrast, students today are more detached and concerned about security and careers. For them, the cause of depression oftens shifts to difficulties with establishing intimacy and achieving personal security.

Another component of depression is deficient self-esteem. Self-esteem has always been a crucial issue in adolescence. During this period of life, the emphasis must shift from wanting external approbation, approval, and acceptance to finding a balance between outside reinforcement and internal affirmation. Kohut (1977) has called the results of this shift "firmness of the self," by which he means that aspirations and goals become perceived as within reach by the self, largely independent of outside reinforcement. However, this form of internal conviction is often lacking in today's college students, even those with considerable achievements, promising future careers, and high status. For a great number of students today, the ideal self is tied to a definite career choice or a wish for financial security. Many have become concerned about externally measured achievement at the expense of self-affirmation. Thus they end up suffering from two related forms of asymmetry. They overemphasize either autonomy or connectedness (usually autonomy) rather than finding a good balance between the two, and they emphasize outside success without searching for satisfaction from inner sources.

As a result, students suffer from loneliness and fragile self-esteem. Indeed, loneliness and self-esteem are the barometers of depression in this age group. Today's students are like lonely voyagers. Their existence feels shallow; they tend to have acquaintances rather than intimates; and their goals do not entail genuine commitment. Though they strive for tangible rewards, they are left with unfulfilling and unsustaining relationships and irresolute ideals.

Many depressed students, in my opinion, have neglected an important process in the formation of identity—namely, knowing how to become or stay involved, as well as how to end an involvement. Schafer (1973) has called attention to this issue in an article pointing out that cohesion with those who are loved is as important as differentiation from them. According to this perspective, genuine maturation is built more on revision and modulation of relationships than on expulsion and rejection. Many depressed students have not learned how to find or keep sustaining attachments.

Unfortunately, aspects of the college or university milieu may compromise the search for fulfilling relationships. Mark Ryan (1980), dean of Jonathon Edwards College at Yale University, has pointed out that "the relentless focus on measurable achievements tends to put a student out of touch with the functioning of his [sic] own psyche" (p. 35), which in Ryan's opinion often leads to dropping out of school to get in touch with both inner life and other people. Because colleges emphasize achievements, students who are seeking to explore a diversity of relationships—who may be seeking to find themselves through finding others—may feel out of place. The result is an increased likelihood of depression.

Students more than ever need wide contact with the complex variety of people who comprise the educational setting. Psychotherapists can play a vital part in this endeavor. Therapists are, as Rockwell (1984) points out, one part of a mosaic of support for students—a mosaic that potentially includes classmates, advisors, lovers, mentors, authorities, and friends. One of therapists' jobs is to repair or complete this mosaic for students.

In addition, therapists can help deliver a message about the importance of connectedness as well as autonomy, of self-affirmation and ideals as well as external success. They should deliver this message in a variety of settings: departmental meetings, residences, classrooms, and workshops. The goal is to help educate students and to change the nature of education. In this way therapists can complement the work they do inside their offices, and help ameliorate the problem of depression in college students.

REFERENCES

Arnstein, R. L. (1984). Young adulthood: Stages of maturity. In D. Offer & M. Sabshin (Eds.), *Normality and the life cycle* (pp. 108–144). New York: Basic Books.

Beck, A. T., & Young, J. E. (1978, September). College blues. *Psychology Today*, pp. 80–92.

Childress, A. R., & Burns, D. D. (1981). Cognitive therapy: The basics. *Psychosomatics, 22,* 1017–1027.

Goldin, L. R., & Gershon, E. S. (1988). The genetic epidemiology of major depressive illness. In A. J. Frances & R. E. Hales (Eds.), *Review of psychiatry* (Vol. 7, pp. 149–168). Washington, DC: American Psychiatric Press.

Kett, J. F. (1977). *Rites of passage.* New York: Basic Books.

Klerman, G. L., & Weissman, M. M. (1982). Interpersonal psychotherapy: Theory and research. In A. J. Rush (Ed.), *Short-term psychotherapies for depression* (pp. 88–106). New York: Guilford Press.

Kohut, H. (1977). *The restoration of the self.* New York: International Universities Press.

Masterson, J. L. (1968). The psychiatric significance of adolescent turmoil. *American Journal of Psychiatry, 124,* 1549–1554.

Nicoli, A. M. (1967). Harvard drop-outs: Some psychiatric findings. *American Journal of Psychiatry, 124,* 651–658.

Offer, D., Ostrov, E., & Howard, K. L. (1981). *The adolescent.* New York: Basic Books.

O'Neil, M. K., & Mingie, P. (1988). Life stress and depression in university students: Clinical illustrations of recent research. *Journal of the American College Health Association, 36,* 235–242.

Rockwell, W. J. K. (1984). Brief psychotherapy with university students. *Psychiatric Annals, 14,* 637–646.

Ryan, M. B. (1980). Doldrum in the Ivies. *Change: The Magazine of Higher Learning,* pp. 33–35.

Schafer, R. (1973). Concepts of self and identity and the experience of separation/individuation. *Psychiatric Quarterly, 42,* 42–59.

Trautman, P. D., & Rotheram-Borus, M. J. (1988). Cognitive therapy with children and adolescents. In A. J. Frances & R. E. Hales (Eds.), *Review of psychiatry* (Vol. 7, pp. 584–607). Washington, DC: American Psychiatric Press.

Walters, P. A., Jr. (1970). Depression. In D. L. Farnsworth (Ed.), *International psychiatry clinics* (Vol. 7, pp. 169–179). Boston: Little, Brown.

8

Anxiety

GERALD AMADA
PAUL A. GRAYSON

Anxiety is one of the themes, like relationship problems, family concerns, and developmental issues, that intersects every other problem area in this book. We expect every student who voluntarily consults us to be anxious about something, at least unconsciously, or else what is the reason for an appointment? Anxiety plays a part as both a cause and a consequence of students' problems. For example, students who are anxious about academics may avoid studies through procrastination, which in the end damages their performance and aggravates their anxiety. A woman who is anxious about her attractiveness and lovability may eat compulsively to quell her fears, but the weight she gains will damage her self-concept further and increase her anxiety. A male's anxiety about his sexual adequacy will impair his performance and thus reinforce his anxiety. With each of these problems, the therapeutic approach requires understanding the role of anxiety and finding constructive ways to cope with it.

The remarks in this chapter therefore bear on virtually every case that comes to the college counseling center. The following sections present causes of anxiety in college students, principles of therapy, and two case examples.

CAUSES OF ANXIETY

Anxiety is defined as "apprehension, tension, or uneasiness that stems from the anticipation of danger, which may be internal or external"; it is characterized by "motor tension, autonomic hyperactivity, apprehensive expectation, and vigilance and scanning" (American Psychiatric Association, 1987, p. 392). In college students it may seize attention suddenly in the form of incapacitating panic attacks, or may reside in the background of consciousness, like noise from the street. Its existence may be known to students, who insistently want it to go away, or it may be so familiar as to go unnoticed and have to be inferred from students' accounts. It may be, or at least appear to be, situation-specific. One graduating senior, for example, was obsessed with what was to him the terrifying prospect of landing a prestigious postgraduate job. His sleep, diet, studies, mood, and relationships deteriorated as he tortured himself with single-minded apprehension about his qualifications and performance on interviews. The more usual pattern, however, is for anxious students to be anxious across the board. Fears expressed in last week's session about taking a test are supplanted this week by fears about going home for Thanksgiving and next week by fears about asking a roommate to pay a phone bill. The details change, but the plot remains familiar.

The causes of human anxiety are as much a subject for social critics and philosophers as for psychologists and psychiatrists. Blame has been attributed to society's overemphasis on competition and individual achievement, the breakdown of ties to the extended family and community, the erosion of traditional values and norms of behavior, and the insidious threat of global nuclear disaster. But even though our era may be particularly an age of anxiety, as W. H. Auden's poem styles us, the human condition has always been shadowed by anxiety. According to psychoanalytic doctrine, every member of our race struggles with the irreducible and inescapable fears of object loss, loss of love, castration, and superego demands and prohibitions (Brenner, 1982). Also within the psychoanalytic tradition, Fenichel (1945) points out that adults never entirely put behind them the helplessness they experienced as infants when bombarded by stimuli they could neither differentiate nor master. Existential theory postulates that none of us is immune from anxiety caused by awareness of death, helplessness against chance, the responsibility to find meaning in our lives, and the recognition that we are ultimately alone (Tillich, 1952).

When we wish to compare and understand the anxiety of specific individuals, it is essential, of course, to make broad diagnostic differentiations. Establishing whether a person's anxiety is associated with incipient psychosis, personality disorder, neurotic conflict, developmental issues, or unusually severe current stressors illuminates its origin and informs the process of treatment. However, very often within the college population, anxiety cannot be assigned to a particular diagnostic pigeonhole; rather, it betokens some combination of environmental, developmental, and psychopathological factors, as discussed in Chapter 1. Thus, a young man in his first semester may have a fear of final examinations (an objectively stressful experience); this may be heightened by underlying ambivalence about separating from his family through succeeding at college (a developmental issue), and also the unconscious wish to fail in order to confirm his deeply held sense of being a misfit (a pathological issue). Ignoring any of these aspects would mean oversimplifying the cause of his distress.

If the broad diagnostic groupings often do not tell the full story, the same can be said for the finer distinctions among anxiety disorders drawn by the revised third edition of the *Diagnostic and Statistical Manual of Mental Disorders* (DSM-III-R; American Psychiatric Association, 1987). In our experience, college students' anxiety problems tend to cross over the boundaries drawn by DSM-III-R among Social Phobia, Generalized Anxiety Disorder, Obsessive–Compulsive Disorder, and Panic Disorder. That is, often the same individuals evidence, concurrently or at different times, signs of fear of scrutiny by others, excessive anxiety and worry about life experiences, persistent unwanted thoughts, and even attacks of panic. However, full-fledged Agoraphobia as defined in DSM-III-R is rarely seen at college counseling centers. The most common DSM-III-R Post-Traumatic Stress Disorder at most counseling centers concerns the aftermath of rape, covered in Chapter 12, although the Mental Health Program at the City College of San Francisco, where one of us (Gerald Amada) works, contains a concentration of international students, some of whom have been traumatized by war and torture.

Let us briefly catalog areas that engender anxiety in college students. One of the most familiar problems at college counseling centers is a generalized social phobia—commonly known as shyness—which involves a fear of and compelling desire to avoid social situations. P. G. Zimbardo (personal communication, 1988), director of the Stanford University Shyness Clinic, conducted a randomly distributed survey in which 40% of college students identified themselves as generally shy, another 15% as shy in particular situations, and another 40% as shy in the past—leaving only 5%, by their own account, free from the problem. Shy students have trouble initiating and maintaining conversations (Pilkonis, 1977). Though they are at times able to form one or two sustaining relationships, their fear of other persons typically causes them difficulty in making friends and forming romantic attachments. For some, the therapist may be their only nonthreatening association. One young man, who was intensely though ambivalently attached to his parents, had been an outsider among peers for his entire life. His only "friends" outside of family were the therapists he had seen since childhood. Leading the same solitary existence at college, he now came to the counseling center to establish in therapy his customary lifeline to another human being.

But shy students are shy in therapy, too. They may avoid eye contact, squirm and fidget, and manifest inappropriate affect such as giggling while discussing painful subjects. They may withhold information or at least not take the initiative in disclosure, or they may speak vaguely or obliquely. Though they frequently complain about receiving too little recognition and respect from others, their low self-esteem makes them acutely uncomfortable if they are commended by the therapist, whom they then view as patronizing or as a poor judge of accomplishment.

The academic arena can rouse social anxiety as well. Many students never raise their hands in class and sit in dread that they will be called on by the instructor. Delivering a speech or exposing their writing to scrutiny can be a traumatic event. A female student of above-average intelligence became panicky and blocked whenever she was confronted with written assignments that required creative expression. She submitted her essays late and displayed a tendency to hedge and underplay her viewpoint, as if she wanted to eliminate herself from her writing. In addition to these public aspects of academic performance, such private aspects as concentration, memorization, and assimilation of written materials can be impaired by anxiety. Test anxiety, often reaching phobic proportions, afflicts vast numbers of students. Often coexisting with test anxiety is procrastination (Rothblum, Solomon, & Murakami, 1986), which involves the self-defeating cycle of fear, avoidance, impaired performance, lowered self-esteem, and renewed fear.

Another focus of social anxiety deserving mention is anxiety and shyness about the body, which is quite common among even attractive, well-formed students. At a developmental stage where many are uncertain about their lovability and appeal, college students naturally focus worried attention on their physical selves. It is not unusual for them to come to therapy dressed in loose-fitting sweaters or coats that disguise rather than reveal their shapes. In fact, a student's arriving bundled up to a session may be taken as a sign of self-repudiation. "I am afraid to show myself," the outfit declares, "because I am inadequate and you will reject me."

Concerns about the body also may be expressed in morbid worries about health (hypochondriasis). Many such students are referred to the counseling center after first seeking medical treatment at the health center. They are sometimes not good candidates for therapy, preferring to monitor and detail their symptoms rather than unearth the causes. Related to these concerns are fears of external danger and death. One student reported fears of choking on food, flying on airplanes, driving a car, riding in a train, and walking on city streets.

On a deeper psychodynamic level, students fear their own impulses. Some fear their tender side—it makes them appear needy or weak. Some fear sexual impulses; perhaps they are attracted to the "wrong" gender or sex act. Many are afraid of hidden hostile impulses, which, according to Horney (1937), are a wellspring of human anxiety. These are the students who lend money to persons they dislike or who keep silent when someone plays an electric guitar at 2 A.M. They are afraid that if they assert themselves they will provoke a retaliatory attack, and they are also afraid of losing control once the genie of self-assertion is let out of the bottle. Outwardly nice and obliging, these students tend to be haunted by daydreams and nightmares of violence, or they may keep hostile impulses at bay through obsessive–compulsive defenses.

Another familiar source of anxiety is the process of change, and particularly the changes associated with the major transitions of college. Every year a handful of shellshocked first-year students and panic-stricken graduating students find their way to counseling centers. Part of what makes these transitions so frightening is the belief of many students that they are crossing the Rubicon, with no turning back. Though this idea is partly grounded in reality (growing up does mean leaving part of one's past behind), its absolutism can be dispelled by therapists' giving encouragement to first-year students to live at home or go home during weekends and to graduating students to spend an extra semester at college. When allowed to proceed at a slower pace, these frightened students tend to reconcile themselves to moving ahead.

This overview of what makes college students anxious is far from complete. Bright persons who turn their ingenuity to finding justifications for worry can always detect new dangers that a therapist has not yet discerned. It should also be stressed that students sometimes cannot name what they are anxious about—their anxiety is free-floating—and almost always they are ignorant of the deeper psychodynamic issues lurking beneath the proximate sources of worry. External dangers are easier to recognize than internal dangers; environmental stressors are more identifiable than developmental and psychopathological issues. Bringing the hidden causes of anxiety to light is one of the purposes of psychotherapy.

PRINCIPLES OF TREATMENT

In theory, diagnostic considerations should determine the disposition of anxiety problems. Psychotic episodes require hospitalization and/or major tranquilizers; entrenched neurotic patterns and personality disorders require long-term psychotherapy; developmental issues (e.g., separation/individuation and identity formation) respond well to short-term, insight-oriented psychotherapy; and environmentally induced anxiety usually warrants only a few sessions. But for the majority of anxious students, whose fears are neither psychotic nor strictly situational but instead stem from a combination of environmental, developmental, and psychopathological sources, this neat scheme breaks down. They generally come to the counseling center because they are anxious about an immediate situation. Whether they then continue in therapy to explore deeper developmental and psychopathological issues has less to do with the existence of these issues than with their rapport with the therapist, their interest and faith in the therapeutic process, the number of sessions the counseling center offers, and so forth.

A modified short-term psychodynamic model fits the needs of most of these students. The City College of San Francisco Mental Health Program, where Amada has worked for 18 years, applies this model to a diverse urban population of community college students. Grayson has employed the model at both a small liberal arts and arts-oriented public college and a small liberal arts private college. Though ideally suited to developmental issues, the short-term psychodynamic model also can be geared to environmental or psychopathological emphases. Students who define their problems as strictly environmental can benefit from the model's accent on finding parallels across situations. By learning how their particular coping mechanisms consistently fail them, they become better prepared to respond to current and future stressors. Meanwhile, college students who are prepared to delve into psychopathological issues may find, thanks to their remarkable capacity for growth, that they can make substantial inroads with this model. At the very least, they can get the ball rolling; they may then continue the process in long-term treatment on or off campus.

The goal of psychodynamically oriented therapy is to unearth the core fears and motives, the central conflicts, with which the anxiety is associated. The assumption is made that beneath the dangers that may be obvious to students lie deeper dangers of which they are incompletely aware. For example, the process of leaving home may be frightening because it is unconsciously equated with the threat of being abandoned by parents, or conversely with the threat of being accused by dependent parents of abandoning them. The prospect of failing a test may unconsciously evoke fears of being chastised by a critical parent, or it may mean that one is doomed to follow in an unsuccessful parent's footsteps. The therapist searches for these underlying meanings by collecting evidence of parallels within and among students' childhood relationships, current dealings with others, and reactions within the therapeutic relationship (cf. Angyal, 1965; Malan, 1976;

Schafer, 1983). Thus, if a student was frightened of her father's anger and acts now as if afraid of the therapist's anger, then one can hypothesize that her current anxiety about dating stems from a generalized fear of angering men.

Of course, short-term work never yields a complete explanation of students' anxiety. Though certain motifs become clear, every student's story contains complications, distortions, and omissions. But complete explanations are not necessary for anxious students to derive relief. It helps merely to bring dark fears and hidden motives out into the open; perhaps they are being admitted for the first time to anyone, maybe even to the student himself or herself. Discussing them with a supportive, understanding adult counteracts one of the darkest fears of all—that one's innermost nature is too strange and reprehensible to reveal to another person. It helps students also to learn that their anxiety is at least potentially understandable; they are not in the grip of quirky, inexplicable forces. And whatever tentative explanations do emerge tend to encourage students to confront their fears. The knowledge a woman gains that her anxiety stems from childhood fears of her father may hearten her to break the pattern. She realizes that perhaps as a young girl she needed to draw back, but she need not do so as a young woman.

This is the essence of the short-term psychodynamic model for treating anxiety problems. In addition to these general principles, there are certain theoretical considerations and practical modifications that must be taken into account when one uses this model with anxious students. These are detailed below.

Deciding When to Take Strong Measures

Students who suffer from acute anxiety often feel and convey a sense of urgency. Wanting to be relieved of anxiety right away, they subtly or overtly demand, "Save me." A key therapeutic task, accordingly, is to decide whether to take strong or even emergency measures to bring them relief. Complicating this task is the possibility of countertransference feelings. When students are desperate, therapists are susceptible to feelings of inadequacy and the concomitant temptation to prove their competence by taking dramatic action. Such countertransference reactions, if not understood and controlled by therapists, obviously may work against students' best interests.

The legitimate reason to institute strong or emergency measures is because students are unable to function without them. Their studies, living situation, or emotional stability is in jeopardy. In these cases therapists may choose to increase the length or frequency of sessions, offer direct advice ("Maybe you should drop the course"), act as agents for the students (arranging housing changes, speaking to instructors), ask the campus physician to prescribe a tranquilizer, or—at the extreme— arrange for hospitalization or a medical leave of absence. When these measures succeed, they reduce students' anxiety to a manageable level, restoring their capacity to function and enabling the regular business of therapy to proceed. At the least, they convey the comforting message that someone cares, is taking charge, and is trying to do something about the problem. Provision of advice, in particular, is often necessary to extricate students from harmful situations or relationships. An anxious young woman may ask regarding a destructive relationship, "How do I leave him?" Sometimes it is appropriate to tell her.

There are risks, however, in departing from usual therapeutic practice and employing strong interventions. Such measures may reinforce students' belief that anxiety is unacceptable and unbearable, that they should be *afraid* of their anxiety (cf. Beck & Emery, 1985). If these steps fail to bring relief, then students may conclude that nothing can help, and their despair will intensify. These measures may also teach students that outside intervention is necessary, that they themselves cannot manage their problems.

The best rule of thumb, then, is to withhold extra sessions, advice, medications, and the like unless and until it is clear that such measures are necessary. Whenever possible, therapists should be calm and patient in their approach; this suggests that students themselves have the resources to ride out and eventually overcome their anxiety. When therapists explain in words and show by example that anxiety is a part of life, not a cause for panic, often students' anxiety will diminish accordingly.

Maintaining Empathy

It is a truism that empathy is essential to all forms of therapy, with all clients, and with all problems. Anxious students can tax therapists' empathy, however. Those who demand relief, as we have seen, can instill in therapists feelings of inadequacy and the incentive to play rescuer. Acutely anxious students also may cause therapists to back away because of the intensity of their need. Those who remain anxious may evoke in therapists an inwardly critical or angry reaction, as if to say, "Enough already!" If students sense any of these countertransference responses, their despair and sense of isolation may be heightened.

A key therapeutic task, therefore, is to retain the capacity to enter into, accept, and mirror anxious students' subjective worlds. Comments such as "I know it must be frustrating to be feeling so bad week after week, even after coming to therapy," demonstrate that someone understands and cares even if he or she is unable to provide a panacea. The interpersonal climate that empathy creates helps ultimately to shake the foundations of students' anxiety.

Encouraging Activity and Assertiveness

Anxious students often perpetuate their problems because of their withdrawal and unassertive behavior. The result is that they do not acquire skills or achieve successes, thereby diminishing their self-esteem and heightening their anxiety. One way to break this vicious cycle is to encourage students to do the very things that frighten them—to assume an active and assertive rather than a passive stance. Doing so initiates a positive chain of events in which students gain skills and successes, bolster self-esteem, and accordingly reduce their anxiety. In pursuing this strategy, therapists may want to employ or even assign the reading of a manual on assertivenss training (e.g., Alberti & Emmons, 1970).

There are dangers inherent in this approach, however. One must not push students toward actions they presently cannot perform. It is also essential that students define success in terms of *trying*, not achieving perfection. The goal is to ask a question in class, not to make a brilliant comment. It is to ask someone out on a date, not necessarily (though it would be nice) to be accepted.

Helping Students to Express Themselves

Anxious students display all manner of difficulties in self-expression. They may be vague, halting, discursive, disjointed, or tangential as they try to explain themselves in therapy. These problems in communication are both a consequence and a cause of anxiety. On the one hand, they reflect both the confusion of anxious students, who often do not know what is happening to them or how it started, and also their fears concerning self-disclosure. On the other hand, problems in communication perpetuate anxiety by suggesting that the causes of suffering are too overwhelming, mysterious, or awful to capture in words. The inexplicable is *ipso facto* a cause of dread.

Therapists should not be impatient with anxious students, who are communicating as well as they can or dare. The task is to be understanding and gentle, yet active in helping them to express themselves more clearly. When students are vague, clarifying questions are recommended, such as "What exactly happened yesterday when you felt upset?" or "In what particular situations are you nervous?" When they fail to complete their thoughts, it helps to ask questions (P: "Yesterday was . . . " T: "How was yesterday?"), or even, if necessary, to finish the thought for them (T: "Yesterday was a bad day, wasn't it?"). When they skip from one problem to another, it is useful to steer them back to the topic under discussion. When they become distracted by a minor point, it helps to direct them to a more pivotal issue ("I notice we haven't talked today about that course that's been worrying you").

Provided they are used with tact and empathy, such structuring questions and comments can help reduce anxiety by conveying that students' problematic situations can be spoken about and understood. In particular, structuring questions and comments can illuminate for students, who often have only a foggy notion of what led up to their present crisis, the events that brought it to pass. Discovering the sequence that preceded an outburst of anxiety contributes to making anxiety understandable, and hence to reducing it.

Identifying Anxiety-Producing Beliefs

Anxious students characteristically entertain irrational, exaggerated, and self-defeating views of themselves, their world, and their efforts. They tend to consider themselves inferior, unable to master challenges. They perceive the world as threatening and hostile, its challenges as frightening. And they believe that it is unacceptable and devastating to fail at these challenges. Such core beliefs engender anxiety. A sound therapeutic strategy is to identify these beliefs, which may be either obvious to students or outside their conscious awareness, and to trace them from their origin to their current manifestations. In this way, the psychodynamic approach we follow dovetails with the cognitive approaches articulated in Beck's (Beck & Emery, 1985) cognitive therapy and Ellis's (Ellis & Grieger, 1977) rational–emotive therapy. Both the psychodynamic and cognitive approaches examine these pivotal cognitive components of subjective experience.

In contrast to Ellis's method, however, we do not advise a strategy of confronting or attacking anxiety-producing beliefs. Doing so may be interpreted as a failure in empathy—proof that therapists do not understand students' feelings of unworthiness and perception of the world as menacing. Furthermore, an attack on beliefs may be perceived as an attack on the self. A better strategy is simply to increase students' awareness of their thinking. What exactly is their opinion of themselves and their world? When do they think this way? What evidence do they use to confirm their beliefs? A related tactic is to have students put down on paper, either during therapy or between sessions, all the negative ideas they entertain. When students' irrational, exaggerated, and self-defeating beliefs are transferred from the private domain of personal thoughts to the more public arena of speech and writings, they themselves may question and gradually modify their beliefs.

Using Relaxation Methods

Though we do not usually employ relaxation methods in our own practice, some anxious students apparently benefit from learning progressive muscle relaxation or deep breathing exercises. Benson's *The Relaxation Response* (1975) may be assigned as supplemental reading. A simple technique is to recommend taking a few deep breaths, perhaps while inwardly reciting the word "relax." Minimal though it is, this method may give students a sense of having some control over their anxiety, which in itself alleviates their mental state.

Applications of the psychodynamic model of therapy and these special modifications are illustrated in the following case examples, which have been altered in certain details.

ANNA: A PSYCHODYNAMIC EXPLORATION

Anna was a 21-year-old student who enrolled at City College soon after emigrating from an Asian country 2 years ago. Her primary expressed concern was a relationship with a man that was causing her acute states of anxiety, which undermined her concentration and lowered her academic standing. Although she was not initially receptive to exploring her motivations, probably because reserve is valued in her culture, her case demonstrates the effectiveness of a patiently applied psychodynamic approach.

In her first session, Anna spoke in a highly self-conscious and rambling manner, discussing the symptoms of her anxiety rather than the actual events that led up to them. It was necessary to ask gently but repeatedly for clarifications; her communications had to be facilitated step by step. Thus, the therapist encouraged her to recount when and under what circumstances she began to experience an increase in anxiety. In response, she vaguely alluded to "boyfriend" problems. He asked what specifically disturbed her about this boyfriend. She said he treated her badly but didn't mean to. The therapist asked in what way he treated her badly. She dodged the question and brought up a neutral topic. Later, sensing from certain clues that she really did want to discuss the relationship, the therapist tried again: "Anna, in what way does this man treat you badly?" Through many questions of this nature, the therapist gradually helped her to express herself and supply the details of her current situation.

The story she told was that a man whom she had dated for only a short time was drunkenly calling her on the telephone and heaping verbal abuse upon her. She said that she tolerated his actions because he was a good person and did not mean to hurt her. As a Christian, she could not justify being angry at him. However, she admitted that worrying about his actions was causing her to neglect schoolwork and was inducing considerable anxiety.

Concluding that Anna's wish to tell about herself outweighed her natural reticence, the therapist proceeded in this first session and in subsequent sessions to employ the basic treatment strategy of searching for parallels among her childhood experiences, her current relationship with the man, and her transferential relationship with the therapist. The investigation disclosed the salience of fear of abandonment, which in turn fueled a fear of her own anger and assertiveness. Anna related that as a child her parents had failed to understand her and responded to her requests for emotional support by recoiling and accusing her of being a crybaby. Fearful of expressing her rage and thereby incurring more disapproval, she withdrew from them and instead sought support by rather indiscriminately attempting to rescue other people from their problems. In her view, if she could somehow help others, they would appreciate and nurture her. It was essential that she please them and withhold any signs of anger, lest she lose them too.

When at the end of her fourth session Anna expressed bitterness at her parents for neglecting her, her display of hostility caused her to be overcome with anxiety. The same dynamics were obviously at the core of her difficulty with her "boyfriend." She was so afraid to confront him and risk losing him that she behaved in an obsequious and fawning manner, which of course only led to an escalation of his abusive behavior. Meanwhile, she also acted indecisively and dependently with the therapist, asking repeatedly what she should do. Though his refusing to give her a solution obviously made her angry, she predictably found it difficult to express these feelings toward him as well.

As the therapist pointed out the common theme in all these relationships, Anna initially reacted with denial and an effort to change the subject, instead asking for advice about what she should do. Later on, the cumulative weight of many interpretations started to have an effect. She began to recognize that her powerful fear of abandonment had led to a lifelong pattern of unassertive behavior and suppression of anger. At first her acknowledgments had a mechanical quality, as if to say, "Yes, that's true, but it doesn't make any difference." Eventually, the insights started to sink in. In one session devoted to her childhood deprivations, she let herself cry intensely and recognize the depth of her unfulfilled need for closeness.

Still, insights alone were not enough; Anna obviously had to take steps to end her relationship with this man. Yet despite her burgeoning self-understanding and his continued harassment, she insisted for some time that she would continue to help him. It is no small matter, of course, to turn one's back on a lifelong pattern of behavior. The therapist here had to walk a tightrope. To give direct advice to drop the relationship—perhaps a good idea with another client—would mean to Anna being assigned to her familiar submissive, dependent role, which would perpetuate her fear of assertiveness. Anna herself had to initiate the break. Yet, at the same time, it was essential that she not be allowed to evade the issue of her self-destructive relationship. The therapist's tack, therefore, was to question her frequently about her thoughts and wishes regarding the man. What did her best judgment suggest she should do? This line of questioning had the effect of encouraging assertiveness while respecting her autonomy.

The behavioral move, when it came, happened suddenly. At the beginning of the fifth session she reported, her voice loud with anger, that she had stopped the man when he tried to taunt her during a chance meeting on campus. She announced then that she wanted nothing more to do with him. When he later tried to call, she immediately hung up.

Having finally jettisoned the anxiety-producing relationship and proved to herself that she could act assertively without catastrophe, Anna was rewarded with reduced anxiety. The remaining seven sessions were devoted to a deeper exploration of her long-standing difficulties with her family and her fears of abandonment and self-assertion. At the termination of therapy, her studies had improved and she was determined to carry on more constructive relationships in the future.

BRENDA: A MODIFIED APPROACH

Brenda's therapy resembled Anna's in important respects. Her current anxiety was traced to its roots through an insight-oriented investigation, and the insights she gained were coupled with encouragement of activity and assertiveness. However, because of the compelling nature of her presenting complaint, the therapist chose to depart more than in Anna's case from the orthodox psychodynamic blueprint. Brenda's case illustrates the flexible approach college therapists sometimes must employ in responding to a student's particular needs.

Brenda's chief concern was mounting dread of delivering a speech in one of her classes. This fear, like Anna's worry about her "boyfriend," could be readily traced to its origins. Indeed, though she spoke in a halting, self-deprecatory manner and rarely established eye contact, Brenda was eager from the start to tell her story. She explained that as a child she had been sadistically ridiculed and teased by her father. Her mother, apparently afraid to intervene, told the girl that the father acted this way only because he wanted the best from her. As a result, Brenda grew up believing that not only would she be subjected to ridicule, but she was wrong to get upset about it; she deserved castigation for her shortcomings. She became a frightened child who cowered when spoken to by adults and hid behind her mother. Later on in school, she felt terrified and self-conscious about speaking in groups, especially among strangers. Determined now to conquer her fear, she had enrolled in a public speaking class. As the week approached for her to deliver a brief speech, however, she was becoming increasingly apprehensive and was seriously considering withdrawing from the class.

The search for parallels among past, present, and transference relationships was for Brenda a tonic experience. She came to understand that the thread of fear of ridicule ran through all her relationships, even patently safe ones, as with the therapist. She had generalized her experience with her father and now expected ridicule from everyone. Though Brenda already suspected as much, having this theme corroborated and illustrated in detail increased her awareness and reinforced her resolve to overcome it. Meanwhile, speaking openly to the supportive therapist provided at least a partial "corrective emotional experience" (Alexander & French, 1946; see also Guntrip, 1971), proving that not everyone, in fact, would demean her. As the sessions progressed, Brenda grew more comfortable and more confident with the therapist.

Had the speech not loomed ahead, this standard psychodynamic approach might well have been sufficient. However, Brenda was still experiencing severe anxiety in anticipation of delivering the talk and was still tempted to drop the course. Since she saw the speech as the acid test of her ability to change, the therapist decided to concentrate on improving her chances for success. Focusing on her anxiety-producing beliefs, he questioned her about her expectations of the event. What images and thoughts came to mind? What exactly did she tell herself about the speech? She responded that speaking before the class would be a catastrophic experience. Her ideas would be poorly formed and jumbled further because of her anxiety; the class would be scornful (if only in silence); and she would end up in tears. At the same time, reason told her that her fears were perhaps irrational or exaggerated. "I know this is silly," she kept saying, as if her fears were shameful.

The therapist's task with this material was delicate. He had to be careful not to join in her denigration of her fears, which would have confirmed her belief that she was ridiculous. Therefore he remarked that her background gave her good reason to expect the worst; furthermore, her fears, far from being silly, were a concern that they both needed to take seriously. But the therapist also wanted to shake the foundations of her anxiety-producing beliefs. Perhaps, he suggested, she was right that her fears were exaggerated. Could she imagine outcomes other than the disaster she predicted? What were more constructive thoughts she might entertain about her performance and the reactions of the class? Through such questions, he invited her to challenge her fears in a nonjudgmental way.

In addition to examining Brenda's cognitions, the therapist decided to teach her methods of relaxation and stressed the importance of breathing deeply before and during the speech. He had her role-play the talk in his office and suggested that she also try it out with her roommate. He instructed her that people can perform in spite of anxiety; indeed, she should expect to be anxious on the day of the talk. Most of all, he encouraged assertiveness—and essentially gave advice—by urging her to follow through on her intentions. The anxiety she was suffering now in anticipation of the speech, he said, was the short-term price to pay for permanent psychological and social rewards. Delivering the talk could be a watershed for her self-confidence and ability to take risks.

It is impossible to say which technique or combination of techniques turned the tide. Perhaps the willingness of the therapist to try different methods in her behalf communicated an involvement that was in itself anxiety-reducing. Whatever the reason, the session after her scheduled speech Brenda came in aglow with triumphant enthusiasm. Despite butterflies from beginning to end, she not only had got through it, but was commended by her classmates and instructor. That session and one other were spent consolidating the lessons she had learned, after which Brenda terminated therapy with a considerable sense of accomplishment.

SUMMARY

Anxiety is a common denominator for virtually every college student who comes to the counseling center. It has many causes, both proximate and psychodynamic; it manifests itself in social situations, academic performance, bodily concerns, and indeed, every aspect of students' college adjustment. A modified short-term psychodynamic approach is recommended for treating the anxiety problems of college students. This approach aims to unearth core fears, motives, and conflicts by searching for parallels among students' past, current, and therapeutic relationships. The insight students gain into the unconscious sources of their anxiety then brings them relief. Working with anxious students calls for certain special therapeutic considerations and modifications within the psychodynamic model. Therapists may decide to take strong measures, encourage activities and assertiveness, help students to express themselves, identify anxiety-producing beliefs, or use relaxation measures. Maintaining empathy can be a particular challenge with anxious clients. The importance of taking a flexible approach within the psychodynamic model is illustrated by the two case studies.

REFERENCES

Alberti, R., & Emmons, M. (1970). *Your perfect right*. San Luis Obispo, CA: Impact.

Alexander, R., & French, T. (1946). *Psychoanalytic therapy*. New York: Ronald Press.

American Psychiatric Association. (1987). *Diagnostic and statistical manual of mental disorders* (3rd ed., rev.). Washington, DC: Author.

Angyal, A. (1965). *Neurosis and treatment*. New York: Wiley.

Beck, A. T., & Emery, G. (1985). *Anxiety disorders and phobias*. New York: Basic Books.

Benson, H. (1975). *The relaxation response*. New York: Avon Books.

Brenner, C. (1982). *The mind in conflict*. New York: International Universities Press.

Ellis, A., & Grieger, T. (1977). *Handbook of rational–emotive therapy*. New York: Springer.

Fenichel, O. (1945). *The psychoanalytic theory of neurosis*. New York: Norton.

Guntrip, H. (1971). *Psychoanalytic theory, therapy, and the self*. New York: Basic Books.

Horney, K. (1937). *The neurotic personality of our time*. New York: Norton.

Malan, D. H. (1976). *The frontier of brief psychotherapy*. New York: Plenum.

Pilkonis, P. A. (1977). The behavioral consequences of shyness. *Journal of Personality, 45*, 596–611.

Rothblum, E. D., Solomon, L. J., & Murakami, J. (1986). Affective, cognitive, and behavioral differences between high and low procrastinators. *Journal of Counseling Psychology, 33*, 387–394.

Schafer, R. (1983). *The analytic attitude*. New York: Basic Books.

Tillich, P. (1952). *The courage to be*. New Haven, CT: Yale University Press.

9

Academic Underachievement

CHARLES P. DUCEY

Learning is the ideal student's passion. When learning has lost its grounding in the student's own desire, or has become a battleground in the struggle to stake out an identity, then academic underachievement (falling short of one's potential) becomes a leading expression of those internal conflicts, particularly in a college setting. In order to treat such academic difficulties, the psychotherapist or counselor must comprehend the significance of learning and achievement in the student's own psyche, family, and culture. Academic difficulties can serve as the unwitting expression of diverse motives, conflicts, or deficits: an attempt to grow beyond a confining set of assumptions; a communication of distress; an underdevelopment of inner resources; an incapacity to take a stand that defines oneself in one's work; a resentment of demanding external or internalized authorities; an unconsciously intentional disruption of an expected career path; a result of depression over loss, neglect, or abuse; or other affective issues. Although "simple" deficiencies of skills or intelligence can of course contribute to academic problems, these difficulties are often caused or accompanied by emotional malaise. Hence, though amelioration of technical skills plays a part in addressing academic underachievement, an understanding of the emotional, characterological, and contextual issues is essential to its treatment.

The thinkers of ancient cultures understood the passionate dimension of education, which our pragmatic society either ignores or officially discourages. The Latin *studium*—"eagerness, zeal, enthusiasm, passionate devotion"—has degenerated into our "study"—a pallid, respectable, dutiful endeavor. For students whose academic problems reflect nonacademic issues, education has taken on a significance that interferes with a passionate devotion to learning, and subverts the ideal aim of "knowledge for its own sake." Students' natural passion for learning has then been compromised by overarching or undermining passions that demand recognition. Insofar as in a college environment the student's self-definition is largely that of a learner, then internal or interpersonal conflicts often appear in the form of academic difficulties. Psychotherapists can respond adequately to the challenge to the extent that they are fully cognizant of these complex dynamics.

SETTING OF THE TREATMENT

The setting within which I operate will give a perspective on the treatment principles and approaches outlined here, although their integration is my own. A clinical psychologist with a psychoanalytic orientation, informed by a developmental, cultural-linguistic, and research focus, I am also the director of an unusual organization whose central aim is to help students develop their intellectual and emotional potential: the Bureau of Study Counsel, a clinical–developmental center at Harvard University. Inasmuch as academic adjustment, psychological adaptation, and social functioning are indissolubly linked and developmentally based, the Bureau addresses external and internal issues that interfere with students' capacity to learn and the general quality of their lives.

The Harvard environment itself obviously exerts a powerful influence on the type of students and problems we encounter, although of course the issues we see can be found to varying extents on any campus. Students who come to Harvard are expected, and expect themselves, to perform excellently in a highly intellectual and competitive atmosphere. These expectations can lead to a variety of academic problems. Students may find that the ways of thinking and learning that served them well in secondary school are now not only ineffective, but possibly detrimental. Private self-doubt may lead them to interpret lapses in their academic performance as an indication of heretofore unrecognized dissimulation; in an environment of intellectual peers (indeed, superiors), they have been "found out," their inadequate performance a telling proof that they are less intelligent than they believed or had led others to believe. They find themselves anxious in the face of internal or external demands for developmental advancement, whether in the form of intellectual independence or commitment to a life direction. Their accustomed cognitive modes of adaptation have become insufficient for emotional maturation, or else they are beset by formerly warded-off conflicts that now invade the once autonomous cognitive sphere of functioning. The resultant crises of confidence are predictable and common, but no less painful for their widespread nature.

PRINCIPLES OF THE TREATMENT

Developmental Assumptions

Students' dilemmas are not simply academic ones in isolation, but reveal a need to reorganize a sense of self. The subjective definition of self is an issue for human beings at all ages; however, the transitional period between adolescence and adulthood confronts individuals with the necessity of consolidating a revised, coherent, and articulated identity, separate from the family of origin, to such an extent as has never occurred before and may never occur again. Difficulties in students' lives may appropriately be understood as representing a developmental struggle toward maturation on one's own terms, and betoken a shift from dependence or spurious independence toward adult interdependence.

The Bureau of Study Counsel has traditionally employed a cognitive–developmental model, in part formulated by its founder (Perry, 1970). The model arises from the empirical discovery of a developmentally based series of "positions" in the construction of the world of knowledge and values during college: from a "dualistic" stance that assumes that there are "right" or "wrong" answers or ways of being or ways of discovering answers, through a "multiplistic" belief in the plurality of knowledge and a "relativistic" recognition of its contextuality, to the development of a "commitment within relativism" that reflects the realization of personal identity and responsibility in a relative world. Students' concerns that emerge as problems in learning or academic mastery have to do with a set of implicit but now confining attitudes beyond which they are struggling to grow. This maturational push may be accompanied by pain and resistance, insofar as students experience a conflict between clinging to a familiar developmental position and moving on to the next position. For instance, students who seek answers from authorities outside themselves find that they are faced in college with the maturational demand and the environmental expectation to think critically and creatively for themselves and claim a personal perspective on their learning experience. The function of study counseling for academic difficulties is therefore a developmental one: to meet students where they are developmentally, to help them find their own voices regarding what is meaningful, and to stay with them as they move beyond dualistic and then multiplistic stances toward their own knowledge and values.

This cognitive-developmental shift is an important aspect of the movement beyond adolescence into adulthood. As students become comfortable with the contextuality and relativity of knowledge and broaden their perspective to include competing or complementary points of view, they alter their relationships to authorities, to peers, and ultimately to themselves. As they relinquish an unreflective faith in authority, they move away from merely conscientious and dutiful study to a definition of themselves and their own goals in a meaningful learning process—from learning for love to love of learning (Ekstein, 1966).

An Integrated Treatment Approach

This cognitive-developmental model often serves as a foundation for an experiential–existential approach to counseling and psychotherapy. Late adolescents' developmental impetus to discover their own beliefs and values, and therefore their "selves," is consistent with the experiential–existential approach, which aims to facilitate students' articulation of their own voice and perspective, independent both of "authorities" and of the tyranny of multiplistic and relativistic thinking. The existential approach pre-eminently utilizes empathy as the way of staying close to the client's experience of self and world. Empathic responsiveness helps students find their voices without their being drowned out by the demands of others or by their own hopes for absolute certainty or fears of absolute anomie or "rulelessness."

Yet insofar as both cognitive and experiential approaches tend to eschew an understanding of emotional, characterological, and unconsciously motivated aspects of personality, they oversimplify the nature of human difficulties. Hence, academic problems that express intrapsychic conflict or unreflective characterological stances call for a psychoanalytic–psychodynamic understanding and approach. Psychoanalytic–psychodynamic treatment aims to bring about a relative harmony among inevitably conflicting aspects of the self, or at least increased acknowledgment of disavowed constituents of the self. The analysand's initial attempt at conflict resolution, which excludes some experience of self, has a totalistic quality that compromises the achievement of other desired goals, such as academic accomplishment. Psychodynamic interventions, such as clarification (of preconscious motives) and interpretation (of unconscious motives), aim at the integration of disavowed motives and thereby the integrity of the self.

These three theoretical streams—cognitive-developmental, experiential–existential, and psychoanalytic–psychodynamic—seem particularly apt for treating the academic difficulties of students who are in a phase of transition from adolescence to adulthood. A treatment that integrates these approaches responds to students' maturational needs to disentangle the sense of self from parental control and parents' internalized presence: Amidst the welter of actual or imaginary pressures, expectations, and demands about who they should become, students feel a developmental push to establish a separate identity, based on their own talents, ideals, and aspirations (Kohut, 1977). In terms of theory, the cognitive-developmental model offers a conception of personality change and transformation; the existential point of view focuses on the phenomenology of identity and change; and the psychodynamic model provides the perspective of personality continuity across different developmental eras. In terms of practice, the cognitive-developmental approach offers explicit training in as yet underdeveloped cognitive skills; the experiential approach emphasizes students' current conscious experience of self and world as the foundation for change; and the psychodynamic approach encourages attention to students' past and future unrecognized motives and unrealized potentials. All three perspectives have demonstrable value for the treatment of academic difficulties.

Significance of Treatment for Academic "Symptoms"

The maturational demand for development into adulthood on one's own terms often makes its disguised appearance as a learning inhibition or a symptom. But because of the developmental and often evanescent nature of such symptoms, college psychotherapists have been loath to diagnose academic difficulties as manifestations of psychopathology, even when certain clear-cut obsessional or hysterical patterns can be identified (Hanfmann, 1978; McArthur, 1961). But if such symptoms are not responded to as unconscious communications of intrapsychic conflict deeply rooted in the student's life experience, such evanescent patterns may take hold and become endemic in the adult personality; adolescent self-defeating behaviors can become adult self-fulfilling prophecies. Therefore, the notion of "treatment" or psychotherapy is not inappropriate as a response to academic difficulties. Even if such failures have subtle adaptive value or even reflect a kind of moral courage (considering their significance as an attempt at self-definition), they are ultimately self-defeating ways of establishing an independent sense of self. Such difficulties call for a broadening of self-awareness through psychotherapy.

Insofar as academic "symptoms" may serve as indicators of internal stalemates of development, they point to neglected but significant aspects of students' past or current life experience that call for recognition. Once such issues are explored and understood, then students can continue their development into adulthood as unique and self-defined individuals. Although it is by no means always necessary to increase students' insight or self-awareness to help them with academic dilemmas, treatment of these dilemmas frequently initiates a more extensive psychotherapy.

ASSESSMENT ISSUES

Fundamental Principles of Assessment

Academic difficulties per se may not lead students to initiate treatment, particularly if they believe they have done their best, or their academic performance is for some reason not a conflictual issue. Nevertheless, there is probably no more accurate barometer of a student's internal "atmospheric pressure" than academic functioning. Particularly in colleges known for academic achievement, difficulties in the learning arena are a sensitive indicator of psychological distress.

The assessment of learning and study problems calls for clinical sensitivity, and should be guided by a few fundamental principles. Since any effective intervention is predicated upon the quality of the working relationship, the first prerequisite is the establishment of an empathic connection with a student. Assessors' empathic responsiveness to students' dilemmas is in itself valuable in reducing anxiety and in helping students to feel understood and hopeful. Second, assessors need to know how to respond appropriately both to the presenting problem and to underlying issues that, initially seemingly tangential and even unconscious, may move to center stage when students start to confide their more private experiences. Third, assessors need to respect students' defenses, which have been instituted to preserve a certain self-experience and self-image, and also to test them for their utility in conflict resolution and for their flexibility. Fourth, assessors need to strike balances between subjective empathy and object evaluation; between "accommodating" to students' horizon of self-understanding and "assimilating" students to their clinical experience with such problems; between responding to students' conscious voices and listening "with the third ear" to the communications from their internal "dispossessed minority voices"; and between following students' lead in the discussion and showing students how to make best use of treatment. Finally, assessors must make treatment decisions and responses based on a match between students' complex needs and the diverse array of available interventions.

Assessors should be responsive to what students are asking for, including ameliorative approaches. But in the ideal assessment students arrive at a deeper understanding of the external and intrapsychic context of their academic problems, while assessors make a comprehensive psychodynamic formulation of the situation and its potential resolution. The final decision about a plan of action depends on this interactional process, as well as these associated considerations: the nature of the presenting problem; the referral source; the unconscious significance of the problem; the student's character structure; the treatment options available; and the personal and professional qualities of the therapist.

Bases for the Decision about Intervention

The nature of the presenting problem has diagnostic significance and aids in the choice of approach and likelihood of resolution. For example, a specific learning difficulty can often be addressed through didactic tutoring, whereas a general collapse in all course subjects bespeaks a more ingrained psychological dilemma and calls for psychotherapeutic investigation. In the latter case, assessors need to determine the chronicity of the problem, for there is a significant difference between a recent academic dysfunction and a protracted failure to meet academic standards. Acute difficulties often respond well to an intensive brief psychotherapeutic approach; protracted academic problems often indicate the need for either extensive therapy devoted to structural character change, or else explicit acknowledgment of the current unsuitability of academic life, and, if need be, "permission" to leave school. (Such an acknowlegment, if appropriate, may serve to sanction students' right to succeed and fail on their own terms rather than those imposed by others. But the assessor must beware of offering this way out of the problem too readily, for a student may hear such "permission" as a "vote of no confidence" in the student's academic motivation or ability. Although students occasionally have an intuitive sense that their maturation will be improved by temporarily leaving school, assessors need to ascertain whether their leaving will be enacted with full awareness and under their own steam, rather than as a self-punitive submission to despised authority, or an excuse for self-denigration, or some other self-defeating compromise of their *joie de vivre*.)

The referral source often has as much prognostic significance as the presenting complaint itself. Self-referred students, who want to do better academically and know they can, are usually suffering acute dis-

tress over an incomprehensible betrayal of their potential, and are therefore highly motivated to understand the disjunction between their ability and performance. Other things being equal, such students have the
greatest likelihood of at least partial resolution of their difficulties
through treatment. On the other hand, students who are referred by
someone else, even seemingly against their will, are by no means necessarily unsuited for psychotherapy. Young people who have learned to
be self-sufficient may balk at the notion of seeking help, and their dramatic failures may be the only way they have of communicating, in a
face-saving way, that they desperately need help. Sensitive therapists
need only indicate clearly that, no matter how these students came in
for help, their need to talk with someone about what they have been
going through is sufficient reason for psychotherapy.

The underlying significance of the academic problem is sometimes
not easy to determine in a brief assessment, but assessors can gain an
intuitive sense of the underlying conflict through dynamically sophisticated and contextually attuned interviewing. A useful question to keep
in mind is the legal *cui bono?*: To whose benefit—or detriment—does
the current symptom redound? For example, if students articulate the
belief that their parents are using their academic achievement for the
parents' own purposes (e.g., enhancement of self-esteem, control, or
libidinal competition), then students may come to understand their academic difficulties as an unconscious plea for recognition of these complicating pressures, and a consequent attempt to reassert their own
independent educational aims. Or if students' parents have imparted
to them their conception of college learning as merely a necessary labor
toward the goal of economic success, is it any wonder that students
may manifest intellectual "blocks" to learning, and incur anxiety or
depression as a result? Or if students have been shepherded, or rather
herded, toward a college or a field that is not of their choosing, but
merely a fulfillment of long-standing family dreams, academic underachievement may be their only way of asserting their own passion for
learning, their own identity. These underlying motives, even if initially
unconscious, are sufficiently common, well understood, and unlikely
to generate intense anxiety when uncovered that their explicit articulation can have dramatic effects on the academic difficulties they have
generated.

The assessment of the developmental level and adaptive quality
of the defenses, and therefore of the character structure, significantly
influences the type of intervention that should be offered to students.
"Higher-level" (neurotic, repressive, inhibitory) defensive styles tend
to result in conflict-based academic problems that respond well to verbal insight-oriented approaches. Obsessional styles, particularly com-

mon and often adaptive in a university setting, point to "superego"-engendered internal conflicts, which can lead to perfectionism, unrecognized rebellion against internalized authority, avoidance of success, or self-punishment as a manifestation of submission to introjects. Although treatment of the underlying character pathology may be in most settings regarded as unduly time-consuming and arduous, relatively isolated habits that are outcrops of this character style, such as procrastination, can often be effectively addressed through time-limited groups or even single-session workshops on time management. Frequently students seek treatment under the impact of a maturational or environmental crisis, when their rigid inhibitory defenses are collapsing. In that circumstance, assessors may determine that counseling can help merely by riding out the crisis with students; though assessors may not know whether the crisis portends more serious disturbance, their very presence is valuable in counteracting students' sense of aloneness in the face of panic.

"Intermediate-level" (characterological, immature, externalizing) defensive styles may be indicated by mood swings, dissociated expression of instinctual strivings, or maladaptive interpersonal relationships. In these instances, academic difficulties may indicate an unresolved struggle against introjected coercive or abusive figures from early life. The recognition of severe character pathology is made more difficult by its manifesting itself in protean forms, including apparently "higher-level" or neurotic conflict over intellectual achievement (Kernberg, 1986). The following indicators suggest its presence: generalized, unbidden, and uncontrollable disruption of ordinary cognitive functioning by peculiar (often sexual or aggressive) preoccupations; assessors' intuitive sense of deception, manipulation, or circumscribed delusional thinking; pathognomomic indications from psychodiagnostic assessment; and evidence, retrospectively reported or observed *in vivo*, of a lack of capacity for fully experienced object relations, an emotional unresponsiveness to self and others. Even when the presence of such pathology is inferred, college psychotherapists often treat it with benign neglect, hoping that interventions less heroic than long-term expressive psychotherapy will help resolve the immediate academic problem. For that matter, these students themselves may balk at long-term therapy. But a positive initial contact, in which students feel responded to and helped in their immediate concern, often leaves the door open for a return for help later, either for specific problems or for acknowledged self-destructive character patterns. The establishment of a continuous positive relationship, in which the abuse and coercion students may transferentially invite are clearly recognized and firmly resisted by psychotherapists, is the foundation for a positive identification that counteracts students' negative introjects.

Occasionally academic difficulties indicate the existence of primitive or psychotic interferences with perception and thinking. Since such severe psychopathology usually manifests itself first in other ways, and its symptoms are more unmistakable than for neurotic and character disorders, the deterioration of academic performance is not usually treated directly in these cases. A combination of environmental manipulation, medication, and therapy may be called for. At such times, academic performance is a comparative luxury, about which one can worry when the immediate crisis has passed.

The availability of treatment options, including the type and extent of professional time, is another obviously influential factor that determines the response to student needs. In any setting, the principle of economy of action is a worthwhile guide: Assessors should offer the treatment option that calls for the least expenditure of student and staff energy and also accomplishes the goal established in the formulation. Of course, if a long-term therapeutic response is not feasible, the imposition upon students of ambitious formulations of unconscious mental functioning has, as Freud put it, "as much influence on the symptoms of nervous illness as a distribution of menu-cards in a time of famine has upon hunger" (1910/1957, p. 225). On the other hand, assessors should avoid merely ameliorative and symptomatic treatment for complex problems: Students see through empty reassurances and objectifying manipulations of their psyches. The wisest policy is an open discussion of available options, a reasoned recommendation of the most probably efficient and effective option, and reality-based (i.e., not crystal-ball forecasting) encouragement, which may function as a "suggestion" (Ducey, 1986) for the success of the undertaking.

In sum, academic difficulties can arise from diverse sources and call for careful and thorough assessment. Not only does such an assessment point the way to an appropriate therapeutic approach, but it also can be therapeutic in itself, and thus serve as the foundation and model for therapy.

FORMS OF TREATMENT

Overview: Application of Three General Approaches

A taxonomy of overt academic difficulties is not yet available, and may not even be feasible, considering the diversity of tributaries that flow into that great stream. We can, however, classify academic problems according to three general treatment approaches: didactic–cognitive techniques, group interventions, and individual psychological counseling or psychotherapy. This rough classification suggests a sequence from cognitive restructuring to emotional experiencing, from remediation of "deficit" to resolution of "conflict," from present focusing to past and future telescoping into the present, and from the publicly crafted persona to the uncomfortably private self. Generally speaking, didactic–cognitive techniques are useful for students whose academic problems can be improved particularly through support of cognitive maturation, and who tend to treat their internal processes behaviorally and objectively rather than emotionally and subjectively. Group techniques offer efficient treatment of common academic problems for which there are developmentally grounded and widely applicable prescriptions, and for which social interaction serves to provide reassurance, morale building, and mutual reinforcement. Individual counseling and psychotherapy show greatest benefit for specific academic problems rooted in students' emotional–motivational life and personality structure.

Didactic and Cognitive Approaches

Accustomed as they are to instruction, students may conceive of any form of treatment as a kind of education and be disconcerted by the relative absence of didactic instruction in psychotherapy or counseling. In a college setting, interventions that have a didactic component work well for students who want this structured approach; who have focal academic problems unconnected with deeper personality issues; who are uncomfortable with their internal lives; or who have specific remediable study or learning deficits. Didactic approaches either directly address specific learning problems or else provide new cognitive perspectives on the learning process.

Students often benefit from peer tutoring by other students who have mastered particular courses. This didactic approach can ameliorate specific deficits or difficulties in such subjects as mathematics, natural sciences, and foreign languages. Since student tutors face issues common to all helpers, they need to be supervised by professional counseling staff for handling difficult situations, reasonable and irrational demands, and countertransference feelings that arise in the tutorial relationship. This supervision can ordinarily be provided in small groups.

The individualized use of study skills counseling and materials offers a cognitive–behavioral amelioration of specific deficits or inhibitions. A typical situation that may call for this approach is a chronic or repetitive learning difficulty that generalizes across courses and seems unlikely to yield to group interventions and other approaches.

For example, students may be inexperienced with organizing their own time; may have writing difficulties; may be unable to offer their own perspective on an analytic paper; or may need help in "examsmanship." For any of these difficulties, they can be helped to develop cognitive techniques and then use practice materials, either with a counselor or on their own. These techniques are also beneficial because they are more efficient and respectful of students' defenses than exploratory therapy; they do not cause students to stereotype themselves as psychologically disturbed.

A sensitive clinical psychologist recognized that a graduate student she was seeing in therapy would not be helped to complete his dissertation by focusing on the difficult marriage that was interfering with his concentration, even though she saw that the writing inhibition and the marital difficulty shared a common pattern of marked performance anxiety and obsessional approach to the world. Instead, she used a careful evaluation of his cognitive style to tailor her interventions to his special modes of thinking and expression. Accordingly, he was encouraged to "think out loud" about his topic, and thus to use her as an intelligent sounding board, to determine whether he could convey his point of view in clear and understandable language. He then wrote down in the session what he had spoken, and his dissertation chapters grew accordingly. Since this student responded well to the concrete and the visible, the clinician cleared a shelf of her bookcase as a repository for his completed chapters; seeing his progress with his own eyes stimulated his ambition and encouraged him to continue. As he became able to make progess on his own, she decreased the frequency of the sessions to once every other week; on the alternate weeks he still came to the Bureau at his usual appointment time and worked alone in another room. His completion of the dissertation, after years of stalling, became a foregone conclusion.

This example illustrates the value of both a sophisticated assessment of the student's writing difficulties and a flexible intervention, responsive to the student's particular character, needs, and dilemmas. Not only does this case illustrate a cognitive–behavioral intervention, but one can also discern an important psychoanalytic principle that influences *any* positive therapeutic experience: the reparative effect of a benign self-object. Thus, in the beginning of treatment the clinician became the mirroring self-object for the student's efforts to make himself understood; next, she was the guarantor and trustee of his dissertation progress, and probably also the idealized embodiment of his own strivings for a successful graduate enterprise; still later, when he wrote his dissertation in a proximate office, her presence was experienced as a symbolic reality in his psyche, which through a "transmitting internalization" fostered the integration of his identity. Thus deficits in empathy from early life were counteracted through a treatment that relied upon neither reflective insight nor emotional expression, but rather the emergence of intellectual achievement. Although the student presumably still had to overcome his obsessional approach to object relations, his success in intellectual accomplishment, after repetitive past failures, provided both a framework for the safe expression of the self and a foundation of hope for the self's further emergence in emotional relationships.

Group Interventions

Groups, workshops, and structured courses are the three group interventions. Time-limited groups focus upon specific issues that are ameliorated by peer support and the sharing of experiences and coping strategies. Workshops are one-time didactic presentations concerned with a specific issue. Structured courses provide ongoing didactic instruction and practice with a more complex issue.

Groups are usually constituted as a time-limited (usually six to eight meetings per semester) and issue-focused series of partly directed discussions. The most popular and successful groups handle a specific academic issue that students are not ashamed to acknowledge, such as procrastination. Group discussions about feeling blocked or taking risks are generally lively and often help relax students who worry unduly about work that, one way or another, usually gets done. Serious obsessional blocking or compulsive ritual, however, does not yield to such brief group experiences and calls for individual therapy. Another well-attended and useful group intervention is assertiveness training, which helps students get over initial anxiety and "stage fright" regarding participating in class discussions, approaching instructors, or talking with the opposite sex. The group itself can serve as a "dry run" for "the real thing"; hence, role play, communication, and behavioral strategies for the management of anxiety are extensively utilized. Support groups for dissertation writers are valuable for counteracting the anxiety, loneliness, and depression common to advanced graduate students, who greet the prospects of sustained effort and completing their education with equal ambivalence.

A group approach also works well for students with "learning disabilities" (Mangrum & Strichart, 1984). The group can supply information about the problem, counteract the withdrawal that often results from shame over a perceived deficit, help students learn skills such as structured time management, and offer ideas about adapting to or getting around limitations. Combining graduate and undergraduate learning-disabled students in the same group has mutually beneficial effects, as older students can increase their sense of competence and self-confidence by offering guidance, while younger students gain both practical suggestions and the perspective that a perceived disability need not stand in the way of postcollege accomplishment. The group leader must conduct a careful balancing act, acknowledging the academic interference imposed by a specific learning disability, yet refusing to reinforce low self-esteem or avoidance of exploring other contributions to poor academic performance.

Workshops offer specific training and practice on topics such as assessment of individual learning strategies, time management, note taking, and examsmanship. For instance, at Harvard we present an opportunity during students' first week of college for a self-assessment of their learning and study strategies. This self-assessment helps them gain a personal perspective on how they best learn, based on their performance on different tasks: a learning typology, in which students' answers to multiple-choice questions about common learning situations serve as the basis of assessing their own characteristic learning style (escape-oriented, dutiful, purposeful, anticipatory, or "voiceful" approach to learning, from Perry's [1970] scheme); open-ended questions about past learning experiences (often deeply emotional in nature); and an experience of grading academic essays of differential quality, to give students the opportunity to assess the sort of analytical thinking expected of them in college. Students enjoy this exercise, and gain a perspective on their own cognitive approaches and on what is expected in college work. Other workshops offer students instruction and practice exercises in managing their time or taking notes and examinations. The exercises are graduated in such a way that students develop the notion that work done with intentionality "sticks" better than a passive and merely receptive attitude toward knowledge. Hence, workshops encourage a transition from dutiful submission to authority to acknowledgment of a personal perspective in one's work.

Courses in learning and study skills are valuable for students who can benefit from a developmentally oriented, didactic approach to learning skills, especially for those unfamiliar with or unprepared for some of the demands of college work. A group didactic approach creates, in the absence of grades, a mutually supportive atmosphere for its members. In addition to promoting the improvement of study skills, such a course can even promote maturation of cognitive development. The Bureau's Harvard Course in Reading Strategies (Perry, 1959), Harvard's oldest continuously offered course (since 1939), provides the skill of "speed reading," but also encourages students' active engagement in the learning process. The course's implicit technique leads students gradually from passive, unreflective reception to active selection, participation, and intentionality; from seeking guidance from an authority to accepting personal responsibility for learning; and from an unrecognized rigid "morality" of study (e.g., a belief that one has to read every text word for word) to a flexible fashioning of learning to one's own ends.

For some students, this change in perspective and attitude generalizes beyond their work to deeply ingrained aspects of personality functioning. One young woman taking the daily, 3-week-long course wrote increasingly negative comments to me about the blurriness of the speed-reading films, their irrelevance, and their speed. She complained that the "horrible fuzzy areas" of the films were impeding her ability to "push myself along" and "force comprehension." Lest I miss the clear message, she ended with the words, "How many different ways can I say this?" I had a brief meeting with her after the class, attempting to reply to the justifiable complaints—the films are indeed old—and to reassure her that anxiety and anger were usual reactions to the course's challenge to tried-and-true ways of reading and studying. I encouraged her to continue, but assured her that it was her choice to do so; I did not address any of the obvious deeper concerns, as I knew that she was returning home to a distant city after the course was over, and that any questioning about her emotional state would be invasive unless she requested my doing so.

After this interchange, I noticed a subtle change in her involvement and responsiveness. Her comments began to focus on how interesting the films were and how much she had learned from the lecture; I also noticed that both her reading speed and comprehension, tested daily, were showing steady and at times dramatic improvement. Near the end of the course she eagerly told me that it had finally "clicked" for her; she grasped the principle of active purpose and choice in the material and was noticing herself putting it into practice without even being aware of doing so. Moreover, she observed that previously she had felt a compulsion to examine and question every little thing that happened during the day, so that large portions of time were spent in rumination. She had not paid attention or given much thought to this behavior, but being pushed by the daily speeding up of the films made her aware that she had been "hanging onto and not letting go of" any word that appeared on the screen. As a consequence, the films seemed to pry her mind free from a habitual behavior. She found, to her astonishment, that she could concentrate *better* if she relaxed and let her mind flow with the film; previously she had been afraid of letting down her guard, of missing something. She realized that her boyfriend and her mother had been pointing out this tenacious behavior for years, in perplexed but sympathetic ways; until now, she had not known what they meant.

Although of course I would not claim that this student's obsessional style was profoundly altered, one troublesome and pervasive symptom seemed to be modified. The joy of beholding change and growth is that, compulsion to repeat notwithstanding, individuals find that they cannot easily go back to a once useful but now superseded solution, once the conflict that gave rise to it is deeply interrupted or resolved: "How're you gonna keep 'em down on the farm, after they've seen Paris?"!

Individual Psychological Approaches

The most extensively used approaches for the resolution of academic problems are individual counseling and psychotherapy. The didactic and cognitive approaches outlined above often evolve into psychological treatment, for a number of reasons. Students' initial anxiety about seeking help may be dispelled through responsive action that emboldens them to probe more deeply into their dissatisfaction; they may use academic difficulties, intentionally or unwittingly, as a kind of "Trojan horse" concealing emotional problems in its belly, or a pass-key to a significant therapeutic enterprise; the didactic approach may be insufficient for the problem, or else, if effective, may open up new perspectives on mental functioning and thus generate unanticipated hope for emotional healing as well. An academic counseling center that does not offer a psychotherapeutic approach must therefore make careful provisions for responding to and referring such students.

Many academic problems can be averted and the need for treatment forestalled by high-quality academic advising, particularly in students' freshman year. A well-designed university curriculum encourages students to sample a wide variety of subjects in order to define their own interests, and a well-established advising system permits them to make the best use of these resources. Through careful attention to educational balance, to an individual's areas of interest, talent, and difficulty, and to the nature of the proposed courses, the academic adviser is in an ideal position to head off insurmountable problems.

Psychological counseling is a response to situational challenges and pressures that interfere with academic functioning. For instance, the pervasive Harvard self-effacing syndrome ("They made a mistake when they chose me") can be significantly defused through the reality testing and support provided by counseling. Specific external interferences with academic functioning, such as difficulties with roommates or instructors, the workload, and adjustment to an unfamiliar environment, generally yield to responsive counseling. Indeed, the very presence of an adult who pays attention to students' needs and concerns can be an important transitional experience, as students move away from parents toward tenure in the adult world.

The term "counseling" is often used to refer to a client-centered or person-centered form of nondirective psychotherapy (Meador & Rogers, 1984), whose aim is to help individuals clarify the relationship between the experienced self and the "conditions of self-regard." Counselors reflect back a (perhaps partly edited and expanded) version of what they hear clients saying, in order to help clients find their real voice and permit them to reflect on their assumptions. In the valuable technical distinctions introduced by Bibring (1954), person-centered counselors use clarification far more than the techniques of suggestion, abreaction, manipulation, or interpretation. In gaining reflective awareness of their assumptions, some of which are based on outmoded and limiting conditions of self-regard, clients are enabled to proceed with their development.

This philosophy of counseling is usefully supplemented by a fundamental cognitive-developmental and psychoanalytic principle: that students' academic problems are the external manifestation of an inevitable developmental change, a struggle to overcome the limiting assumptions of a soon-to-be-superseded stage (such as the basis of knowledge in authority). Within this framework, "resistance" to academic work and external demands is a sign of integrity, of students' striving for a self-defined identity. Therefore, counselors do not attempt to overcome resistance, but rather to help students to understand and respect the message they are unwittingly giving themselves in their struggles. Once the integrity of resistance is acknowledged, the resistance will have outlived its usefulness and need no longer be used as an expression of self. By reframing an apparent failure as a disguised success, counselors release students to some extent from the burdens of self-blame and self-denigration implied in the term "resistance." By the same token, students benefit by having their strivings treated respectfully by a transference figure, and by expanding their awareness of their own subtle motivations.

For example, a young woman was failing dramatically in a basic chemistry course that she should have been able to handle. Her attitude seemed to be that if she did not try she was not really failing, and therefore her vulnerable self-esteem was not threatened. Her academic adviser, a counselor, was too sophisticated to take a simplistic view of academic problems. This counselor did not ignore the student's inveterate proclivity to "forget" her advising appointments or to crowd them out with other time demands and activities; she also refused to make the usually sexist assumption that the young woman had a "science disability." Instead, the counselor made active efforts to engage the student in nonthreatening ways. This was no easy task, as the student avoided contact, and was also becoming unpopular on campus because of her "spoiled brat" attitude, inconsiderateness, and provocative behavior. She was on the verge of being shown the door on both academic and behavioral counts.

The counselor kept abreast of the student's activities, invited her out to lunch, showed concern for her well-being, and forbore to criticize her for her "resistance" or her occasional "acting out," even when her behavior brought her to the attention of the dean's office. The counselor tacitly recognized these behavioral problems as pleas for psychological help. When the student acted as if nothing were wrong, the counselor confined herself to wondering aloud about the disparity between what the student was saying and what she was doing. This mild comment bore fruit, and the student herself gradually wondered about the contradiction.

Through persistent, quiet demonstration of her availability and responsiveness, the counselor finally engaged the recalcitrant student in a genuine conversation about her current academic and life dilemmas. The emerging tale showed why the student had been at once so reluctant to talk and yet so devoted to making her initial year a disastrous spectacle. The young woman's mother had job duties beyond her technical expertise. The mother's peculiar solution, imbued with symbiotic overtones, was to send her daughter for scientific training to Harvard, in the expectation of her eventually joining the business and in the meantime offering educated advice. The mother had her heart set on her daughter's living out what she herself had not been able to do. But she turned this desire into a demand by threatening to discontinue tuition payments unless the daughter complied, and by threatening her husband with divorce unless he supported her. Since the young woman had to take chemistry, the only escape she saw was to fail; she was indeed succeeding in failing.

Counseling helped the student gain a clearer understanding of the situation. She saw how her conflict between conscious dutifulness as a daughter and unconscious uncompromising rebellion lay behind her inadequate academic performance. With the unspoken command and the silent struggle out in the open, the mother called the counselor, who obtained her daughter's permission to talk with her parents. The counselor used the opportunity to suggest to the mother, "You of course want the best for your daughter," with the implication that "the best" would be respect for her own choices. This suggestion from a concerned college administrator helped temper the mother's controlling behavior. The counselor also encouraged the student to discuss the situation openly with her parents. This step always requires courage, as it is not easy to challenge a parental dictate, whether explicit or implicit, rational or irrational. The student did so directly but refrained from accusations and criticism of her embattled mother, whose psychological health was apparently precarious.

The airing of the situation had positive effects, at least on the daughter's education. The mother temporarily withdrew her threat to pull her daughter out of school, perhaps because her designs were obviously unappealing when exposed to the clear light of day. In standing up for herself and speaking openly to her parents, the young woman began a transition from being an apparently immature, passive–aggressive, and acting-out adolescent to a more self-possessed, grown-up young woman, who could know what she wanted and achieve it through assertion rather than failure and disruption. Gaining self-confidence through her actions, she discovered the possibility of compromising with her mother's wishes, now that they were no longer framed as rigid and arm-twisting demands. She succeeded in an appropriate chemistry course in the second semester.

In this case, the counselor took several steps that helped resolve the young woman's repetitive self-defeating behaviors. First, the counselor refused to take a passive stance of waiting for the student to ask for help; assertively but in a nonauthoritarian way, she continued to reach out to her despite discouragement. Had she responded passively to the student's *apparent* wishes (e.g., to fail in school, to miss advising appointments, to engage in disruptive behavior), she would have helped perpetuate the student's pattern of overt narcissistic demandingness and covert abysmal self-esteem, and would have encouraged her to escalate her already dangerously out-of-control behavior in order to have her impossible entrapment noticed. Second, the counselor communicated to the student that they could openly discuss conflict and the emotional significance of action, something that did not happen in the student's family of origin; they could air covert and festering problems and thereby help resolve them. At the same time, the counselor's concerned attentiveness, which indicated that an adult could be on her side and act unselfishly in her interest, was probably also unprecedented in the young woman's experience. Third, the counselor's openness and assertiveness provided the student with a model for direct dealing with problems rather than passive, self-destructive submission. Indeed, the student herself showed concern about growing up to be like her mother, and implied that the counselor offered a different model for being a female adult. Fourth, the counselor improved the family situation by suggesting that "of course" the mother wanted what was best for her daughter, thereby providing the psychologically disturbed woman with a positive model of mothering. As a result of these interventions, the young woman was able to extricate herself from her dilemma. She saw that her parents, whatever their own psychological issues, loved her and could be encouraged to want the best for her. She was able to continue her education and begin a less ambivalent developmental transition to adulthood, now that she no longer had to make the impossible choice between subordinating herself to external demands and harming her mother.

The boundary between counseling and individual psychotherapy is easier to draw in theory than in practice (Perry, 1955); the latter term is derived from a different theoretical tradition that defines its activity in terms of "cure" of the suffering "patient" (from the latin *pati*, "to suffer or endure"). Even when psychotherapy is shorn of inappropriate medical connotations, as (ideally) in psychoanalytic and existential approaches, it remains an enterprise in which patients, who feel "passive" (also from *pati*) in relation to their suffering, are helped to integrate "passion" (also from *pati*) into their sense of self. Insofar as "patients" feel at the mercy of their "symptoms," unable to act, think, or feel differently, then they experience themselves as trapped and unfree: "He that is not free is not an *agent*, but a *patient*" (John Wesley, circa 1780).* The aim of psychotherapy is the transformation of a patient into an agent—that is, from one who "suffers" into one who "does" ("agent," "active," and "action" are derived from the Latin *agere*, "to do").

The distinction between counseling and psychotherapy, at least in theory, involves a differential emphasis regarding the proper stance and activity of the professional in relation to the client (May, 1987a). The person-centered counseling tradition recommends staying close to clients' conscious experience and relying mainly on clarification, and cautions against getting ahead of or going beyond clients' understanding of their life situation, lest counselors succumb to the temptation to offer their own stereotypes and predilections in place of their clients' wishes and ways of understanding. By contrast, the psychotherapeutic tradition declines to comprehend communications only at face value and to "accompany" patients in their conscious experience only. Unlike counselors, psychotherapists who address academic dilemmas pay more attention to students' intrapsychic world of the imaginary and the symbolic than to actual external pressures and demands upon them, to their "study skills," or to their cognitive-developmental position; they attend not only to students' spoken voices, but also to the unspoken, the unfelt, the disavowed, and the unconscious. Assuming that the integration of this realm of experience will in itself renew a sense of agency,

*Quoted in Anthony Powell (1979), *Agents and Patients*, New York: Warner.

psychotherapists augment clarifications with empathic interpretations of as yet alien experience (Binstock, 1986).

This orientation means that the realm of the alien is explicitly invited into the relationship, rather than being left (politely or brusquely) outside the door. What had seemed irrelevant to the discussion of academic problems—the student's childhood and early adolescent experience, dreams, irrational thoughts, intrusive emotions, transference—may now take center stage. Current anxieties about academic performance may begin to be seen as uncannily like past experiences; current self-defeating behaviors in the academic realm are recognized as repetitions of earlier, unremembered ways of behaving. Steadfastly adhering to the goal of integration of all components of the self, psychotherapists keep their attention focused on disowned aspects of the self and life experience, unwilling to support the panoply of avoidances and defenses students direct against their own emotional life.

The interventions discussed previously differ from psychotherapy in holding out the comic and romantic promises of altering reality: If the academic problem is due to environmental demands, accommodate to them or change them; if due to poor study skills, improve them through education and practice; if due to inexperience, then just wait until inevitable development takes place. Psychotherapy, by contrast, assumes a tragic and ironic vision of reality: The past creates the present, and is impossible to change (Schafer, 1970). But psychotherapy can change an individual's relationship to the past.

Psychotherapy for academic difficulties is not different in principle from that for any condition, once the determination has been made that psychotherapy is the most appropriate response. Psychotherapists initially find out whatever they can about the meaning of the problem to students, the situations and contexts within which it manifests itself, the familial significance of achievement, parental responses to academic failures, and parental treatment of students' needs and desires in general. As students come to recognize that their academic problem is the tip of the iceberg, a symptom of broader and deeper malaise, the investigation of how their life is going in general usually proceeds naturally. Meanwhile, psychotherapists privately notice areas of silence, conflict, abstruse communication, unexpected passion, and the other signs of unconscious or ego-alien experience.

A senior woman in a seriously depressed state came for treatment for an unaccountable pattern of "snatching defeat from the jaws of victory," and for superficial but uncontrollable self-cutting. Throughout college, she had always started a semester with a strong showing that indicated she might be a star of her classes; around midterm she would falter; and ultimately, because of an incapacity to study for final exams, she would do abysmally. She was saved from academic probation by virtue of her earlier good grades. Her quick intelligence was apparent, but her language seemed unusually cluttered by such words as "stupid" and "imbecile." She claimed not to notice how commonly she used those words until I pointed them out to her; but gradually she came to realize that such verbalizations formed a steady but unnoticed intrapsychic "background radiation" that accompanied any intellectual behavior.

Reconnaissance of her life history depicted her family as afflicted with usually covert tensions between a bright but somewhat ne'er-do-well father and an angry and bitter mother; they praised and seemed to prefer her older sister, and pampered a younger brother. My initial interpretations of her denigrating inner voices as her parents' words intrigued her, and yielded scattered memories of tendentious comparisons between her own and her sister's academic performance. These themes were apparently pushed aside when the student called me in a suicidal panic on a weekend night. In our next few, more frequent sessions, she recounted her growing disturbance about her marijuana smoking and about an unsavory and dangerous-sounding boyfriend, an older man who owned a gun and was pressing her to take more potent drugs.

Relying on the deepening trust implied by the student's articulation of long-standing self-destructive patterns, I was able to ally myself with her struggling self against hostile, destructive introjects. In practice, this aim translated into upholding her right to be happy and to oppose the mistreatment perpetrated by others and by her own internal assaults. I also refused to join the chorus of inner voices that made her academic failures a proof of her stupidity. Dream work and close attention to her associations suggested that her academic difficulties had the apotropaic function of helping her ward off an unspecified danger that would ineluctably occur were she to succeed. Hence, I took the ironic stance of justifying her underperformance: "No wonder you didn't do what you're capable of: You kept your talents well hidden, and outwitted the demons once again!" In thus articulating an obscure and unspoken subjective experience, I intended not only to make sense of her self-defeating behavior, but also to "smuggle in" praise of her intellect that would never have gained her assent—and may have earned her suspicion—if expressed directly.

This explication of the wisdom and dignity of her academic symptoms, in conjunction with implicit sanctioning of her protecting herself against both her sociopathic boyfriend and her introjects, gradually led the way to fresh interpretation of her past. The vague "introjects" resolved themselves into their original models, and a story of both physical and emotional abuse emerged. The parents had awesome, awful fights both in front of and involving the little girl. She was exposed to systematic derogation of her abilities until she felt intense confusion and ambivalence about intellectual achievement; for instance, she longed to escape from school, and yet at home longed to escape to school. She recalled bizarre memories from adolescence of her father's chasing and hitting her with a broom, and of her mother's throwing onions and trash into the bathtub while the young woman was taking a bath. From this flood of memories, which brought a flow of tears, a plausible explanation emerged for the symptom of snatching defeat from the jaws of victory: Whenever in early life she threatened to be successful, her competitive, depressed, and self-despising parents turned on her and persecuted her ruthlessly. Through projective identification, they cast her as the representative of despised parts of themselves. Therefore, to protect herself and yet fulfill their expectations of failure, she had to stop herself from succeeding. Discussion of these themes aided her intrapsychic differentiation from parents and introjects, and enabled her to end the harmful relationship, use of drugs, and self-mutilation. Several years of follow-up have indicated lasting change, ever-increasing maturation, and general life satisfaction, even though she has not (yet) used her intellect for sustained accomplishment.

This case illustrates the goal of psychoanalysis, as Freud forcefully formulated it over half a century ago: "Where it was, there shall I come to be" (1933/1964, p. 80). That is, the realms of our experience in which we feel like passive sufferers and victims of forces beyond our ken and control ("it") must be claimed as integral aspects of ourselves ("I"), if we are to release ourselves from unnecessary suffering and take an active stance in relation to our lives. We accomplish this aim by attaching words to the unknown and by giving voice to the unspoken, the privately endured, the passively suffered. When words are given to the unspoken, then "events—external, impinging, foreign—are transformed into experience, that is, into things we are and do, and thus we can appropriate our own history" (May, 1987a, p. 5).

It is an essential aspect of psychotherapy that the alien aspects of the self be communicated to someone who is able to hear and respond to the underlying message of the repetitive symptomatology. The "compulsion to repeat" painful experiences, which is intrinsic to all undue emotional suffering (Freud, 1920/1955), is a determined attempt to gain active control over traumatic, passively endured events and relationships. In the form of automatic and unreflective habits of thought, feeling, and action, the compulsion to repeat lasts until someone hears the unrecognized and unspoken meaning of one's suffering, and responds to it in a way that does not perpetuate the need to suffer. Psychotherapists do not provide a corrective emotional experience per se, as Alexander and French (1946) claim; nor can they function as substitutes, stand-ins, or "better" mothers or fathers; nor can they, of course, alter the actuality (or often even the experience) of the past. Instead, they can effect intrapsychic or structural change. They can reverse the self-imposed, long-standing psychological thralldom (the narrowing of thought, freezing of feeling, or inhibition of action) that patients have endured because of chronic unresponsiveness to their needs and wishes. Parents' unresponsiveness is usually not malicious, but an indication of unmet narcissistic needs of their own. The children's project to make parents into something they were not and could never be is their own impossible narcissistic aim. The enslavement of their present life and happiness to this aim is counteracted by psychotherapy, which releases them from continuing preoccupation with past victimization and enables them to assume responsibility for their own ways of adapting to early experiences (Ducey, 1987). Once this freedom from bondage has taken place, the natural outcome is a broadening of thought, a deepening of feeling, a widening of the possibilities of action, and, in general, an expansion of the horizons of the self.

Hence, psychotherapists need not be concerned over the impossibility of altering the past. The preponderance of suffering is not necessary or inevitable; unacknowledged allegiance to unnecessary suffering results from the inveterate human proclivity to refashion the intrapsychic world to make the past not have happened. Such a project, far from accomplishing mastery over the past, allows the past to master oneself; thereby are the assumptions and demands from the past superimposed on the present and future. Freud's early psychotherapeutic intention of "transforming . . . hysterical misery into common unhappiness" (Breuer & Freud, 1895/1955, p. 305) could hardly be regarded as pessimistic, its mordant quality notwithstanding, particularly when he went on to assert that renewed psychological health will better arm the person against that unhappiness.

The merits of psychodynamic psychotherapy for addressing the academic problems of college students may be inferred from psychotherapy outcome research. Psychodynamic therapy (as compared with behavioral, cognitive, humanistic, developmental, and cognitive–behavioral approaches) was found consistently through meta-analysis of published studies to be the most powerful for enhancing work or school achievement (Smith, Glass, & Miller, 1980, p. 97). Brief psychodynamic psychotherapy (Gustafson, 1981; Malan, 1976a, 1976b, 1979) seems maximally suited to college psychotherapy, not only because of the predictable interruptions and built-in time constraints at college (May, 1987b), but also because intellectually active, curious, and highly motivated college students are ideal patients for brief insight-oriented psychotherapy (Hanfmann, 1978). In general, psychodynamic psychotherapy has been found in the outcome research studies of the highest quality (Beutler, 1979) to be appropriate for patients who have complex symptoms, employ internalizing modes of defense, and have an internal locus of control. Accordingly, students who are psychologically minded and whose academic difficulty has a psychodynamic or emotional etiology should benefit from this approach. Students who are not psychologically minded and who lack certain study skills or require further maturation are better candidates for the cognitive–didactic and group approaches.

CONCLUSION

Academic difficulties are sensitive indicators of students' general psychological well-being, and cannot be abstracted from the context of their level of development, adaptive style, psychodynamic conflicts, social functioning, family expectations, and situational demands. A clinically sophisticated assessment can aid the decision about the most appropriate approach to choose from the diverse array of responses available in college counseling or treatment centers.

Three types and numerous subtypes of interventions can be identified. Individual didactic and cognitive approaches, such as peer tutoring and study skills counseling, are particularly suited for students who have specific and remediable academic problems. Group interventions, such as issue-focused groups, workshops, and courses in study strategies, create an atmosphere of joint noncompetitive learning, mutual support, increased interpersonal self-confidence, promotion of maturation, and beneficial exchange of information; these approaches help students whose need for social interaction or didactic instruction is paramount. Individual psychological treatment—counseling or psychotherapy—is appropriate for the resolution of situational challenges or interactional or intrapsychic conflict. Appropriate interventions enable students to recover their passion for learning as well as for life's other rewards.

ACKNOWLEDGMENTS

I would like to express my appreciation to Abigail Lipson, Deborah Pilgrim, and M. Suzanne Repetto for their substantive and extensive contributions to this chapter; to Paul A. Grayson and Kate Cauley for their close and repeated readings and careful revision of the manuscript; and to Barbara A. Ducey for her depth of insight into the psychotherapeutic process, which continually influences my clinical thinking and practice.

REFERENCES

Alexander, F., & French, T. M. (1946). *Psychoanalytic therapy.* New York: Ronald Press.

Beutler, L. E. (1979). Toward specific psychological therapies for specific conditions. *Journal of Consulting and Clinical Psychology, 47,* 882–897.

Bibring, E. (1954). Psychoanalysis and the dynamic psychotherapies. *Journal of the American Psychoanalytic Association, 2,* 745–770.

Binstock, W. A. (1986). Clarification: Clinical application. In M. P. Nichols & T. J. Paolino (Eds.), *Basic techniques of psychodynamic psychotherapy: Foundations of clinical practice* (pp. 265–286). New York: Gardner Press.

Breuer, J., & Freud, S. (1955). Studies on hysteria. In J. Strachey (Ed. and Trans.), *The standard edition of the complete psychological works of Sigmund Freud* (Vol. 2, pp. 1–305). London: Hogarth Press. (Original work published 1895)

Ducey, C. P. (1986). Suggestion: History and theory. In M. P. Nichols & T. J. Paolino (Eds.), *Basic techniques of psychodynamic psychotherapy: Foundations of clinical practice* (pp. 21–55). New York: Gardner Press.

Ducey, C. P. (1987). Odipus am Scheideweg der Zivilisation [Oedipus at the crossroads of civilization]. In H.-P. Duerr (Ed.), *Die wilde Seele: Zur Ethnopsychoanalyse von Georges Devereux* (pp. 124–139) Frankfurt am Main: Suhrkamp Verlag.

Ekstein, R. (1966). *Children of time and space, of action and impulse.* New York: Appleton-Century-Crofts.

Freud, S. (1955). Beyond the pleasure principle. In J. Strachey (Ed. and Trans.), *The standard edition of the complete psychological works of Signmund Freud* (Vol. 18, pp. 7–64). London: Hogarth Press. (Original work published 1920)

Freud, S. (1957). "Wild psycho-analysis. In J. Strachey (Ed. and Trans.), *The standard edition of the complete psychological works of Sigmund Freud* (Vol. 11, pp. 221–227). London: Hogarth Press. (Original work published 1910)

Freud, S. (1964). New introductory lectures of psycho-analysis. In J. Strachey (Ed. and Trans.), *The standard edition of the complete psychological works of Sigmund Freud* (Vol. 22, pp. 5–182). London: Hogarth Press. (Original work published 1933)

Freud, S. (1964). Analysis terminable and interminable. In J. Strachey (Ed. and Trans.), *The standard edition of the complete psychological works of Sigmund Freud* (Vol. 23, pp. 216–253). London: Hogarth Press. (Original work published 1937)

Freud, S. (1964). An outline of psycho-analysis. In J. Strachey (Ed. and Trans.), *The standard edition of the complete psychological works of Sigmund Freud* (Vol. 23, pp. 144–207). London: Hogarth Press. (Original work published 1940)

Gustafson, J. P. (1981). The complex secret of brief psychotherapy in the works of Malan and Balint. In S. H. Budman (Ed.), *Forms of brief therapy* (pp. 83–128). New York: Guilford Press.

Hanfmann, E. (1978). *Effective therapy for college students.* San Francisco: Jossey-Bass.

Kernberg, O. (1986). *Severe personality disorders.* New Haven, CT: Yale University Press.

Kohut, H. (1977). *The restoration of the self.* New York: International Universities Press.

Malan, D. H. (1976a). *The frontier of brief psychotherapy.* New York: Plenum.

Malan, D. H. (1976b). *Toward the validation of dynamic psychotherapy.* New York: Plenum.

Malan, D. H. (1979). *Individual psychotherapy and the science of psychodynamics.* London: Butterworths.

Mangrum, C. T., & Strichart, S. S. (1984). *College and the learning disabled student.* New York: Grune & Stratton.

May, R. (1987a). Boundaries and voices in college psychotherapy. *Journal of College Student Psychotherapy, 1,* 3–28.

May, R. (1987b). The scope of college psychotherapy. In R. May (Ed.), *Psychoanalytic psychotherapy in a college context* (pp. 57–100). New York: Praeger.

McArthur, C. C. (1961). Distinguishing patterns of student neuroses. In G. B. Blaine & C. C. McArthur (Eds.), *Emotional problems of the student* (pp. 54–75). New York: Appleton-Century-Crofts.

Meador, B., & Rogers, C. (1984). Person-centered therapy. In R. J. Corsini (Ed.), *Current psychotherapies* (3rd ed., pp. 142–195). Itasca, IL: Peacock.

Perry, W. G. (1955). On the relation of psychotherapy to counseling. *Annals of the New York Academy of Sciences, 63,* 396–407.

Perry, W. G. (1959). The student's use and misuse of reading skills: A report to a faculty. *Harvard Educational Review, 29,* 193–200.

Perry, W. G. (1970). *Forms of intellectual and ethical development in the college years.* New York: Holt, Rinehart & Winston.

Schafer, R. (1970). The psychoanalytic vision of reality. *International Journal of Psycho-Analysis, 51,* 279–297.

Smith, M., Glass, G. V., & Miller, T. I. (1980). *The benefits of psychotherapy.* Baltimore: Johns Hopkins University Press.

10

Substance Abuse

PHILIP W. MEILMAN
MICHAEL S. GAYLOR

Substance abuse and substance dependency problems in young people exist in far greater numbers than is generally recognized. According to national statistics, approximately 13% of college-age males and 5% of females suffer from alcoholism, while another 10% of males and 6% of females in this age group suffer the effects of alcohol abuse without having moved into dependency (Williams, Stinson, Parker, Harford, & Noble, 1987). Given that individuals with abuse and dependency often experience significant life difficulties, and given that problematic chemical usage often presents as other forms of psychopathology, it would not be unreasonable to conclude that as many as 20–30% of cases seen at a college mental health facility may involve problematic use of alcohol or other drugs.

It is also likely that undiagnosed chemical use accounts for a significant percentage of cases where symptoms are not resolved in therapy. A case in point was the student couple who came in for marital counseling, complaining of continual "time management problems." Despite the best efforts of the therapist, no progress was forthcoming in treatment. A year after the treatment was terminated, the wife telephoned to ask for "biofeedback" for her husband. She felt that he needed stress management because he was using marijuana to handle the pressures of his academic work. Further telephone inquiry revealed that they both used marijuana daily, though her husband had expressly prohibited his wife from mentioning marijuana usage in the therapy a year before. It is little wonder that their "time management problems" were not resolved.

Clearly, a major issue in the psychotherapy of substance abuse is the clinician's ability to recognize the disorder. When it *is* recognized, it is then sometimes considered a symptom of or secondary to an underlying psychological problem, rather than a problem in its own right. Such a perspective may be learned during the therapist's training, where the topic is traditionally given scant attention compared to intrapsychic processes. As a result, the philosophy that emerges is that problematic chemical usage is a symptom that will cease when the underlying problem is resolved. Sometimes, of course, it *is* a symptom, but often it is the primary problem.

Even when the clinician is sensitive to substance abuse issues, there are further difficulties in diagnosing the problem. First, denial, minimization of problems, and rationalization all form a significant part of the clinical picture. Someone with an untrained ear can miss the import of such statements as "I only had a couple of beers," "I can take it or leave it," "I've gone for months at a time without drinking," or "I only drink on weekends." Second, even the seasoned professional may overlook the possible causative role of substance abuse in panic attacks, sleeping problems, depressive disorders, and psychotic symptoms because of its uncanny ability to masquerade as other psychiatric disorders.

When we speak of the "psychotherapy" of substance abuse, we are really talking about the *management* of such cases so that psychotherapeutic processes can take place. Although the therapy itself shares some elements in common with the treatment of other college mental health problems, the management of these cases is very different. It may require the use of leverage, which college therapists have traditionally been hesitant to use. Examples of leverage include raising the possibility of an involuntary medical withdrawal and thereby motivating an unwilling student to undertake treatment; making readmission to college after a medical withdrawal contingent upon inpatient rehabilitation; urging a dean to mandate a student's participation in an alcohol program; and conducting an alcohol "intervention," which is described later in this chapter.

Before turning to clinical issues, let us consider some of the important developmental functions that alcohol may serve in the college setting: (1) It facilitates an association with a peer group; (2) it allows students to try out new and different identities without a commitment to these momentary choices; (3) it provides a sense of belongingness at a time when students want to be connected, but may not know how to achieve this; (4) for better and for worse, it facilitates sexual experimentation; and (5) it allows a release of tensions resulting from academic pressures and developmental issues, including the separation from home.

In dealing with alcohol problems, we often ask students to moderate or give up their usage. In so doing, we should always keep in mind that we are asking students to be different from their peers and to give up some of the positive developmental aspects of alcohol use.

A CONTINUUM OF
SUBSTANCE USE PATTERNS

Let us describe a continuum of substance use practices, so that we can put abuse and dependence into a larger context. Alcohol is used here as a model, for two reasons. First, alcohol is the drug of choice at most colleges (Medical News and Perspectives, 1987). Second, alcohol is the drug about which we know the most. Once we have identified typical usage patterns found with alcohol, the reader can easily extrapolate these to other drugs.

At one end of the spectrum, we have abstinence; at the other end, we have chronic daily usage and late-stage alcoholism. In between these endpoints, there are patterns of "normal" drinking, alcohol incidents, and "problem" drinking, otherwise known as alcohol abuse.

Abstinence

Abstinence refers to complete nonuse of alcohol. Individuals choose to be abstinent for any number of reasons. Some people prefer other beverages and simply do not enjoy alcohol. Others want to be "in control" over their behavior and thinking, and feel that they lose control when they drink. Still others are the offspring of alcoholic parents and are frightened about the effects of alcohol. They feel instinctively or are intellectually aware that they are "at risk" for developing alcoholism (Goodwin, Schulsinger, Hermansen, Guze, & Winokur, 1973; Goodwin et al., 1974). Finally, an abstainer may have recognized that his or her previous usage was problematic or dependent in nature, and has chosen abstinence as a solution. In assessing a client, it is important that a clinician explore reasons for abstaining, as the reasons may prove to be of clinical significance. Approximately 30% of the general population does not drink, according to the National Institute of Alcohol Abuse and Alcoholism (NIAAA) (1980). However, the number of abstainers in the college setting is much lower (Wechsler & McFadden, 1979); a recent survey at an Ivy League college found that fewer than 4% of students were nondrinkers (Meilman & Gaylor, 1987).

"Normal" Drinking

"Normal" or "social" drinking is hard to define except by differentiating it from abusive drinking practices. Perhaps it should be called "non-problematic" drinking behavior. Here we see individuals who drink in moderation; whose behavior is appropriate; who avoid drinking as a way of coping with stressful situations; and who show none of the early warning signs of alcoholism, such as intoxication, blackouts, fights, accidents, and appearances on campus police reports. Published data from the NIAAA (1980) show that 50% of the adult population of the United States consumes only 20% of the alcohol, suggesting that most people's drinking falls into this category.

Alcohol Incidents

We can differentiate "alcohol incidents," or negative consequences arising from alcohol use, from "alcohol abuse" (problem drinking) in that alcohol abuse implies a degree of chronicity (American Psychiatric Association, 1987, p. 169). According to Kinney (1987), the descriptive term "alcohol incident" should be used when a pattern of negative consequences has not been established and the situation appears to be an isolated event. A single incident of driving while intoxicated or one blackout (a period of amnesia for a drinking episode) in an otherwise unremarkable history would be categorized as an alcohol incident. With repeated and multiple alcohol incidents, behavior is more accurately defined by one of the terms listed below. The destructive power of alcohol incidents should not be underestimated, however, as even a single episode of alcohol misuse can have devastating consequences.

Problem Drinking

The NIAAA statistics cited above also demonstrate that 20% of the American population consumes 80% of the alcohol. When the data are broken down even further, 7% of the population consumes 50% of the alcohol (NIAAA, 1980). These figures suggest that most, if not all, of the 20% who are heavy drinkers are drinking abusively.

Problem drinking entails a pattern of use with negative consequences and multiple incidents. Although all alcoholics abuse alcohol, not every abuser is an alcoholic. Careful assessment is needed to differentiate the two groups. Problem drinkers have not made the transition into dependency, and may or may not make that transition in time.

The revised third edition of the Diagnostic and Statistical Manual of Mental Disorders (DSM-III-R; American Psychiatric Association, 1987, p. 169) uses the diagnosis Psychoactive Substance Abuse as a residual category for drug and alcohol problems that do not meet the criteria for dependence. It is defined as a condition where an individual continues to use a substance despite knowledge that usage causes or contributes to problems, or where an individual uses the substance in situations that are physically dangerous (e.g., driving a car while intoxicated). Examples would include a college student who, on several occasions, has been taken to the emergency room for alcohol poisoning but who demonstrates no other symptoms, or a monthly user of cocaine whose only ill effect is missing a day of classes due to the withdrawal or "crash."

When students demonstrate certain substance use symptoms, repeatedly or in combination, they should be carefully evaluated to see whether their behavior qualifies as "abuse" or, even more seriously, "dependence." These symptoms include accidents and injuries, promiscuity, reckless driving, social isolation and withdrawal, academic problems, missed classes, memory problems, hoarding of drugs, and preoccupation with use. Other symptoms include using up a drug or alcohol supply in one sitting, working to assure a steady supply, spending substantial amounts of money on substances, using them to feel confident in social situations or to relieve anxiety, being unable to predict behavior when using, having family members or friends express concern about one's use, having fights and arguments, and experiencing a loss of self-respect (Dartmouth College Health Services, 1987). These symptoms are "red flags" indicating abuse at the very least, and possibly dependence.

Alcoholism

Most of us have a personal definition of alcoholism. Some people would describe alcoholics as persons who cannot hold a job. Others describe skid row derelicts. Some say that alcoholics drink every day. Tellingly, people with undiagnosed alcohol problems often carefully construct their definitions so as to exclude their own behavior. For example, a student who says, "Alcoholics are people who drink in the morning," probably has limited his alcoholic drinking to afternoons and evenings. Another student may say, "Alcoholics are people who can't control their drinking," because she has stopped her alcoholic drinking for a 3-month period. This exclusionary reasoning is part of the process of denial. Because of denial, students with alcholism do not readily come forth and ask for help. Therefore, clinicians must carefully assess students to see whether they fit objective diagnostic criteria.

The hallmark of alcoholism is "loss of control." This refers to loss of control over the amount of alcohol consumed, as well as loss of control over behavior. "Loss of control" does not mean that the alcoholic experiences this reaction every time. He or she could drink on 10 different occasions and function well on 9 of them. If, however, on 1 occasion out of every 10 there is a loss of control over the quantity of alcohol consumed as well as over behavior (e.g., leading to property damage and a visit to the local emergency room for treatment of injuries or alcohol poisoning), then alcoholism is probably indicated.

In the process of assessment, it is important to consider a complicating factor with college students. In an older adult population, an individual who has a fight when drinking, experiences a blackout, or throws up can be said to be out of control. This conclusion is clear-cut because the demand characteristics of adult living require holding a job, meeting family obligations, paying a mortgage, and similar responsibilities. However, the demand characteristics surrounding college drinking often exert pressure for students to *be* out of control. In college, there are few responsibilities, usually no children to be parented, no mortgages, and often no pressing academic obligations, while at the same time there is peer pressure to drink to excess. It has been estimated, for example, that 33% of college students have experienced a blackout, a clear form of loss of control. Yet one-third of the college population is not alcoholic. Thus, problematic behavior may represent alcoholic loss of control, or may be, in the eyes of peers, an expected and even desirable state of being. The differing demand characteristics in the college setting and in the working world can affect drinking behavior and make a difference in the diagnosis.

The terms "addiction," "alcoholism," and "drug dependence" all describe a relationship with a substance in which the chemical is becoming the centerpiece of a person's life. Although he or she may not know it yet, the student cannot function comfortably without it. The relationship with the drug is strong, and for some it may be the most significant relationship they have. A case in point was a female graduate student, who, when her defenses were down, said with great affect to her therapist, "Pot loves me." The therapist made the interpretation that marijuana was always there for her, always with a predictable soothing effect, in contrast to her abusive father, her manipulative mother, and her stormy marriage.

It is this relationship that we are describing when we talk about addiction. In the beginning, usage is generally recreational in nature and is experienced as pleasurable. With continued use, a dependency may develop that is at first psychological. As the nervous system adapts to having quantities of the drug in the system, the addiction also becomes physical. There may be both physical and psychological signs of alcoholism (Skinner, Holt, Schuller, Roy, & Israel, 1984), but the diagnosis can be most readily made by observing a patient's behavior. DSM-III-R (American Psychiatric Association, 1987, pp. 166–168) contains a carefully delineated set of criteria for making a diagnosis of Substance Dependency, and is far superior to previously published guidelines. When three of the following symptoms have existed for at least a month, or have occurred on a repeated basis over a longer period of time, the diagnosis can be made: (1) The substance is used more than the individual intended; (2) the person struggles to maintain control of usage; (3) much time is spent in obtaining, using, or recovering from a substance; (4) there is frequent intoxication or withdrawal, or physically hazardous use (e.g., while driving); (5) use has an impact on work or lifestyle; (6) use continues despite the knowledge that it causes problems; (7) significant tolerance to the substance has developed; (8) withdrawal syndromes occur when initially attempting abstinence (except possibly with marijuana, hallucinogens, or phencyclidine [PCP]); and (9) alcohol or other drugs are used to ward off withdrawal symptoms.

Much has been written about alcoholism as a disease. Whereas some believe that alcoholism is related to habit, social demand characteristics, and public policy (Dreger, 1986), others consider its physiological basis (Royce, 1985). Some view the condition as chronic, progressive, and lethal, maintaining that the construct "disease" is an appropriate model for describing these characteristics (e.g., Johnson, 1980). Others feel that the word "disease" is appropriate for some types of alcoholism but not others; the latter are more reflective of cultural norms concerning alcohol use (e.g., Jellinek, 1960).

The vast majority of substance abuse professionals subscribe to the disease model. The disease model is clinically useful because it can facilitate a movement into treatment by removing obstacles—notably the stigma of "weakness," as well as the blame, guilt, and self-hatred that many alcoholics feel. To say to someone, "You need treatment for your disease," is far more palatable than saying, "You are an alcoholic and need to straighten out your life." The disease concept also gives the family, which is often profoundly affected, a structure with which to understand the condition. The family is then often able to respond with compassion, firm limits, and some degree of detachment, which might not be possible otherwise. Finally, the disease concept makes addicts' continuing difficulties with willpower more understandable to themselves and others.

No matter which model is used, three points are clear. One is that, left untreated, the vast majority of alcoholics will die prematurely (Johnson, 1980, p. 1), whether through cirrhosis of the liver, suicide, automobile wrecks, assaults, or accidents arising out of poor judgment. Second, dependency on one mood-altering drug implies dependency on other mood-altering drugs. Alcoholics generally cannot use sedatives, hypnotics, narcotics, tranquilizers, stimulants, or hallucinogens without risking major life problems and a perpetuation of an active addiction. Third, active drinking tends to block any progress that alcoholics try to make in other areas of their lives. This has serious implications for therapy and is addressed later in this chapter.

Before turning to referral, assessment, and treatment, we should note two important concepts that are described later in detail: "denial" and "impairment." Denial is the inability to recognize difficulties that substances cause; impairment refers to the cognitive deficits, health problems, and behavioral difficulties that result. Just as substance use falls on a continuum, so do denial and impairment. The degree to which they are present affects decisions throughout the referral, assessment, and treatment process. Since much of the impairment that substance abusers experience is physiologically based (e.g., memory loss, impaired judgment) rather than psychologically based, clinical work with these students requires a somewhat more directive approach than that found in traditional psychotherapy.

REFERRAL

Students with substance abuse problems can come to the attention of campus mental health workers in a variety of ways. Most directly, the student can be self-referred. An example is the young woman who presented herself after being shocked to discover a male student in her bed the morning after an alcohol-induced blackout. Another student came in after reading a campus brochure about drugs. Fearful that he might be cocaine-dependent, he was in fact in serious need of help.

"Friendly" Referrals

Sometimes peers become concerned about problematic chemical usage in one of their classmates. Likewise, resident assistants often consult about students in the dormitories. Peers and resident assistants are perceived as "friends" who do not carry the weight and threat of higher authority figures. Sometimes deans, faculty, administrators, coaches, and support staff also make "friendly" referrals to the counseling center that carry no requirement of a follow-through.

Occasionally, referrals come from parents. There is no set way to handle such referrals, but it is often helpful to have an initial meeting with both the student and the parents to obtain a complete picture of the problem. This meeting also minimizes the possibility that the clinician will be placed in the uncomfortable role of intermediary if the student and the parents disagree about the problem or even its existence.

A referral may also come from the physicians at the campus health service. In our own setting, we follow up on all cases admitted to the infirmary for alcohol- and drug-related medical problems. One of the more interesting cases was that of a student hospitalized in the infirmary for complaints of fatigue, anxiety, depression, dizziness, and profuse sweating. The student, a varsity football player, was fearful that he either had a brain tumor or was "going crazy." A neurological examination and all other medical tests proved negative. However, the student gave a history of daily heavy drinking for the previous 6 months, which he had discontinued 36 hours prior to the infirmary admission. This student was experiencing an alcohol withdrawal syndrome. He was reassured about his symptoms, enrolled in an alcohol education program, and provided with individual counseling.

In-House Referrals/Assessments

As noted at the outset, 20–30% of all cases coming to a college counseling center may involve problematic use of alcohol and other drugs. Given this percentage, it is reasonable to screen all incoming cases for substance abuse (Kinney & Meilman, 1987). However, there are some students already in therapy in the college counseling center who should be carefully evaluated. These include students with panic attacks, sleeping problems, eating disorders, chronic pain, and psychotic symptoms. It is not uncommon for students with panic attacks to self-medicate with alcohol. Although liquor may help at first, tolerance develops in time, and then the anxiety re-emerges. To compensate, the student increases usage and eventually is caught in an addictive, leapfrogging usage pattern. A case in point was the graduate student who said that sipping beer helped him manage his anxiety and panic attacks. Further inquiry revealed that he had been "sipping" a dozen 12-ounce beers nightly for a year and a half. When he stopped drinking, he went into a withdrawal syndrome manifested by profuse sweating and mood swings. Significantly, his panic attacks subsided approximately 3 weeks after he stopped drinking, and they did not return during the 6-month follow-up period.

Students who present with sleep disorders should also be evaluated for their consumption of medications and alcohol, since both may be used as sleep aids. Likewise, students with eating disorders should be carefully evaluated, since these diagnoses appear to have characteristics in common with substance abuse disorders, and they often go hand in hand (Brisman & Siegel, 1984; Jones, Cheshire, & Moorhouse, 1985). Even if they are not alcohol-dependent, bulimics who abuse alcohol will find it difficult, if not impossible, to make headway in psychotherapy. Students with chronic pain syndromes should be evaluated, as these patients are frequently addicted to prescription drugs such as tranquilizers, sleeping pills, and narcotic analgesics (Davis, 1984). Finally, students with thought disorders should be carefully assessed, as some self-medicate with alcohol, whereas others may have actually precipitated or may perpetuate their psychotic symptoms by using hallucinogens.

Mandatory Referrals

Mandatory deans' referrals are often appropriate. At our own institution, there is a policy that after an alcohol-related incident appears on a campus police report, a dean can ask the student to be evaluated or to face disciplinary charges. In fact, students always choose to be evaluated. A release is then signed, and after the evaluation, recommendations are made to the student and the dean as to the need for further treatment. The dean can then choose to mandate the recommendations or not. In actuality, the dean's choice will largely depend on information the clinician provides.

This policy applies to relatively minor behavioral infractions, such as public intoxication and reports that a student was transported by campus police to the emergency room because of an alcohol overdose. With serious breaches of campus conduct codes that require disciplinary action, sometimes students are also required to undergo assessment and treatment. Examples of serious infractions include a student, who, on a drunken rampage, ransacked a dining hall, and another student who totally demolished his own car as well as a parked car while driving down fraternity row under the influence of alcohol.

There is a myth that people with alcohol and drug problems have to *want* to get help in order to get better. This is clearly untrue. Forcing the issue sometimes leads to proper evaluation and treatment. During the treatment process, students are confronted with their own behavior, often come to realize their difficulties with chemical substances, and develop motivation to deal with the problem. Left to their own devices, many students will never deal with their difficulties, and others will only recognize them after years of pain. Forcing the issue may also save a life, as we are dealing with a potentially lethal condition (NIAAA, 1986; West, 1984). A most moving acknowledgment of this occurred with a young man who previously had purchased heroin and cocaine from unsavory characters on the Lower East Side of New York City. At the termination of therapy, the patient shook the therapist's hand and said, "I'm sure I would be dead or killed by now if you hadn't forced me to deal with my problems. You saved my life."

ASSESSMENT

The initial therapeutic task is establishing a correct diagnosis. With substance use practices, this essentially means determing whether the individual (1) has no substance abuse problem, (2) has experienced an alcohol or drug "incident" only, (3) is a problem drinker or user, or (4) has moved into actual chemical dependency. Establishing a diagnosis is important because treatment depends upon the diagnosis. For example, drinking in moderation may be an acceptable goal for dealing with problem drinking but not for alcoholism, which requires a different approach.

Sometimes the diagnostic process is easy; at other times, it is difficult and the end picture is unclear. This can happen because the student expresses an unconscious denial of substance abuse problems and literally has no awareness of his or her difficulty. At other times, a student's outward denial may reflect attempts to lessen the pain and embarassment of being discovered. At still other times, the data may not be clear enough to establish a firm diagnosis.

When diagnosis is difficult, we employ "rule out" diagnoses (e.g., the diagnosis "psychoactive substance abuse, rule out psychoactive substance dependence") until more information is available, or we make referrals for second opinions. Another possibility is to monitor the student's problems over a period of months or even years. Finally, one can ask to meet with family and friends to collect more data, since significant others can often provide a clearer picture than the student.

There are a variety of individual interview techniques and screening instruments that assist in making a diagnosis of substance abuse problems. Essentially, these methods look for markers such as negative consequences of substance use, expressed concern by self or others, and evidence of physical dependence. The degree to which these markers are present determines the location, or diagnosis, on the continuum of substance use practices described earlier. The techniques ask about markers rather than about substance abuse itself, because most individuals deny chemical problems. Thus, questions such as "Has anyone ever complained to you about your behavior when you were drinking?" are more useful than "How do you act when you drink too much?"

In answer to the first question, students might laugh and respond that their friends have said they are loud and obnoxious, but in response to the second, they would be more likely to say that their behavior when drinking is "no problem." The important marker here is the effect on the environment, as described by others.

Screening Techniques

There are numerous instruments designed to assess substance use problems. Three of the most commonly used tests are the CAGE, the Michigan Alcohol Screening Test (MAST), and the Trauma Scale.

A set of four questions known by the acronym "CAGE" (Ewing, 1984; Mayfield, McLeod, & Hall, 1974) looks at some behavioral, external markers of alcohol abuse. The four questions are carefully worded to elicit information about those markers:

- Have you felt you should   *Cut down* on your drinking?
- Have people   *Annoyed* you by criticizing your drinking?

- Have you ever felt bad or   *Guilty* about your drinking?
- Have you ever had a drink first thing in the morning to steady nerves or get rid of a hangover?   (*Eye-opener*)

The usefulness of the CAGE is twofold: First, it provides a short semistructured interview that yields significant data. Each of the questions can be followed up regarding times, places, events, and experiences. Second, the CAGE is scorable. Two or three positive answers create a high index of suspicion of alcohol problems. Four positive answers are considered pathognomonic of alcoholism.

Another well-known screening instrument is the MAST (Selzer, 1971). The MAST consists of 25 items that are answered "yes" or "no." The questions can be put in the form of pencil-and-paper test that takes no more than 3–5 minutes to administer, or the questions can be asked as part of a clinical interview. Based on the MAST score, a subject can be placed into one of three groups: (1) nonalcoholic, (2) suspect, or (3) alcoholic drinker.

The Trauma Scale is another useful instrument. Recognizing that physical trauma frequently accompanies alcoholism, Skinner et al. (1984) developed a five-question test that is sensitive to problem drinking. The questions are as follows:

Since your 18th birthday, have you . . .
(1) had any fractures, or dislocations of bones or joints?
(2) been injured in a traffic accident?
(3) had a head injury?
(4) been injured in an assault or fight?
(5) been injured after drinking? (p. 848)

A positive answer to two or more questions should alert the clinician to the likely presence of alcohol abuse or excessive drinking.

Interview Techniques

As noted by Weinberg (1974), assessing substance abuse by interview is a fine art. Weinberg focuses on alcohol abuse, but the suggestions he makes can easily be applied to abuse of other substances. He recommends introducing the subject in a straightforward manner by asking, "Now I'd like to learn a bit about your use of alcohol and other drugs. Do you drink at all?" Because alcohol problems are manifested in one or more areas of a person's life, the clinician should then cover a series of major topics, including the impact of substance use on family relationships, marriage and/or significant friendships, social life, legal problems, physical health, self-esteem, and occupational functioning. In the case of college students, occupational functioning includes academic work, campus employment, and summer employment. In addition, the clinician should seek to determine the role of alcohol in recreational activities, and should look for the possible development of tolerance and withdrawal phenomena.

In doing all of this, the clinician should make use of highly specific, factual questions that are difficult to answer evasively. For example, Weinberg suggests following up the question, "Have any of your relatives suggested it might be better if you drank less or quit?" with the inquiry, "What exactly don't they like about your behavior when you drink?"

At this point, the clinician needs to look for denial in the form of evasiveness, minimization, or rationalization. Active alcoholics usually have a well-developed denial system that protects them from acknowledging an alcohol problem. For example, in response to the question, "Has anyone ever said that drinking might be causing a problem for you?", the nonalcoholic will respond with a straightforward "no." The alcoholic, however, denies by saying, "I can quit any time I want to—I can handle it myself." In response to the question, "Have you ever had to consider cutting down on your drinking?", the nonalcoholic replies, "No, except when I'm trying to lose weight," but the alcoholic will say, "There's no problem for me—I can take it or leave it" (Weinberg, 1974).

It is possible to hear denial in such statements as "I only drink on weekends," "I only drink at social events," or "I never drink alone." Such statements indicate that on some level the individual experiences concern about drinking and accordingly has begun to make rules about it. Normal drinkers do not make rules; they simply choose to drink or not to drink on any given occasion, based on what is appropriate at the time.

Statements that appear to minimize drinking as an issue are also suspect—for example, "I've quit for months at a time," "I don't drink half as much as my friends do," and "I only had a couple of beers." Likewise, evasive and qualified answers are suspect (e.g., "not as a rule," "practically never," "not really," "nothing worth mentioning," "probably not," "no more than anyone else," and "nothing recently"). It is a good idea to plan out in advance one's responses to these qualified denials. For example, if the student says, "I wouldn't say so," the clinician can ask, "Who *would* say so?" Or if the student says, "I don't know," the clinician can ask, "*What* don't you know?" or "Who *would* know?" To "practically never," the clinician can ask, "When *does* it happen?"

Attempts to persuade the interviewer that there is not a problem, alibis and rationalizations, and hostility directed toward the interviewer are other telling signs. For example, a student rationalized his father's concern about his drinking alone at home in the kitchen at 5:00 A.M. by saying that he was drinking in order to help himself fall asleep. One student was so skilled at rationalization, denial, and minimization that the psychologist who interviewed him had two distinct impressions: first, that the student was definitely alcoholic, and second, that there was not a single shred of hard data on which to base the diagnosis! In order to make sure that he was not imagining the diagnosis, the psychologist secured a second opinion that confirmed his first impression.

Second opinions are one way to determine a diagnosis when the clinical picture is not clear. Another possibility is to interview roommates, friends, lovers, spouses, and/or parents. In some cases these interviews may be the best sources of information. Normally, college mental health professionals go to great lengths to keep the therapeutic relationship individual and private. In substance abuse cases, however, outside information is often necessary in order for evaluation and treatment to be clinically effective. The clinician needs to exercise careful judgment so as to protect confidentiality while at the same time obtaining needed information. Sometimes this can be done with a signed release. At other times, deans, parents, and friends of students will voluntarily come forth with information. As such, there is no violation of confidentiality.

Of course, not all individual interviews are filled with denial, rationalization, and evasiveness. Some are straightforward and make a diagnosis possible even after one interview. Getting the student to accept a diagnosis is usually the next step.

ACCEPTING THE DIAGNOSIS

Some students readily accept the diagnosis or even know beforehand where they fall diagnostically. They are then ready for therapy. For other students, it is not even necessary to present a diagnosis. The clinician can simply talk about the students' misuse of drugs or alcohol and then make the transition into treatment.

For still other students, it may be helpful to describe in detail the continuum presented earlier, including the DSM-III-R criteria for Psychoactive Substance Abuse and Substance Dependency. In describing points along the continuum, it is useful to avoid the emotionally charged words "alcoholic" and "addict"; students who might be willing to consider themselves "alcohol-dependent" are often unwilling to accept the label "alcoholic." With respect to alcoholism, it is perhaps best to describe the characteristics of the disorder and ask students whether or not the description fits, rather than focusing on the label.

Once this is done, the student and the clinician can state their individual judgments as to where on the continuum the student falls. If there is agreement, the student can move directly to therapy. If there is disagreement, almost always the student places himself or herself closer to the "normal drinking" region of the continuum than does the clinician. Usually, the student's unrealistic assessment is due to denial. One student, for example, drank approximately 15 drinks per day, had been in trouble with the dean's office because of alcohol abuse, had had numerous blackouts, and had also been arrested several times on drunk driving charges, yet insisted he was a normal drinker. His response was this: "Your CAGE and your MAST and your fancy statistics don't mean a thing. I know where I am with drinking, and I don't have the problem you think I have."

This response is helpful diagnostically, though not therapeutically. Such a student's denial system is far too intact for him or her to see the problem realistically. At this point, the clinician can provide education through readings, discussion, and audiovisual media; he or she can refer the student for a second opinion, hoping that there will be strength in numbers or in a different approach; or the clinician can refer the student to an alcohol education program, either voluntarily or by means of leverage. If a second opinion has been requested and obtained, the clinician can then meet with the student and the consultant to allow for follow-up and continuity of care. Recommendations can then be made and presented to the student.

Some universities have intensive alcohol education programs on their campuses, and these can be utilized to help break through denial. Where such formal programs are not available, a clinician can make use of the many films and books about substance abuse that are commercially available (see, e.g., Hazelden Foundation, 1987), in addition to ongoing individual discussions.

If a student still does not accept the diagnosis, any number of routes can be taken. The clinician can choose to let the situation go, or he or she can opt to monitor the student through outside sources (e.g., other students or the dean's office) and make contact if and when it is useful. Before letting the student go, the clinician can plant some seeds by asking the student to specify how bad things would have to become in order for him or her to say there was a problem and be willing to seek help.

Alternatively, students who cannot accept a diagnosis may be willing to self-monitor their behavior in regard to drugs and alcohol and come in if they feel the need. In other cases, students may agree to come in periodically to check in and review their usage patterns. If this option is chosen, usually reminders (nudges, really) are needed from the clinician. Yet another possibility usually reserved for dependent students is to offer them a novel experiment. This entails their setting a limit on drinking or drug use and seeing whether they can actually stay within that limit over a period of months. Violations of the limit are defined as indications of loss of control and therefore as dependency indicators.

There are many variations on this experiment, such as having students drink their self-imposed limits every day for 3 weeks, never any more and never any less. Conducting the experiment this way "collapses" the monitored time period required, because it is difficult for an alcohol-dependent individual to maintain control when drinking a set daily amount. The student is informed that abstaining or drinking less than the limit invalidates the experiment, and it has to be attempted again.

Usually students who are drug- or alcohol-dependent will fail the experiment, and thus it is helpful in demonstrating loss of control. In the unlikely event that the student does control usage during the experiment, the clinician should point out that this does not rule out dependency and that ongoing monitoring should continue.

In choosing any of the options described above, the clinician should keep in mind four general principles: (1) Take the student as far as it is reasonably possible to go without harassment; (2) voluntary participation is generally better than involuntary participation; and (3) more is better than less when it comes to interactions with the student. Finally, (4) remember that it is not absolutely necessary that a student accept a diagnosis, especially when there are other issues that need to be addressed.

Even if a student cannot accept a diagnosis, every discussion or confrontation concerning alcohol and drug issues heightens the discomfort that a substance abuser feels. The discomfort may not be immediately apparent, but the effect is cumulative. Although any one interaction may not produce the desired result, many interactions may help the abuser to realize the problem a month, a year, or even 10 years later.

FORMAL "INTERVENTION"

As described by the Johnson Institute, the term "intervention" is a method of moving a patient directly into treatment, bypassing the process just outlined (Johnson, 1980, pp. 48–61). The formal alcohol intervention is a meeting involving family, friends, employers, and other concerned individuals who confront the addicted individual and ask him or her to enter treatment immediately. It is a last-resort technique for situations where the individual needs inpatient treatment but denies the problem and has refused previous requests to seek help. In our own setting, we conduct approximately three interventions per year.

During an intervention, the therapist or designated speaker will state that everyone deeply cares for the student and therefore must talk about what is happening because of alcohol and/or drugs. This is followed by a recitation of observed drug- or alcohol-affected behavior that is given in the form of facts rather than opinions. It is nonjudgmental in tone. Each speaker indicates that he or she wants the patient to get help immediately and describes the natural consequences, if any, that will occur if the situation does not change. For example, a lover may need to end a relationship, or parents may feel that they are unwilling to pay further college tuition if the student continues abusing substances.

If the intervention has been carefully executed, the patient may well accept the recommendation for immediate help. This means that the clinician must have made arrangements, in advance, for a bed in a residential treatment facility. If the patient refuses to enter treatment, then that student can be asked what he or she *would* be willing to do. Sometimes the patient will volunteer to attend Alcoholics Anonymous (AA) or Narcotics Anonymous (NA), or may say that he or she will quit on his own. This is acceptable, provided that the student agrees to go into residential treatment immediately if abstinence is not maintained. It should be noted that those present at the intervention will hold the student to that agreement.

Because emotions run high during an intervention, it is recommended that there be professional staff members present to confront hostility and manage other problematic moments. It is also recommended that professional staff members do "apprenticeships" with experienced intervention leaders before offering this kind of service to students.

Sometimes an intervention fails in its goal of moving a person into treatment. However, it should be remembered that any confrontation will make the patient increasingly uncomfortable about his or her chemical use, so that the cumulative effect of others' complaints, over time, may ultimately lead to an acceptance of help. In this sense, the intervention has not failed.

TREATMENT

There are a variety of treatment options available for students. These include educational approaches; AA, NA, or similar group experiences; outpatient psychotherapy; and inpatient treatment. Proper management involves tailoring the particular treatment to the particular problem for the individual student.

In cases of alcohol and drug incidents, educational approaches, including discussions about dosage (e.g., blood alcohol levels) and drug effects, may be utilized. Students should be encouraged to evaluate their usage in accordance with their new understanding. If necessary, the clinician can help students to evaluate their usage over time.

Education and monitoring, with the goal of moderation or elimination of use, are clearly appropriate for substance abuse. The clinician should understand that even moderation of usage represents a herculean effort, as it means changing a college lifestyle, friendship networks, and recreational activities. A self-monitoring program by means of a daily drinking (or drug) diary often helps the student and the clinician identify usage patterns and high-risk situations. Ideally, the educational and behavioral approaches described here are supplemented with individual psychotherapy to look at issues that relate to drug and alcohol misuse. In therapy, the student should be told that unchecked substance abuse will block progress on other issues. It is also important to discuss not only the present difficulties relating to alcohol and drugs, but also the student's "at-risk" status for developing a chemical dependency problem. In order to help the student learn more about substance dependence, attendance at meetings of AA or NA can be recommended, although it should be recognized that the student may not comply because of initial fear or embarrassment.

In some substance abuse cases, a prescription can be made for a temporary, immediate halt in usage, and the student will accept this recommendation. In a recent case, a student who was in serious academic trouble was given such a recommendation as an "experiment." Two weeks later, he reported that his friends found him easier to handle and that he had not binged on alcohol when upset, as he had in the past. This gave him 2 extra days for studying that would have been lost to intoxication and recovery from intoxication. This experiment turned out to be a major learning experience for the student and was a good starting place for his therapy.

Substance dependence is more difficult to handle. If at all possible, treatment should include weekly outpatient psychotherapy and AA or NA attendance. There are two goals of treatment: the maintenance of sobriety, and the effective handling of troublesome issues and emotions. Although a few behavioral psychologists have taken the position that it is possible to teach some alcoholics to drink socially and responsibly (e.g., Marlatt, 1983), the consensus is that controlled drinking is realistically possible only for alcohol abusers who have relatively few drinking problems and who are not alcohol-dependent ("Treatment of Alcoholism—Part II," 1987).

In therapy with chemically dependent students, it is critical to deal with a number of issues. The first issue consists of the obstacles to sobriety, which must be identified, understood, and overcome. "Slips" or relapses into substance use are likely to be frequent in the initial stages of treatment. These are best labeled as learning experiences, so that patients can begin to explore in therapy the situations and emotions that make them vulnerable to use. This process can be expected to take a period of months.

As patients begin to achieve lengthier periods of abstinence, new and often troubling emotions will emerge. The reason for this is simple. For years, these individuals have been anesthetizing their feelings; drugs and alcohol have been used to drown sorrows, to celebrate joyous events, and to have fun. Real emotions, real feelings, rarely have been experienced. Now that the chemicals are gone, the feelings reemerge, which is confusing and sometimes frightening. In discussing this phenomenon, a chemically dependent person explained that when he initially became sober, he once experienced an uncomfortable feeling and found himself searching through his now cleaned-out medicine cabinet for something to take. As he did that, he made a remarkable discovery about the source of his discomfort: His bladder was full! Up to that point, he had been so unaware of his feelings and bodily sensations that he literally could not differentiate among needing to urinate, having a headache, or feeling depressed.

In addition to rediscovering emotions and sensations, newly recovering individuals also experience "flare-ups," or periods of intense irritability, tension, or depression for no apparent reason. For example, a patient may report a short-lived episode of intense depression that has no precipitating cause and that is uncharacteristic. The therapist needs to explain such experiences as part of the process of recovery and as indications that the patient is actually getting better, not worse. Of course, mood swings will also occur for actual situational or environmental reasons. It is important to differentiate these latter experiences from "flare-ups," which are thought to be more physiologically based (Weinberg, 1975).

Next, there may be intense anxiety. Having begun to come face to face with the bankruptcy of their old ways, patients may feel ashamed and guilty about past deeds. Beyond this, they are struggling to figure out new ways to handle old problems, which were previously handled by drinking or taking drugs. They have few if any sober experiences to use as reference points; figuratively speaking, it is as though they are learning to walk for the first time. An axiom of therapy with chemically dependent people is that their development stopped when they began to use drugs and alcohol. It is not unusual to be conducting therapy with a 35-year-old graduate student, for example, and find oneself helping that person deal with early adolescent or even preadolescent developmental issues. Sometimes at this point in therapy, the simplest and most common sensical therapeutic suggestions appear as great revelations to the patient; these are often the reference points that the student is missing within his or her own experience.

This therapeutic work presupposes that students' anxiety levels are within manageable limits; that their behavior is largely under control; and that, for the most part, sobriety is possible. When this is not the case, inpatient treatment should be considered. For example, a chemically dependent student in crisis about maintaining sobriety was initially comforted by her stay in the college infirmary. However, as days went by, her anxiety level became higher rather than lower. Her therapist therefore recommended that she enter an inpatient, 4-week rehabilitation program. Afterward, when she returned from this treatment, she was improved and her anxiety level was reduced to the point at which therapy was possible on an outpatient basis.

Students who return to campus from inpatient treatment will have significant aftercare needs. These include the need for individual therapy as well as group support. Here is another way in which AA or NA attendance can be especially helpful. Ordinarily, the newly recovering student has such significant and overwhelming needs for support that the therapist cannot possibly meet them all. The student's contact with the AA or NA network spreads out these needs over a large number of people, so that no one person or therapist is overwhelmed. At the same time, the student is likely to meet one or more kindred spirits with whom contact will be especially meaningful and helpful.

AA is essentially a support group for people trying to maintain sobriety. Based on a 12-step format, the program helps individuals overcome denial, acknowledge the destructive power of alcohol, and rebuild their lives. Meetings are available in most localities 365 days a year. If a student-oriented AA meeting exists on campus or can be established, this is especially useful. It is also helpful for the clinician to network with the "key players" among the student AA group in order to have contacts for other interested students.

The student's AA attendance can be invaluable to the clinician in helping students address certain issues. For example, it is useful to ask, "What do the people in AA say?" in response to questions such as "Is it okay to get sexually involved with someone now?", and "How do I calculate my length of sobriety if I slipped this week, but otherwise haven't drunk for 3 months?" Since AA members are full of witty and insightful answers, the therapist should not feel compelled to respond to all of the complicated questions that recovering students ask. Deferring to AA wisdom also helps integrate AA with the student's therapy.

Throughout this discussion, the term "recovering" has been used in place of "recovered." This reflects our belief that recovery from chemical dependency is an ongoing process and that relapse is possible at any time. Recovery takes a long time: The first 3 months of sobriety are almost always problematic, and patients' adjustments are usually shaky for the first 6 months. It generally takes 1 or 2 years of counseling and group support for recovering students to get their bearings and achieve a more comfortable sobriety. Even so, problematic issues will continue to surface over even longer periods of time.

Because recovery is ongoing, therapy should be terminated with an "open door," so that the student can return if the need arises. Before terminating therapy, however, the therapist should discuss the dangers of mood-altering drugs other than those previously used, including sedatives, hypnotics, tranquilizers, stimulants, narcotic analgesics, bowel preparations, and antihistamines, as well as illegal drugs and alcohol.

Readings on this topic and resources for answering specific questions should be presented to the student before termination.

ACKNOWLEDGMENT

We wish to express our appreciation to Jean Kinney, MSW, Executive Director of the Project Cork Institute, Dartmouth Medical School, for her review and critique of this chapter.

REFERENCES

American Psychiatric Association. (1987). *Diagnostic and statistical manual of mental disorders* (3rd ed., rev.). Washington, DC: Author.

Brisman, J., & Siegel, M. (1984). Bulimia and alcoholism: Two sides of the same coin? *Journal of Substance Abuse Treatment, 1,* 113–118.

Dartmouth College Health Services. (1987). *Drugs.* Hanover, NH: Author.

Davis, J. C. (1984). Analgesic and psychoactive drugs in the chronic pain patient. *Journal of Orthopaedic and Sports Physical Therapy, 5,* 315–317.

Dreger, R. M. (1986). Does anyone really believe alcoholism is a disease? *American Psychologist, 41,* 322.

Ewing, J. A. (1984). Detecting alcoholism: The CAGE questionnaire. *Journal of the American Medical Association, 252,* 1905–1907.

Goodwin, D. W., Schulsinger, F., Hermansen, L., Guze, S. B., & Winokur, G. (1973). Alcohol problems in adoptees raised apart from alcoholic biological parents. *Archives of General Psychiatry, 28,* 238–243.

Goodwin, D. W., Schulsinger, F., Moller, N., Hermansen, L., Winokur, G., & Guze, S. B. (1974). Drinking problems in adopted and non-adopted sons of alcoholics. *Archives of General Psychiatry, 31,* 164–169.

Hazelden Foundation. (1987). *Educational materials 1987.* Center City, MN: Author.

Jellinek, E. M. (1960). *The disease concept of alcoholism.* New Haven, CT: Hillhouse.

Jones, D. A., Cheshire, N., & Moorhouse, H. (1985). Anorexia nervosa, bulimia, and alcoholism—association of eating disorder and alcohol. *Journal of Psychiatric Research, 19,* 377–380.

Johnson, V. E. (1980). *I'll quit tomorrow.* New York: Harper & Row.

Kinney, J. (1987). *Alcohol use and alcohol problems: Slide Unit 8.* [Slide presentation]. Timonium, MD: Milner-Fenwick, Section A.

Kinney, J., & Meilman, P. (1987). Alcohol use and alcohol problems: Clinical approaches for the college health service. *Journal of American College Health, 36,* 73–82.

Marlatt, G. A. (1983). The controlled-drinking controversy: A commentary. *American Psychologist, 38,* 1097–1110.

Mayfield, D., McLeod, G., & Hall, P. (1974). The CAGE questionnaire: Validation of a new alcoholism screening instrument. *American Journal of Psychiatry, 131,* 1121–1123.

Medical News and Perspectives. (1987). Alcohol and athletics don't mix—can the players now learn to say "nix"? *Journal of the American Medical Association, 258,* 1571–1572, 1578.

Meilman, P. W., & Gaylor, M. S. (1987). *Dartmouth College 1987 alcohol and drug use survey.* Unpublished data, Dartmouth College.

National Institute of Alcohol Abuse and Alcoholism (NIAAA). (1980). *The public health approach to problems associated with alcohol comsumption: A briefing* (DHHS Publication No. ADM 80-994). Rockville, MD: Author.

National Institute of Alcohol Abuse and Alcoholism (NIAAA). (1986). *Toward a national plan to combat alcohol abuse and alcoholism: A report to the United States Congress.* Rockville, MD: Author.

Royce, J. E. (1985). Alcoholism: A disease? *American Psychologist, 40,* 371–372.

Selzer, M. L. (1971). The Michigan Alcoholism Screening Test: The quest for a new diagnostic instrument. *American Journal of Psychiatry, 127,* 1653–1658.

Skinner, H. A., Holt, S., Schuller, R., Roy, J., & Israel, Y. (1984). Identification of alcohol abuse using laboratory tests and a history of trauma. *Annals of Internal Medicine, 101,* 847–851.

Treatment of alcoholism—Part II. (1987). *Harvard Medical School Mental Health Letter, 4*(1), 1–3.

Wechsler, H., & McFadden, M. (1979). Drinking among college students in New England. *Journal of Studies on Alcohol, 40,* 969–996.

Weinberg, J. R. (1974). *Interview techniques for diagnosing alcoholism.* Center City, MN: Hazelden Foundation.

Weinberg, J. R. (1975). *Ten tips for counseling recovering alcoholics.* Center City, MN: Hazelden Foundation.

West, L. J. (Moderator). (1984). UCLA conference. *Annals of Internal Medicine, 100,* 405–416.

Williams, G. D., Stinson, F. S., Parker, D. A., Harford, T. C., & Noble, J. (1987, spring). Demographic trends, alcohol abuse and alcoholism: 1985–1995. *Alcohol Health and Research World, 11*(3), 80–83, 91.

11

Adult Children of Alcoholics

SHEILA CUMMINGS

I used to stay quiet and out of his way at night. My mother, sister, and I would avoid the family room where he would be lying on the couch and drinking. Then I would hear him grumble and I'd have to go in. He'd be lying there having just vomited in the ashtray, on the floor, all over. I'd have to clean it up, never saying a word, and then fix him another drink. Then I could go back to the room where my mother and sister were and resume what I was doing.

The speaker was Ann, a 22-year-old college student. What was most striking in her account of her father's drinking was the lack of any affect while she spoke. She had graduated from high school at 16, had graduated from college at 20, and was on her way to becoming a psychiatrist in medical school. She presented as sweet, good-natured, bright, and independent—a model student who talked as if she were unaffected by growing up in a family where her father was alcoholic. But it was a lie. She wanted me and the world to believe this lie so she could continue to believe it also.

Early research on adult children of alcoholics (ACOAs) characterized them as having glaring behavioral problems. These studies told us that children of alcoholics were overrepresented in the health and legal systems, and were already delinquent, antisocial, hyperactive, socially inappropriate, and academically low-achieving (El-Guebaly & Offord, 1977). But this research studied only the most obvious and visible victims. Without taking into account alcoholic family dynamics, and particularly the role of denial in the family system, the research missed those children of alcoholics who adapted differently—those who went unnoticed through the school system and quietly entered college. They missed victims like Ann.

With the rise of family therapy and Alcoholics Anonymous (AA), and with society's emerging awareness regarding alcoholism, we know today that ACOAs do make it to college; in fact, they comprise 15–25% of all college students (Berkowitz & Perkins, 1987; Woodson, 1976), which is proportionate to their numbers in the general population. Furthermore, in a recent survey of my own, I found that 22% of all college students entering treatment are ACOAs, and they apparently use emergency services at a higher rate than other students. Recent writings have also explicated the family dynamics and roles that characterize alcoholic families. Wegscheider-Cruse (1981) and Black (1981), in particular, have delineated roles that children play in these families that seem pertinent to understanding ACOAs in college. For example, the "hero," the "responsible one," and the "caretaker" are students we are more likely to see in college mental health settings than the "scapegoat." College students who are ACOAs have been damaged, but their pain is not readily apparent.

ACOAs are a population at risk. They are at risk for developing alcoholism, marrying alcoholics, or developing other problems such as depression and eating disorders. There is a need for innovative models for understanding and treating them in the college setting. This chapter explicates the family experience of ACOAs; describes commonalities in the way they feel, think, and behave; and considers various treatment issues.

THE FAMILY ENVIRONMENT

Alcohol is America's drug of choice. It is visible, it is sanctioned, it is encouraged. What is the effect of growing up in a family where alcohol use crosses over into abuse? As Sharon Wegscheider-Cruse, herself an ACOA, comments in *Another Chance* (1981, p. 78):

> The crises that blackouts and loss of control bring are dramatic, but they are not any more damaging to health and self-worth than the sanity eroding effects of living day to day with a chemically dependent person. The price of adapting to the alcoholic's erratic behavior is very, very high. . . . There is *no* healthy way to adapt to alcoholism.

Valliant (1983) has likened growing up in an alcoholic family to growing up in a Nazi concentration camp. Middleton-Moz and Dwinell (1986) refer to the alcoholic family as being a "depressogenic" environment. One of the main points these authors emphasize is the chronic nature of the trauma ACOAs have lived through. The dynamics of the dysfunctional alcoholic family—its tension, chaos, and unpredictability—become internalized and normalized so that the children have little awareness of the traumatic nature of their background.

One reason ACOAs are unaware of their plight is because alcoholism often is not directly apparent. Children, in particular, do not experience alcoholism per se, but the altered behavior of their alcoholic parents. As one student commented, "It wasn't the alcoholism of my father which affected me the most, but his violence." Another said, "I never connected my mother's behavior with her drinking until I got to college. And then it wasn't until therapy that I connected her treatment of me with how I am now."

Usually the development of alcoholism is slow and gradual, evolving over years. The more a parent becomes addicted to alcohol, the more the family becomes "alcohol-centered" rather than "child-centered." Steinglass (1980) claims that alcohol becomes the central organizing principle of the family. Wegscheider-Cruse (1981) adds that "the alcoholic's personal goals are to maintain access to alcohol, avoid pain, protect his or her defenses and finally deny that any of these goals exist" (p. 81). Thus the focus of the alcoholic is on his or her addiction rather than on the developing needs of the child. "Good enough" care gives way to preoccupation with alcohol, while care from the other parent (the alcoholic's spouse) is diminished by the stress of being with an impaired partner. The end result is that ACOAs have an aborted childhood that cannot ever be made up for.

Inconsistency and unpredictability of behavior are two of the most salient aspects in an alcoholic family. As one student remarked, "What was most predictable in our home was how unpredictable it was." The alcoholic parent may be quite "normal" in between drinking periods and then become quite irrational when intoxicated. During sober times, the parent may even attempt to make up for past failures by being too attentive, at times intrusive, and making promises that dissolve during drunken states. Children feel buffeted by the chaos, unclear roles, and changing limits. It is most disconcerting and confusing that the affection they need and the irrationality they fear come in the same package. It is also confusing, especially for middle-class children, that a parent who is competent in the outside world is irrational and incompetent at home, or that a parent who outwardly maintains a family by providing food, clothing, and shelter is not also emotionally available.

Children react to this inconsistency in several ways. They may think, "If Mommy and Daddy really loved me, they wouldn't drink. There's something wrong with me." Thus they attempt to impose order on a chaotic world. They may attempt to shield themselves from inconsistency and unpredictability by learning not to want so that they will not feel disappointed. They also may resent society, relatives, and neighbors for knowing and yet allowing the abusive and neglectful behavior to continue. They then come to believe that no one can be a source of help or comfort.

Alcoholism always strongly affects the marital relationship. It decreases inhibitions and allows more aggressive impulses to emerge, and alcoholics' spouses are often angry at alcoholics for not meeting their needs. Thus tension and argumentativeness are common, as are broken homes and divorce. Children often feel responsible for their parents' marital problems. Their parents are the fabric of their lives; for their marriage to fail is experienced as inner rupture. A child therefore may try to become a buffer between the parents, or may attempt to be a substitute partner for the nonalcoholic parent. Whatever the strategy, children are never truly free from the marital discord.

CLINICAL CONSEQUENCES

Affects

Several characteristic affects of ACOAs can be identified: denial; alienation from others; an inner sense of deprivation and rage; and low self-esteem, shame, and guilt.

Denial is one of the most striking features of ACOAs. Some students deny parental alcoholism itself, whereas others acknowledge alcoholism but do so without any real emotion. As one student said, "After you come to admit you're a child of an alcoholic, isn't that all there is to it?" Another student, who did identify herself as an ACOA, recounted horror stories of violence, abuse, and name calling, but without showing any affective reaction. She was articulate and glib, but had yet to deal with the emotional consequences of parental alcoholism. The same could be said for every member of an ACOA group I have run on a university campus. For many students, the lack of affect is tied to psychophobia, a deep-seated fear of taking emotional factors seriously.

Children learn denial because it is in the family system, where so much pain is being anesthetized both by alcohol and by the parents' use of denial. Denial is also rewarded. To belong to the alcoholic family—to feel as if they fit in—the children must adopt the ways of thinking and perceiving that characterize the family, even if it means sacrificing their own thoughts and perceptions. Brown (1985) calls this denial in the service of attachment. Denial of feelings is also learned because emotions are equated with being out of control and irrational as the alcoholic parent, or with neediness. Neediness is a vulnerability that children of an alcoholic family cannot afford to experience, since in their experience needs are never met.

A second characteristic affect is alienation from others. Winnicott (1965) said, "Feelings are object seeking. Feelings evoke responses from others and build connections; they are what all people have in common." ACOAs deny not only feelings, but their connections with others as well. Inwardly they feel alienated, different, and unacceptable. They doubt their capacity to love and be loved; they wonder whether they really care about others or whether others really care about them. One married student said that his notion of an ideal vacation was to go off on a mountaintop by himself and read. His attitude was "I don't need you. You don't have any effect on me." Another said she would cringe whenever her boyfriend said he loved and needed her. She could not stand his becoming intimate because it evoked her own neediness, which she had disowned.

A third set of affects consists of deprivation and rage. ACOAs usually arrive at our doors appearing self-sufficient and mature—a legacy from their experience as children, when they were expected to be like little adults in order to compensate for deficits in the parents. They came to have an exaggerated sense of self (Winnicott's [1965] "false self"), which became the bulwark of their self-worth. Inside, though, they felt inadequate to the task of taking care of a sick parent; they felt deprived. Bowlby (1980) calls this being self-sufficient in an insufficient way. A student vividly recalled sitting as a 12-year-old on the beach with her younger brother and knowing that she must kill him and herself. She felt depleted. Having rescued her alcoholic mother from a suicide attempt 4 years earlier and raised her brother since he was born, she had few internal supplies left for herself, and felt a despair that no one could be a source of comfort or caring. She felt 30 years old at age 12. She had been deprived of her childhood.

Eventually, feelings of deprivation result in rage. But anger tends to be equated with violence and recklessness in the experience of ACOAs. As one student remarked, "Being angry is being like my father," who was often violently out of control. ACOAs often do not know *whether* they are angry, *when* one should be angry, or *how* to be angry. In group settings one sees them trying to control each other's expressions of anger and dissatisfaction, for fear they will get out of control. Often students contain their anger in rage-filled thoughts and fantasies, which spill over into chronic dissatisfaction with and criticism of themselves and others. One student, who was emotionally controlled and somewhat isolated, could talk matter-of-factly about wanting to kill his alcoholic father when he was aged 7, and he often had rageful fantasies while driving his car. Occasionally, such anger may burst out when stress is high or defenses fail, and ACOAs then may experience a brief episode of uncharacteristic and disorganizing rage. At these times, they fear that their rage will make them crazy.

Finally, ACOAs suffer from low self-worth, shame, and guilt. Though they present a competent exterior, they feel damaged and defective inside. Their outwardly mature stance is praised and rewarded in school and society, but they talk about being "found out" or feeling like a "sham." They play the role of "hero" or "responsible one" and head straight to college, hoping thereby to heal their families of pain and shame, but inwardly they feel inadequate. Such feelings come about because their self-esteem is based on a futile fight against their parents' drinking. "For," as Wegscheider-Cruse (1981) says, "he or she, as successful as they [sic] might be in the outer world, is losing the only battle that counts. . . . They have not 'cured' the family" (p. 108).

These negative feelings impede separation and bind ACOAs to their families. To leave a sick family and become truly successful and satisfied is tantamount to betrayal and abandonment. Thus ACOAs face a dilemma. If they stay with their families they will "go down with the ship," but if they leave they are deserting the persons they love.

Cognitions

Brown (1985) believes that specific thinking disorders characterize alcoholic families. For example, the cause–effect sequence is distorted so that children are blamed for the parents' drinking behavior, and alcohol is seen as a solution to all problems. Four additional aspects that characterize ACOAs' thinking can be identified: confusion about normality, extreme thinking, inverted identifications, and faith in willpower.

First, ACOAs are confused about normality. According to Woititz (1983), they have to "guess at what normal is" (p. 3). They certainly have no map of normality based on their own home situation. For example, one student in an ACOA group reported, "We didn't have a refrigerator for 1½ years even though we had the money for it." Another said, "We had all these appliances but none of them worked." ACOAs therefore must look outside the home to learn about typical families. They may turn to TV for clues; *The Brady Bunch* may be cited as an example of normal family life. They also may turn to idealized fantasies about the world. These fantasies, which may concern an all-giving mother or lover, may be the only alternatives to their painful reality, and thus ACOAs continue to believe in them despite disappointments when the fantasies inevitably fail to come true.

The second cognitive feature is thinking in extremes—black or white, all or none, good or bad. This tendency is due to ACOAs' use of massive denial and to the extreme conditions in their childhood families. ACOAs see others in simplistic terms—a tendency that inevitably leads to feelings of disillusionment, since very few people are totally worthy or trustworthy. All-or-nothing thinking also precludes ACOAs from defining and reorganizing problems into smaller and thus more attainable steps, and therefore they perceive themselves as continually failing, even when they are not. ACOAs attempt to live up to extreme standards. Typical statements they make to themselves are "I must be in control at all times," "I must be perfect or I am nothing at all," "I must be all-giving," and "I don't need anthing." These extreme goals guarantee failure.

A third cognitive characteristic, inverted identifications, represents an attempt to resist identification with an impaired parent. The thinking goes: "If mother was X, then I'll not be X." For example, one student perceived her alcoholic mother as a slob, so she became a compulsive cleaner who acted in control at all times. An uneasy feeling would develop within her if she even was tempted not to clean; a single break, she felt, would make her lose control forever and become an alcoholic. Though such thinking is an attempt to separate from parents, it of course leaves ACOAs as bound to parents as if they were directly trying to emulate them.

The fourth cognitive characteristic of ACOAs is faith in willpower. In contrast to their alcoholic parents, who lost the battle with themselves over and over again, ACOAs believe that they can control anything if they try hard enough (Brown, 1985). The family situation contributes to this sense of omnipotence. Alcoholics tend to externalize, and children make convenient targets for blame and responsibility. Consequently, the children grow up feeling that they should control the alcoholic parents' drinking and behavior. For ACOAs, the sense of omnipotence allows them to have a sense of control and predictability; they feel they can make things better. But a negative consequence is that they blame themselves unjustly. They internalize the "badness" of their families, and assume that their parents' drinking and the ill-treatment they receive is their fault. Moreover, they develop a faulty notion of their own powers and limitations.

Behaviors

ACOAs present as self-reliant and perfectionistic. Though socially poised, they are actually somewhat secretive and detached. They also may abuse alcohol themselves.

The self-reliance ACOAs display grows out of the unreliability of their parents. Because their own needs have not been met, they learn to become their own caretakers and eventually play this role with others, sacrificing their own needs for nurturance in the process (often in an unhealthy way, turning to fantasy, food, drink, and self-destructive activities). ACOAs also try to compensate for their family backgrounds by achieving some special status: Perhaps if they are good enough, then their parents will be happy and stop drinking. This course leads ACOAs to feel measured by what they *do* rather than who they *are*, which motivates them to try to perform ever better, to live up to perfectionistic standards. If they can be perfect, they feel, they will gain love from others and defend themselves against criticism. One student who received only an A– on an exam called the emergency service that night; that "minus," signifying imperfection, was devastating to her. Not only do ACOAs try to be perfect, but they search for perfect others. These others, they unconsciously hope, will make up for love lost in the past and be an antidote for negative self-feelings. The search for a perfect other, like the pursuit of perfection in oneself, is of course doomed to be futile.

Secrets play a special role for ACOAs. Although many were told that there was nothing wrong in the family, the concurrent message was "Don't tell anyone." They learned, therefore, to keep to themselves what was going on within the family, to hide facts from people and not bring friends into the home. Originally, keeping secrets made them feel "okay" and "normal"; secrets were intended to thwart rejection by others. Ironically, as the children grow older, the secrets once intended to preserve relationships now have the effect of keeping people at a distance. Blocking so many avenues that might lead to the secrets makes ACOAs guarded and deprives them of the chance for genuine relatedness.

ACOAs also unconsciously sabotage their relationships. Often they do this when they feel good and therefore unconsciously fear that disappointment is soon to follow, as in the past. Their uneasiness and feelings of alienation lead them to control the situation by making disappointment happen; in this way, they are not caught off guard.

A student recounted how she and her boyfriend were having a pleasant time at dinner. But when her boyfriend made a minor gaffe, she became withdrawn, and later she expressed anger about his lack of caring and refused to accept his apology. Although the evening had been enjoyable up to that point, she unconsciously preferred to retreat inside herself; then she need not trust or depend on anyone. By withdrawing, she was in control and could not be hurt.

The price of these behaviors is self-imposed isolation—a prison of one's own making. ACOAs report walling themselves off from others, literally locking themselves in their dorm rooms, because they feel distressed and unfit for company. Their isolation then reinforces their sense of being social misfits. One student said, "I'm miserable when I go out on weekends. I'm either feeling so out of it or I'm so busy figuring out how to please others that I have no time to enjoy myself. My real self is locked back in my dorm room. When I go back there I'm lonely but comfortable." ACOAs try to hide their attachments to others, since as children their desires for closeness were usually thwarted. Being vulnerable means becoming hurt.

Another behavior ACOAs must worry about is the possibility of alcoholism in themselves. There are startling statistics behind this concern: 25–50% of all alcoholics are children of alcoholics (Cotton, 1979). Sons are more likely to develop drinking problems, whereas daughters tend to develop depression and to marry alcoholics, thereby becoming mothers to potential future alcoholics (Russel, Henderson, & Blume, 1985).

A recent survey I conducted revealed that 65% of all users of student mental health services who claimed that they were "concerned about their own drinking" were ACOAs. On another campus, it was found that ACOAs were four times as likely as other students to have drinking problems, three times as likely to have drug problems, and more likely to have irresponsible behavior and negative outcomes from alcohol (Claydon, 1987). Another study showed that children of alcoholic parents (especially children from families where both parents were alcoholics) were younger than children of nonalcoholic parents when first intoxicated, had more pretreatment problems, and showed a more rapid course between first intoxication and admission to treatment (McKenna & Pickens, 1980).

These findings may in part reflect genetic susceptibility to alcoholism. In addition, ACOAs may drink because it makes them feel as if they belong to the family or fit in with friends. Drinking bolsters denial, it is reinforcing, and it helps assuage negative emotions. No wonder many children of alcoholic parents develop drinking problems of their own.

TREATMENT ISSUES

Assigning Students to Group Treatment

Many ACOAs are reluctant to join groups. Group interchanges mean revealing secrets, betraying one's family, and admitting to a painful and shameful reality. But inwardly these students hunger to meet people with similar experiences. Once they admit to parental alcoholism, they want to find out what it was like for others and to validate their own feelings. Thus group work is effective for ACOAs and is often the treatment of choice.

Groups provide an opportunity for a wide array of curative factors to take effect (Yalom, 1975). Two such factors deserve special mention in connection with ACOAs. First, it is virtually impossible for students to remain in a group and keep their denial intact. Students must make the admission, "I am an adult child of an alcoholic," with all that entails. The group experience evokes the expression of deep feelings that students have tried to deny. One group member remarked, "In my individual therapy I can get away from feelings, but it's harder when there are eight people. Someone is always showing feelings here." Group members are apt to confront one another's denial. When a student claimed he was different from the others because his father was not alcoholic until the student was 12, another responded, "I thought that was true for my mother, too, but I only *recognized* it at age 12. Actually, she was having problems way before that."

Second, students tend to recognize and work through interpersonal issues that they could not cope with in their families. Other members may squash or foment conflict, withdraw or intrude, talk irrationally or act inconsistently, just as members of their families did. Thus, the group provides rich opportunities to relive old experiences and to learn new, effective ways to relate to others.

When deciding whether to assign an ACOA to a group, to individual treatment, or to both, the therapist should consider the following:

1. When alcoholism or problem drinking is a primary diagnosis, individual treatment—and probably a special inpatient or outpatient alcoholism program—may be required first. One does not want an active alcoholic in an ACOA group situation.

2. Severe psychopathology such as borderline conditions may require too much attention and disrupt the group experience for others. Again, individual treatment is the treatment of choice.

3. Although denial is to be expected, a student must at least admit to having an alcoholic parent. This is necessary for him or her to bond with others and share in disclosing shameful experiences. If the student does not do this, he or she will be unable to identify with the group, and individual treatment is then needed to address the shame and denial.

Taking the Problem Seriously

Whether students are in group or individual treatment, one of the most fundamental principles for therapists is to recognize the impact of growing up in an alcoholic family. Some therapists underestimate the problem. Their ears may perk up when students say, "My mother was schizophrenic," or "My father molested me for 5 years," but they are less concerned when they hear, "My father drank a lot." This reaction by therapists only serves to reinforce students' denial.

Therapists' countertransference feelings or ignorance may make them treat ACOAs' experiences as more normal than they are. Therapists may have issues of their own concerning their drinking or family members' drinking that they are afraid to acknowledge, or they may be personally unfamiliar with and therefore insensitive to alcohol problems. They may also underestimate the problem because of students' facade of maturity. Therapists should be aware of the false front—of these persons' ability to hide feelings and often act more socially poised and older than they are. Thus, therapists must walk a thin line. They want to remove the stigma and shame from alcoholism, but they also need to raise students' consciousness as to its horrors. They must not add to students' denial with their own.

Being a Reality Figure

Reality is a casualty in the alcoholic family, distorted to fit the needs of the parents. Therefore it is important for the therapist to be a reality figure. Direct references to alcoholism are helpful: "You keep speaking about your mother's moods, but it seems as if you really mean she was drunk." Students may wince, but they realize the therapist is going to speak honestly and to validate their feelings and perceptions. One group member said, "We rationalize a lot. That's what we were taught. I was told things like, 'Don't talk to your mother at night.' No one explained it was because she was always drunk then."

Part of being a reality figure is to answer questions first rather than to follow the usual therapeutic practice of exploring the reasons behind the questions; after the questions are answered, an exploration can take place. ACOAs are not used to getting straight answers. It is also important to give accurate information about social reality. One female student was shocked when the therapist commented that it is harmful to a child's growth to have to break up quarrels between her parents. She had thought that her role was normal and therefore felt guilty about leaving home and no longer being a buffer between them. Therapists should not be reluctant to explain social reality to ACOAs.

Dealing honestly with feelings and experiences is the best antidote for these students' depression and alcoholism. Therefore, therapists should confront interferences with the expressions of students' true selves. They should be advocates for honesty and reality—rare commodities in the alcoholic family.

Offering the Right Kind of Empathy

Although it is important to empathize with the child inside the college student, a therapist should not come across as too sympathetic. ACOAs are likely to experience overt displays of concern as intrusive and engulfing, and will stiffen up and reinstate defenses. One student was telling about being locked in his room every night at age 3 with a key around his wrist. His parents were either drinking or working, and he would entertain himself until he went to sleep. When the therapist expressed strong feeling for the abandoned 3-year-old, the student immediately dismissed it as "no big deal." He wanted empathy for his tough, self-sufficient side, not his abandoned side.

Although students must eventually find their lost, needy selves before they can continue their growth, the order of empathy is important. First the therapist should align with the "survivor," the adaptive side of the child—for example, by pointing out that the child's defenses were sane responses to an abnormal family situation. Then the therapist can empathize with the abandoned self:

ANN: Our house was so dark, dank, and depressing—always smelling like a bar—smoke and alcohol. So I used to try to sneak quietly out of the house. I'd be real quiet so my father wouldn't see me. If he saw me, no matter what, he'd react. He was always gruff. I'd get out to the garage and feel exhilarated to be free, but it would only last a minute. I'd have nowhere to go, I would feel lonely, and then I'd have to quietly sneak back in.

THERAPIST: It was pretty clever of you to be so quiet. It gave you more freedom and protected you from his irrational outbursts.

ANN: Yes, but now I'm being punished for being so careful and quiet. People don't gravitate to me. I'm too controlled and quiet (*crying*).

THERAPIST: So what once worked for you—perhaps saved you in some literal ways—now might trap you, cut you off from others, and it hurts.

ANN: I want to change, but it's so hard. And maybe the rules will change again. They've changed once, you know.

THERAPIST: . . . I can see how hurt and betrayed you feel right now.

It takes time for persons like Ann to admit to their own feelings of hurt and need. Her crying in this session was a new experience that had been made possible by letting her open up at her own pace. Her usual pattern, common for ACOAs, was to cry for others but not herself. As one group member said, "I can feel more myself by going through you."

Recognizing Individual Differences

ACOAs show considerable variability. Many factors need to be considered when working with a particular student. One is the quality of parenting. Was the alcoholic parent unavailable, or violent, or intrusive? How did this person act when sober? Was the nonalcoholic parent unavailable, angry, exhausted, overcompensating, or erratic? Such issues determine students' self-concept, patterns of behavior, and expectations from others.

Gender issues need to be considered. Was the alcoholic parent the father or the mother? Usually the alcoholic is the father, the son's major identification figure. However, children of either gender who have alcoholic mothers rather than alcoholic fathers tend to have especially disturbed interpersonal relationships.

Age of onset is also important. How old was the child, and what developmental issues was he or she dealing with, when the parent's alcoholism became manifest? The earlier the onset, the more severe the consequences. When did the child know that there was a problem? Did anyone talk about it then? These issues determine the extent of denial the student must break through.

Birth order, according to Wegscheider-Cruse (1981), determines the role an ACOA will adopt. The first-born will often be the "hero" or "responsible one," identifying with the enabler (the codependent); the second-born may become the "scapegoat" and develop an addiction; and the third-born often becomes the "lost child."

Finally, significant others are an important factor. What other persons, if any, was the child able to find as substitutes for parents? The ability to find nurturing others is a favorable sign for mental health.

Handling Denial

One of the first issues in treatment is to assess and address the student's denial. Students who deny even that their parents were alcoholic seek treatment regarding other issues and make no mention of parental alcoholism. Their presenting complaints tend to be vague and at times somaticized. Sometimes they seek help because of an eating disorder, which is often linked with having an alcoholic family background (Claydon, 1987).

If the therapist suspects parental alcoholism, the following questions may uncover it:

- Has the drinking of either parent ever created any problems for you?

- Were your parents often unavailable?
- Were they often aggressive?
- Has any family member or close relative ever expressed concern over either parent's drinking?
- Has the drinking of either parent ever created problems in their relationship?
- If not, were there problems in their relationship due to other causes?

Students also may deny emotional reactions to their parents' drinking by minimizing, discounting, or ignoring feelings; by using fantasies and intellectualization; or by drinking themselves. Frequently, the rationalizations the alcoholic once gave to maintain drinking are the same ones the child now gives as to why feelings must be avoided:

ALCOHOLIC: I can't cope unless I drink.
ACOA: I can't cope if I let feelings out.

ALCOHOLIC: I'll quit tomorrow.
ACOA: I'll deal with these issues when I graduate.

Students may defend their use of denial: "What good is it to feel? Doesn't experiencing feelings make me feel worse than ever?" A good therapeutic response to all such defenses is to point out that the patient's attempted control over feelings does not really work: "You talk as if you can control how you feel, and yet it seems that you've been plagued by your feelings anyway. Maybe giving them a voice will help you to be released from them." The therapist may then explain how unexpressed feelings underlie depression, social isolation, poor grades, or other presenting complaints: "You've come in because of difficulty connecting to people. To feel connected, first you must feel. You are denying yourself relationships, and perhaps that is why you are depressed." Another useful tack is to explain that denial of feelings was a once necessary expedient that has outlived its usefulness.

Wood (1987) claims that often ACOAs come into therapy in order to make their image stronger: to be better looking, to be more pleasing to others, to cope better with isolation, to lose weight, and so forth. The goal is to become perfect through therapy and not to have to deal with underlying issues centered around parental alcoholism.

At times students use the therapist's word "understanding" as a synonym for control. They say, "I want to understand this," or "Why did that happen?", in an effort to control or get rid of their feelings. No sooner have they experienced a fleeting feeling than they say, "What do I do with it?", as if one *does* something with feelings. At the start of a second session a student said, "Well, when do I start seeing results?" Translation: "When does therapy help me get rid of these uncomfortable feelings?"

Often students believe that feelings must lead to immediate, destructive action; impulsiveness was typical of their families. A student may think, for example, "If I'm angry I must scream at him, and he'll scream back, and then he'll leave." Thus the only way to control behavior is to stifle the underlying feelings that might prompt the behavior. In response, the therapist can ask, "If you weren't so concerned about consequences, how would you express what you feel?" The therapist may explain that feelings do not have to lead to destructive experiences, and discuss with students appropriate behaviors for their strong feelings. Safe expression of feelings can be an important aspect of group work:

> SUSAN: Today I've been fighting off tears all day. I went swimming and could hide my tears in the water. . . . If I start to cry here, then everyone will.
>
> LOUIS: I don't know about other people, but that would be too emotional for me.
>
> THERAPIST: It sounds like "too emotional" means being out of control.
>
> IRENE: Well, earlier I didn't want Alice to start crying, so I comforted her instead. I told her I was sorry for whatever was upsetting her. I apologized so that no one would be upset.
>
> THERAPIST: It's as if no one can get angry and still be good friends.
>
> SUSAN: I don't know if my anger will be accepted here. It feels so out of proportion. I don't know how to be pissed off. I don't know what to do when something horribly unfair is happening to me, so I try to control other people's anger.
>
> THERAPIST: I'm wondering if we are also discussing whether we can get mad at one another here in the group.

Handling Students' Fear of Abandonment

Helping students break through denial leads to guilty feelings about betraying the family. But underlying this concern is a deeper fear, defended against all their lives, that they have been abandoned—in effect, orphaned. Students now realize that their alcoholic parents may die actively alcoholic and they never will have known them. It is at these moments of profound recognition that therapists will hear clients say,

"No, it wasn't *that* bad." This reinstatement of denial is an effort to stay connected to their families, at least in fantasy, and to defend against the feelings of abandonment. It is helpful to interpret this denial as a desire to feel close again to their families, while explaining that doing so requires sacrificing feelings, perceptions, and needs. Giving up part of oneself is always the cost of denial. It is also important to point out that there are other people available with whom students can be honest and truly themselves—a lesson that is particularly relevant for group work.

Handling Students' Wish to Rescue and Encouraging Their Grieving

Another consequence of breaking through denial is activating student's wish to rescue family members. Denial has enabled students to leave home and go to college. They have pretended to themselves that theirs are healthy, functioning families that they can safely leave. As denial is challenged during therapy, however, students are strongly tempted to return home, like moths to a flame. Their fantasy is rekindled of curing their alcoholic parents in order to have loving caretakers at last. Or they may want to rescue other family members, as did the student who, upon learning more about alcoholism, canceled her vacation plans in order to fly to her brother's house. She had given up on her parents and was transferring her efforts to her brother, who was denying his parents' and his own drinking.

Therapists need to help students come to terms with their own powerlessness over their families' problems. Students must detach themselves from their families and mourn their own lost childhoods in order to engage in a healthier existence and select healthy partners. As denial breaks down and students admit the truth that in fact they did not have happy childhoods or loving parents, they tend to have strong emotional reactions. Depressive affect, defended against for years, starts to surface. Therapists should explain that this response is inevitable and necessary; students need to grieve for their lost childhoods and the needy selves that did not get enough love and attention.

Another reaction is anger. A student may express resentment at either the alcoholic or the nonalcoholic parent. Anger is directed at the nonalcoholic parent for not providing protection and nurturance, not stopping the spouse's drinking, or not leaving the chaotic situation. These feelings may eventually be projected onto the therapist, who should give the student the full opportunity to express them.

Handling Students' Counterdependency

Therapy is experienced as threatening for ACOAs, because it pulls for the neediness they have so long defended against. One way they try to control their dependency needs is to bounce in and out of treatment. Thus one outwardly mature, self-identified ACOA declared after two sessions that she had gained from therapy and it was time to quit. Other ways these students combat the neediness is to come late or leave early, miss sessions, or treat the therapist not as a real person but strictly as a paid professional. Or they may simply discredit the need for therapy. One student said, "I don't want help. I've been on my own since eighth grade. I didn't get help when I needed it, and I don't believe in it now." To counteract these fears of neediness, therapists should help ACOAs talk about their anxiety regarding coming for help.

Therapists also need to help these students make more accurate judgments about their needs. They should explain that having a need does not necessarily mean it is overwhelming or that it will not be fulfilled. Therapists also should point out when students use self-destructive methods—for example, procrastinating or making graduation difficult—as an excuse to have some dependency needs met through continuing in the role of student. In general, therapists need to help ACOAs, who were experts at parenting parents and are experts now at helping others (they often become therapists themselves), to acknowledge their own needs and admit to being the patients.

Understanding Transference Issues

ACOAs' pervasive stance toward therapists tends to be one of wariness. They particularly distrust the phrase or even the attitude "Trust me," because it puts the therapist into the position of the alcoholic parent who broke many promises. In general, therapists become in students' minds substitutes for the parents, and as such they are always potentially like the alcoholic. Therefore ACOAs keep therapists at a distance by denying that the therapists are persons who have needs, feelings, and reactions. Then they can talk, but not to real, and hence dangerous, persons. Such a view of a therapist does not allow for the development of a real attachment, which is needed for the ACOA's self to emerge.

At the same time, ACOAs project onto therapists their longing for the idealized parents they never had, and their rage at not having them. These feelings tend to be unconscious. It is as if a student has a secret relationship with his or her therapist that is kept safely out of view and harm's way. One ACOA at the end of therapy showed little reaction to the loss of the relationship. When asked about this, she replied, "Oh,

I already went off for a few days and cried about that. I'm good at going off alone and mourning." Although always looking for a mother in her relationships, she would never show this side in order to protect herself from disappointment.

Addressing these issues is most appropriate in long-term therapy and group work. For short-term treatment, dealing with students' denial and emotional constrictiveness is more pressing.

Identifying and Confronting Students' Self-Defeating Behaviors

Therapists must help ACOAs give up the compulsive pursuit of perfection so that they can be free to be "ordinary." This goal may be accomplished simply by explaining that achievement is not necessary to earn love, nor is it the same as love. The goal also may be accomplished through the experience of acceptance that the therapist provides. Therapists also must call attention to students' lack of involvement in relationships, including the therapeutic one. A therapist can point out that even though a student may be physically present in therapy, a group, or a relationship, the student's real self has been withheld for safekeeping. "Now may be the time," the therapist may say, "to venture out and test with your senses whether people can be trusted." In counteracting students' isolation, therapists may help them to avoid the all-or-nothing thinking that tends to stand in the students' way, such as "Unless I receive total approval when I speak, then I will never reveal myself again."

Another important therapeutic goal is to help students learn to identify healthy relationships. As young children they were maltreated when they looked for love, and therefore they have never experienced genuinely loving attachments; they believe that suffering is part of intimacy. Consequently, they let themselves get hurt in exchange for a modicum of acceptance. Therapists can help them to identify the difference between loving and nonloving acts by having them focus on their feelings: "How does it *feel* to you when he or she treats you like that?"

Assessing and Treating Drinking Behavior

ACOAs may be concerned about their own predisposition to alcoholism, whether they have a problem or not. However, they are not good judges of how much is enough. They may compare their current weekend drinking to the advanced alcoholism they witnessed in their parents, and conclude that they have no problem. Sometimes they switch to another substance, such as marijuana, to convince themselves that they are free of their parents' problem.

Therapists should carefully assess students' drinking practices. The best approach is to be straightforward, telling students that they are at risk and suggesting that they may have found at times that they are drinking or using drugs excessively. A particular danger signal of alcoholism is loss of control after a couple of drinks. If this has happened, students need to be informed that they may well have a drinking problem of their own.

Of course, 20-year-olds are reluctant to give up their drinking or drug usage, and ACOAs in particular often use a system of denial that enables them to drink without awareness of consequences. But even if therapists are unable to arrest students' drinking, they can chip away at the system of denial and raise students' consciousness, so that later in life students will perhaps be ready for treatment.

REFERENCES

Berkowitz, A., & Perkins, W. (1988). Personality characteristics of male and female children of alcoholics. *Journal of Consulting and Clinical Psychology, 56,* 206–209.

Black, C. (1981). *It will never happen to me.* Denver, CO: Medical Administration.

Bowlby, J. (1980). *Attachment and loss* (Vol. 3). New York: Basic Books.

Brown, S. (1985). *The treatment of adult children of alcoholics.* Portola Valley, CA: IAHB.

Claydon, C. (1987). Self-reported alcohol, drug and eating-disorder problems among male and female collegiate children of alcoholics. *Journal of American College Health, 36,* 111–116.

Cotton, N. S. (1979). The familial incidence of alcoholism. *Journal of Studies on Alcohol, 40,* 89–116.

El-Guebaly, N., & Offord, D. (1977). The offspring of alcoholics: A critical review. *American Journal of Psychiatry, 134,* 357–367.

McKenna, T., & Pickens, R. (1980). Personality characteristics of children of alcoholics. *Journal of Studies on Alcohol, 44,* 688–700.

Middleton-Moz, E., & Dwinell, L. (1986). *After the fears.* Pompano Beach, FL: Health Communications, Inc.

Russel, M., Henderson, C., & Blume, S. (1985). *Children of alcoholics: A review of the literature.* Buffalo: New York State Division of Alcoholism and Alcohol Abuse, Research Institute on Alcoholism.

Steinglass, P. (1980). A life history model of the alcoholic family. *Family Process, 19,* 211–226.

Valliant, G. (1983). *The natural history of alcoholism.* Cambridge, MA: Harvard University Press.

Wegscheider-Cruse, S. (1981). *Another chance.* Palo Alto, CA: Science and Behavior Books.

Winnicott, D. W. (1965). *Maturational process and the facilitating environment: Studies on the theory of emotional development.* New York: International Universities Press.

Woititz, J. G. (1983). *Adult children of alcoholics*. Pompano Beach, FL: Health Communications, Inc.

Wood, B. (1987). *Children of alcoholism*. New York: New York University Press.

Woodson, A. (1976). *Parental drinking questionnaire*. Unpublished manuscript, University of Wisconsin, Madison, WI.

Yalom, I. (1975). *The theory and practice of group psychotherapy*. New York: Basic Books.

12

Sexual Problems

GEORGE C. HIGGINS

There is probably no area of life that is less under the control of the reasoning portions of the personality than sexuality. Sexual behavior is often determined by urgent erotic impulses, controlled only by the equally unthoughtful emotional prohibitions of guilt or shame, with reason used only after the fact for purposes of rationalization. Specific sexual acts often are not chosen by a person, but are the result of the relative strength of a lustful affect pitted against a prohibiting affect; the struggle between these sets of affects is carried out without the benefit of cognitive processes even faintly resembling reasonable thought. The general goal of therapy for sexual issues with college students, regardless of the presenting problem, is to help students use reason and thought in sexual areas—to equip them to make actual decisions about their sexual lives, rather than to be controlled by the strongest affect present during some erotic event.

The comments in this chapter are directed to the general therapist who deals with a wide vareity of student problems and who does not have special training and experience in treating persons with sexual difficulties. It is assumed that the major counseling population is 17- to 22-year-old undergraduates who are unmarried and childless, and whose complaints about sexuality or sexual orientation are the concerns of reasonably healthy persons. These students have developmental problems concerning sexuality that can be modified spontaneously with supportive psychotherapy and age.

Healthy students, however, are not the only ones who come to college counseling centers with chief complaints in the sexual area. Students who present themselves with sexual problems are frequently pathological in other ways (often seriously so), and their sexual complaints are symptoms of the dominant pathology. Psychotherapy for this group must focus on the major disorder, especially if the disorder is psychotic in nature, which it often can be. Although sexual issues will undoubtedly be a focus of discussion and treatment in therapy with these students, and some of the material in this chapter may be of use, these comments are not meant as a guide for therapy with persons who have serious concomitant psychopathologies in addition to sexual concerns.

GOALS OF THERAPY

Regardless of the reason a student seeks therapy for a sexual issue, there is one fundamental goal for sexual counseling with undergraduates. That goal is to transform sexuality from a taboo topic, about which students do not think critically, to one in which they bring to bear their problem-solving skills. It is important, furthermore, for the therapist to help students expand their problem-solving skills for sexual problems.

Therapy about sexual issues should free students to pursue information about sex that aids them to make accurately informed decisions about their sexual lives. Therapists are often pressed both by their own convictions and by outsiders to help students behave sexually in ways considered to be consistent with "mental health." Most sexual problems, however, are not as much a matter of doing "wrong things" as of making decisions using "wrong processes." The main impediment to making healthy sexual decisions is that decisions about sexual matters are often made without critical thinking. The assignment of sexual decision making to the area of cognition is the principal goal of sexual therapy.

For responsible decision making, students need access to reliable facts about sexuality. To help students obtain facts easily, it is advisable to have bibliographic sources readily available either in the counseling office or in the institution's library. A small suggested general bibliography is appended to this chapter, but information in the area of sexuality changes rapidly, so any library needs continuing revision.

Since general therapists cannot be experts on all facets of sexual functioning and problems, they should develop expert referral resources with whom they maintain personal contact. When a student is referred to an outside professional, it is imperative for the college therapist to talk with both the professional and the student to be sure that the nature of the referral question and its treatment are well understood by all parties. It is also wise for referral professionals to have access to the collegiate therapist, since the realities and pressures of the undergraduate milieu are often poorly understood by those who are not continually involved in it.

Although the basic goal of sexual therapy may be easily stated, achieving it is more difficult. One reason for the difficulty is that probably no topics arise in therapy about which less can be said definitively than those involving sexuality. Few areas of human life evoke such high levels of emotionality, destroying individuals' ability to gather simple empirical evidence. Students will report as pleasurable and continue some sexual behavior that actually makes them feel uneasy, because it is considered appropriate or laudable behavior by a peer group. Countless students, both women and men, force themselves into physically and emotionally unpleasant sexual misadventures on the grounds that they must be the only virgins remaining on their campuses—a state perceived as horrible. Conversely, students often enjoy acts but then distort and deny the reality of their enjoyment. College men who have had homosexual experiences maintain that the experiences were disgusting and unpleasurable, in spite of the fact that it is virtually impossible for a male to function sexually with even minor distractions, let alone in a situation that is disgusting. These men ignore evidence concerning homosexual acts that might inform their ideas about homosexual persons—evidence they have gathered themselves. Therapists must help students learn to understand the data of their own experiences.

OBSTACLES TO TREATMENT

Three major obstacles to achieving the goal of sexual therapy, which can arise from both student and therapist, are sexual value judgments, discomfort using sexual vocabulary, and sexual attraction during therapy.

It is commonplace that all therapists are laden with values of which they must be aware. In the area of sexuality, however, the multiplicity of values, the intensity with which they are held, and their subtlety of expression make therapy almost different in kind. Some therapists have deeply held religious beliefs and values about sex, which are not necessarily antitherapeutic. However, when these values markedly affect the therapist's attitudes toward the sexual behavior a student wishes to discuss, the therapist's position must be made explicit before therapy begins. Regardless of whether a therapist is offended by or advocates the use of contraceptives or premarital sexual intercourse, if the therapist conveys strong personal preferences, the student may feel discouraged from talking openly and candidly about his or her feelings and from seeking unbiased information. The therapist may, contrary to the goal of therapy, become yet another force in the student's life reinforcing the idea that sexuality cannot be openly studied and reasonably considered. In such a case, a student should be referred to a therapist who has no stake in the decision the student may make.

The use of language is a matter of great importance in sexual counseling. From infancy sexuality is shrouded in mystery, and this is nowhere more apparent than in the vocabulary children are taught. Though they learn the correct words to identify most objects with which they come in contact, including parts of their bodies, the collection of euphemisms for sexual organs would make a fascinating and lengthy dictionary. Consequently, even in these times—supposedly after the sexual revolution—even very bright and verbal students often do not possess a sufficiently extensive vocabulary to discuss sexuality cogently. Therefore, therapists must listen to and occasionally use sexual euphemisms, or else get information of poor accuracy. If therapists consistently correct their clients' language, they will convey disapproval—not of the students' poor vocabulary, but of the very act of talking about sex. This, of course, may defeat the fundamental goal of sexual counseling.

Some therapists use scientific vocabulary at all times when discussing sexuality with students, intending in part to teach students a more sophisticated manner in which to discuss sex and to provide them the language with which to do it. The intention is laudable, and when it works it allows students greater latitude to discuss sexuality with people in addition to the therapist. But the use of sophisticated vocabulary often backfires. Students may be inhibited about discussing sex if they believe that only Latin and Greek root words are permitted. Frequently they will not understand the therapist's words, and they will be embarrassed to say so. Students may receive the impression that the therapist only understands scientific vocabulary, giving them a sense of hopelessness about communicating with the therapist if they use the vocabulary they know. Finally, the therapist's avoidance of slang vocabulary may give the impression that the therapist is uncomfortable discussing sexuality at all. However, therapists should also avoid indiscriminate use of slang, which may make them seem condescending or offensive to students.

Because the developmental levels of college students' sexual behavior are so varied, when they use the term "sex life" in therapy, it is necessary to inquire into it thoroughly. Nothing must be assumed. For example, students are apt to say that they have no sex life if they have never practiced coitus, but they may have had considerable noncoital sexual activities (e.g., masturbation, reading erotic literature for stimulation, or precoital sexual activity with a partner including mutual orgasm). The students are not lying; they understand "sexual activity" to be only intercourse. Conversely, therapists will often encounter students who complain that their sexual drives are leading them into a wanton and depraved sex life, when, in fact, they are referring to having kissed more than one person or having masturbated twice in the semester.

Therapists must check the meaning of all sexual words students use to be sure that the meaning intended is the meaning conveyed. A student, for example, said to his therapist that he had never "masturbated," and the failure to do so was puzzling, given everything else the student had said about himself. Later, when discussing his inhibition, the therapist used a common euphemism for masturbation. The student instantly said that he did indeed "jerk off" quite frequently, and he explained that he thought the word "masturbation" referred only to nocturnal emissions. To be absolutely clear about what a student means when using a sexual word, the therapist should ask for a description of the act. Two outcomes in addition to clearer understanding will become apparent if this advice is followed. The first is vastly improved therapeutic communication. When a therapist makes it clear that talking about sexual matters in concrete terms is not wicked, the decrease in anxiety and guilt experienced by the student is often great enough that information will flow more freely and candidly. Second, therapists will learn a great deal that they do not find in books. Most of us discover that, at least in the realm of sexuality, there are indeed more things than we ever thought possible in our philosophies, experiences, and imaginations.

A new problem concerning therapeutic sexual vocabulary is the resurgence of a puritanical attitide toward language that has occasionally appeared in academia as part of the otherwise laudable campaign against sexual harassment. Since the definition of "sexual harassment" includes use of language that makes the workplace uncongenial, some sexual harassment grievance committees have concluded that even in therapy language must conform to a standard set by the most prudish person in the student body. In some places charges have been brought against therapists for too intimate questioning of clients and for the use of language that is "inappropriately" sexual and intimate. The possibility of having such an action brought against oneself can inhibit probing a student's use of language to elicit the information necessary to do realistic and effective therapy. Each therapist must decide whether to be cautious to avoid accusations of using offensive and inappropriate language, or to risk these accusations in the search for more effective therapy. The balance is not easy to find, but certainly therapists cannot counsel effectively on any matter, especially sexuality, unless they are sure that they understand what their clients are saying. In the area of sexuality, this requires checking for specific meanings. There is no substitute for asking for details to be sure that a therapist and a student understand each other.

Another major problem is that students' primary emotional attachments are still to their parents, and their sexual feelings toward parental objects are not yet fully under personal control. The dread of incest usually controls specific sexual urges toward their parents per se, but it does not control these impulses toward therapists, who are often seen by students as parent figures. I suspect that no clients develop sexual attachments to therapists more readily than college students.

If a short time limit is imposed on the therapy, sexual transferences do not fully develop, and goal-directed therapy can be accomplished without complication. If, however, a counseling center allows the time necessary to do long-term work, sexual transferences will develop, which will allow for more complex therapeutic exploration. The opportunity for sexual countertransference problems is great, too. Therapists who cannot tolerate being the object of clients' sexual feelings will actively interfere with students' free exploration of sexual feelings in the transference, whereas therapists who have unfilled sexual or self-esteem needs may use the therapy relationship to satisfy these needs by consciously or unconsciously acting out in ways ranging from flirting with students to expressing affection and sexual feelings. Both situations are potentially disastrous: The focus of therapy is lost, and the relationship between the therapist and the student serves the therapist's needs rather than being used to advance the student's ability to deal cognitively with issues of sexuality.

THE GENERAL THERAPEUTIC TASK

The general therapeutic task is to help students understand their sexuality. It is to increase their knowledge and not to prescribe their behavior. With better knowledge, students should be better able to determine their own behavior responsibly. This task implies that the therapist has at least a basic understanding of usual adolescent sexual development.

Adolescent Sexuality

During adolescence, an individual normally develops from the reasonably sophisticated personality and social structure of late childhood to

the even more sophisticated and complex personality and social structure of the adult, with the added complication that personal relationships are accompanied by adult sexual drives. During this time, persons
outside the family replace or gain equal status with parents as the primary persons of importance. Most frequently, an alliance with a person of the opposite sex from outside the family becomes the central
relationship.

Adolescence begins with puberty, a biological event that increases
the strength of both sexual and aggressive drives, and ends with formal acceptance into adult society, usually in the form of a job or a career.
The increased drive levels at puberty create incestuous and hostile feelings toward parents that provoke a withdrawal from them as the central persons in the child's life; instead, strong bonds with sexual feelings
are made with persons outside the family. Finally, a psychological position is reached where the young adult establishes a fairly stable personality structure, with sexuality integrated within it, and with stable
relationships that serve personal as well as sexual needs.

Adolescence is closed by a social event that serves as a formal
acknowledgment that the adolescent is an adult. This event is usually
acceptance into either gainful employment or an apprenticeship. The
arrival of adult sexual maturity is traditionally signaled by marriage,
which is supported by social customs and expectations. This transition
from adolescence to adulthood was once swift and clearly defined. As
recently as 1925, vagrancy in a 16-year-old was considered a problem
great enough to merit comment in a book about adolescence (Aichhorn,
1955). The problems today's college therapists see, however, occur
because the transition now comes later and is less clearly defined.
Though marriage was never the close of adolescent sexual development
for persons pursuing a college education, going to college was once
accepted as an apprenticeship sufficient to close adolescent social
development. Nowadays, however, going to college is so common that
it is not a special marker serving as a social rite of passage from adolescence to adulthood; it does not signify the attainment of a notable maturity either to society or to the adolescent. For most students, college
is just the next grade in school. Consequently, much behavior that therapists see in college students can be understood as similar to that of
latency-age children who are psychologically practicing adult life, but
with the difference that college students are practicing adulthood with
mature bodies and mature drives. (The preceding discussion has been
drawn from Blos, 1962, 1979; Engel, 1962; Hopkins, 1977; and Lorand
& Schneer, 1962.)

Sexual History

General sexual therapy sometimes may be accomplished simply by taking a careful sexual history. If conducted skillfully, history taking will be experienced as a nonthreatening discussion of the student's sexual activities, and it will serve as a model for thinking about sexual issues. It is important to be thorough in the history taking. Topics discussed should include early sexual experiences such as childhood bathing habits, nudity at home, sexual education obtained and from whom, parents' attitude toward sexuality, and the sharing that took place or did not take place between child and parents concerning sexual matters in the family. Masturbation history and fantasies are often the largest part of the sexual history of a college student, and much sexual anxiety is often bound up in the fact of masturbation and in the thoughts that accompany it. Incestuous, homosexual, and other troubling thoughts may have crept into masturbation fantasies, and it is reassuring to have a significant adult talk about such matters without shock or disapproval. The therapist may also gain information that is difficult to elicit in another context. Many nascent neuroses may be aborted by a simple comment from a therapist that "taboo" thoughts during masturbation are not unusual and do not necessarily indicate the presence of a sexual disorder.

A review of childhood sexual activity often allows the student to bring up problems that may have festered for years. A suicidal male student was able, with mortification and horrible self-condemnation, to reveal that as a child he had on two occasions peeked at his mother while she was taking a bath. The student's mother was now dead, so he could not ask for forgiveness from her. The relief he experienced by mentioning the event to the therapist, who assured him that such an action was not unusual in early childhood, moved him from his suicidal position. The reassurance was made possible because of the systematic review of his childhood sexual experiences.

Direct review of current "normal" sexual functioning can also be therapeutic. Often there are conflicts about an ongoing sexual relationship: "Should I be having this relationship at all? Am I performing well? Why don't I like oral sex? Do we have to 'do it' every night to be normal?" These and a myriad of other questions are of concern to college students. Allowing a student to raise them makes them fair topics to be thought about and discussed rationally with the therapist, the sexual partner, other personal or religious counselors, peers, and parents.

It is difficult for many students to discuss even what they consider normal sexual behavior, so it is important to question students directly about what they may consider "unusual" behavior. Concerns about oral and anal sex acts, homosexuality, incest, bestiality, pedophilia, and other possible experiences may surface, allowing the therapist to incorporate them into the therapy. Asking a student in a neutral tone of voice about any of these topics will often get a thoughtful answer, as will simply asking, "Are you concerned about what you consider to be unusual sexual acts or thoughts?" When asked this question directly, one student revealed and discussed an extended sexual liaison with an aunt that she had kept secret for years.

When a therapist allows students to discuss sexual material, students often reveal memories or concerns that they have kept isolated because no one ever allowed them to become part of a serious discussion. Often they pretend to themselves that the events never happened; simply mentioning them in the presence of a nonjudgmental therapist is often enough to allow the healthy personality to integrate the experiences. This type of inquiry may also reveal material of a pathological kind that might otherwise have been concealed, presenting the therapist with the opportunity to treat the pathology directly.

Since permission to talk is so crucial to successful sexual therapy, counseling services that limit the number of sessions should be cautious about imposing the limits rigidly when dealing with students who are discussing sexual topics. To terminate a case of this kind and refer the student elsewhere may be interpreted by the student as an indication that the problems are too grim to be discussed in a college counseling center. The new therapist may not have the same success in facilitating talking, and the student who has spent psychic effort opening up to the first therapist may not be willing to do so again easily, especially since the result the first time was that the student was passed on to someone else.

COMMON PROBLEMS

Because of the ability of the sexual impulse to enter into so many different areas of life, it is impossible to discuss all the problems that come up in sexual therapy. The issues chosen for discussion here reflect current concerns of young people as recently expressed to me in my practice. New topics and new therapeutic interventions will inevitably arise in the future.

Value Problems

Differing sets of social values impinge upon the child throughout development. College is not the first time that a peer group's values may have clashed with parental values. It is often the first time, however, that students may do something contrary to their parents' values with reasonable freedom from discovery. The therapeutic problem is that students often have not yet clarified their own personal values; their behavior is often an uncomfortable compromise or alternation between two sets of values, neither of which is fully theirs (D'Augelli & D'Augelli, 1977; McCary & McCary, 1982).

A question often posed by students is whether to become involved in a genital sexual relationship. It is not, of course, the therapist's job to decide; the therapist's job is to clarify the issues important to each individual student. The therapist should convey to students unambiguously that whether to be sexually active or not is a real question without an arbitrary answer. Too often students are caught between two or more sets of expectations, and they seek to discover which one is "correct." The therapist is approached as the authority who will bless one set of expectations with the *imprimatur* of mental health. The therapist instead must authorize the student to decide the matter thoughtfully for himself or herself.

Therapists should be sure that students review their parents' expectations, if those expectations are at issue, and help students to anticipate the consequences of meeting or failing to meet their parents' expectations. Students often make decisions in order to defy or please their parents, rather than on the basis of their own beliefs about sexuality. A student may also decide about a sexual relationship in order to please or defy a peer group. The therapist must not always assume that the peer group is urging its members to be sexually active and that the parents are opposed. All possible pressures exist; therapists who aid students to think through issues not only must avoid pressing their own values onto students, but must also avoid assuming that stereotypes hold. For example, a woman student was pursuing a religious path of which her mother did not approve, and her mother was overtly pressuring her to be sexually active. Clarifying the student's motivations in this case was the proper therapeutic task. The student needed to understand the motivation for her sexual choices and for her religious involvement, in order to discover whether they were actual choices or were instead strategies in a struggle with her mother.

Relationship Issues: Performance, Contraception, Abortion, and Disease

A frequent subject of sexual counseling in the college setting is "the relationship" between two students. Sexual issues in "the relationship" usually involve performance, contraception, abortion, and disease.

Since these issues involve physiological components, a close relation-ship with a medical setting is recommended. It is not, of course, the responsibility of the psychological therapist to dispense medical infor-mation, nor should it be attempted. However, the therapist should be a well-informed layperson, and the counseling office should have printed material about sexual functioning available for students who are interested. The suggested bibliography appended to this chapter covers most necessary topics.

Sexual performance is brought to the college therapist most often in the form of complaints by men about erection and ejaculation diffi-culty and by women about orgasmic failure. Unless a therapist is spe-cifically trained in the remediation of such sexual performance problems, it is wise not to attempt to treat them. Sexual drives are plastic and unruly, and it is easy to worsen a problem if a therapist has not been clinically trained in the treatment of sexual performance disorders (Masters, Johnson, & Kolodny, 1982, p. 396). The therapist can provide literature and referral help, and can support the idea that these are treat-able disorders, not signs of some moral or character failure.

Once the choice to be sexually active is made, students must choose whether to use contraception or not, and if so, which form of contracep-tion to use. Questions about the commitment to the sexual partner are also central: whether to be monogamous; what kind of relationships are possible with other people; and how time will be allotted among other friends, schoolwork, activities, and the partner. Finally, questions about pregnancy, parenthood, and the interruption of pregnancy often arise.

With respect to avoiding pregnancy, the largest problem I have found facing college therapists is the reluctance of many students to consider using contraception. They need to justify their sexual activity on the grounds that it is spontaneous, love-driven, and therefore pure. The idea of gathering information about contraception, of having a phys-ical exam, and of deciding in a thoughtful manner how to avoid a preg-nancy is often considered "first-degree" fornication, morally or religiously wrong. They assume it is better to avoid thinking about it and pretend that "it happened" in the passion of the moment. The job of the therapist is to make informed thinking possible and desirable, to dispel the myth that no decision has been made, and to let the stu-dent see that the moral or religious questions and the sexual act should be thought of together and beforehand. Students need to acquire as much control as possible over their choices.

When a student decides to use contraception, the therapist may encourage mutual discussion between the partners, rather than letting them assign one to be responsible. When medical consultation is necessary, encouraging both members of the couple to seek advice together aids the development of healthy attitudes toward sex. To this end, it is useful if the college psychotherapist cooperates with the college medical health service to encourage the provision of couples counseling about sexual matters, including contraception, and to provide well-coordinated mutual referrals between the services. When the services are separate, it is very important for psychological counselors to keep the relationship between their department and the medical department in good repair. It is inexcusable to deny students a smooth, cooperative relationship.

Abortion is never an easy issue, regardless of religious belief, and the therapist should be willing to support a couple during the contemplation and/or aftermath of a pregnancy termination. This is an area in which therapists may have to be more active than usual. Students often believe that an abortion will not have any untoward effect on them. In my experience, this is never the case, and to insist that there be some counseling about abortion will never be wrong. Sometimes the father believes or acts as if he has no role or responsibility in the matter, when he may be quite helpful to his partner. At other times the man is treated as if he indeed had no legitimate interest in the situation, with the implication that his only interest was in the sexual act, he is at fault, and now he should stay away. Men frequently also need therapy in this situation, especially if it can help combat the notion that they have no role or responsibility in sexuality other than a lustful one. If religious beliefs are at issue, students should be encouraged to seek religious counseling, too. In general, avoiding any relevant issues in this difficult area is a mistake. As many issues as possible should be identified and addressed before the choice is made.

Another troublesome issue occurs when a partner in a relationship contracts a sexually transmitted disease. The therapist must be most alert to whether in the student's mind the disease confirms the stereotype that sex is bad, that the disease is a punishment for indulging in a forbidden activity. Guilt and shame can occur not only when the disease is the result of a partner's contracting it from someone else, but also when it is due to, for example, a yeast infection. Once again, it is the therapist's job to turn the situation from paralyzing emotions to judgment and coping. And here again, it is good to have a solid relationship between the psychological counseling service and the medical service.

Power and Abuse

Power is often an issue in sexual relationships that crops up in subtle as well as obvious ways. The most discussed power issue in sexuality is when a man forces a woman to submit to a sexual act to which she has not given consent—forcible rape. Rape is not restricted to genital intercourse; any sexual act constitutes rape if both partners are not consenting (Czinner, 1970). College therapists are required on occasion to talk with both the victims of rape and the perpetrators. It is difficult to keep a cool head and an open mind when dealing with sexual issues in general; in cases of rape it is very difficult.

How to deal with victims of rape has been well studied (see Brownmiller, 1976; Notman & Nadelson, 1976; Sutherland & Scherl, 1970). If a rape crisis facility is available, its services should be offered to the victim. Prompt and skillful intervention after rape can diminish negative psychological consequences for many, although it should be kept in mind that some victims seem to do better if left on their own (Masters et al., 1982, p. 435). The choice should be the student's. If trained help is not immediately available, the major therapeutic emphasis in the interim is to maintain the victim's self-esteem. It is typical in sexual assault of all varieties for victims to believe that they are the villains (Brownmiller, 1976). This is especially true if there was any pleasurable feeling during the nonconsensual sexual activity. Even when there was no pleasure, questions inevitably arise about whether a victim was too open to the perpetrator or took unnecessary chances. As clearly as possible, the victim needs constant reassurance that the choice to have sex should always be mutual, and that a person who has that choice taken away is always a victim.

When conducting therapy with either women or men concerning sexual abuse, it is necessary to be painstaking when exploring whether choice was present and whether permission was given. Too often victims believe permission was given when it was not. Both men and women fall easily into stereotyping male and female sexual behavior as that of the hunter and the hunted, respectively. They both tend to excuse abusive sexual behavior as a normal expression of male sexuality and to misperceive abuse of women when it occurs. Illustrative of this misperception was an occasion when two male students undressed a female student to the waist, made her dance, and then encouraged her to remove the rest of her clothes while they sprayed her with soda spurting from a shaken bottle. She did not report the incident to a disciplinary administrator. It was brought to the attention of a dorm advisor by a third party, a friend of the woman to whom she had described the affair with annoyance but not with outrage. The dorm advisor then called the counseling department. The situation was seen by all, including the victim, as a psychological issue and not as the rape it was. But, regardless of what the victim thought, choice was not present. She was raped.

Power in the sexual area does not lie only in the hands of men. The power of normative values is subtle but profound, and in the area of sexual behavior the pressure may be as great on men as on women. The therapist must be keenly alert to men who are unaware that they have been forced into sexual behavior of which they disapprove. It is assumed that a man always enjoys a genital sexual experience, that he is always able to perform successfully, and that no sexual opportunity should ever be turned down. A man who has reservations about sexual activity can be goaded into it subtly by being asked, "What's the matter?" or pointedly by saying, "What's wrong—are you gay?" For example, a student with a deep religious commitment and a chronic mixed bipolar mood disorder was approached by two female students one evening in his room while he was playing his guitar. They asked him to continue playing, and while he did they opened his pants and performed fellatio. He described the incident to his therapist as "fantastic" and "wonderful," but within 4 days he was hospitalized with a major depressive episode marked with an almost delusional sense of religious punishment for having engaged in sinful sexual behavior. Neither he, the perpetrators, nor his therapist characterized the incident or dealt with it as one of abusive sex based on power. As this case illustrates, men, too, do not always consciously experience sexual events as abusive even when they are, even though they may experience them psychologically as negative. Therapists must remember that normative power can be directed toward men as well as women, and that men may also need aid to understand and to protect themselves from it. All sexually active students need to understand that they can be victims, and that they should guard against surrending their control over sexual behavior.

Impulse Disorders

At some time every college therapist is approached by a student whose chief complaint is a diagnosable impulse disorder, such as voyeurism, exhibitionism, sadism, masochism, fetishism, pedophilia, or even necrophilia. In a small counseling service, the therapist may find it necessary to render service to these persons because of the lack of a specialized backup service. The primary fact about these disorders is that there is little evidence that the objects or activities causing sexual excitement in an adult can be changed. Since most of the impulse disorders are distasteful to society, and many are also illegal, a student with such a disorder would have changed long ago if change were easy.

The best therapeutic approach is first to help a student understand how entrenched the orientation is, and then to focus on how the student may still live his or her life without acting on the unwanted impulses, even though the impulses will undoubtedly continue to be present. It is usually very difficult to get undergraduates to believe that everything is not changeable by willpower alone. Most students and many well-meaning therapists believe that these orientations can be outgrown or that techniques are available to eradicate the impulses. This is rarely true. A useful approach is to help students think of their orientation as a handicap—as a condition that is likely to be of long standing, but one that is not of their choosing, so they need not feel guilty about it. In spite of this handicap, they can choose a more usual sexual life if they wish. Though the impulses cannot be banished, it is not obligatory to act on them; a student can find ways to control or divert the troublesome sexual urges.

Because the impulses do not go away, therapy with these individuals can be a long process. The students need to try various methods to avoid acting on their impulses, to evaluate their successes and failures with these methods, to modify their approach, and to try again. The therapist could suggest, for example, that students who have pedophilic feelings and have volunteered as Big Brothers or Big Sisters should work with their little brothers or sisters only in a group setting, or suggest to voyeurs that they avoid driving home from school when it is dark through places where they have previously committed voyeurism. Since the target impulses are often scorned by society, the afflicted students are often self-punitive. They give up therapy easily, interpreting any failures in their attempts to control their behavior as a confirmation of their worthlessness. To achieve a successful result, it is necessary to combat self-degradation, which requires that the therapist be patient, confident, and reliable.

Three problems arise. The first two have been discussed previously: The therapist's attitude toward the behavior must be accepting, and a time limitation must not be imposed on the therapy. The third problem is that some of the behaviors for which students seek help are unlawful, and sometimes therapists have legal obligations. This is particularly the case with pedophilia, where many jurisdictions require reporting of some sort when a therapist has some legally specified type of knowledge of a pedophilic act. This presents a thorny therapeutic problem, since many pedophiles can be helped. If there is a requirement that a patient must be reported to an authority in case of a relapse, either the patient may not tell the therapist the truth about a relapse, which disrupts therapy, or therapy may end when the therapist reports the patient and the patient is arrested. Therapists should know the laws of their jurisdictions and should consult with their own or their colleges' attorneys about what is permissible in their practice. They then should make it clear to their clients how dangerous information will be handled in therapy.

SEXUAL IDENTITY ISSUES

In the past decade and a half, issues of sexual preference and sexual identity have been in the forefront of both scientific and public scrutiny. In this section, I discuss heterosexuality, homosexuality, transvestitism, and transsexuality. The college psychotherapist is mainly called upon to do two kinds of therapy in regard to these issues. The first is to aid students who are in some fashion unclear about or unhappy with their sexual identity. The second is to provide psychotherapy for homosexuals, transvestites, and transsexuals who are not in conflict about their sexual orientation; it is essential here not to make changing their orientation a tacit goal of therapy. In order to achieve either of these goals, a therapist needs to have an understanding of the nature of the sexual orientations and of the underlying order that exists among them.

Definitions

In the simplest sense, "heterosexual" describes erotic attraction between persons of the opposite gender, while "homosexual" describes sexual attraction between persons of the same gender. "Transsexual" describes persons whose subjective sense of gender is different from their biological anatomy, and "transvestite" describes a preference in clothing and grooming that is contrary to that usually expected for the person's gender. Unfortunately, these simple definitions are not very useful therapeutically, because different conditions frequently have the same clinical manifestations. For example, both a homosexual and a transsexual may be sexually attracted to persons of the same biological sex, and both a transsexual and a transvestite may desire to cross-dress. Since appropriate therapy requires a clear diagnosis, the therapist must rely on definitions that are not solely dependent on clinical appearance. It is premature to be definitive about these matters; new facts are discovered each day, and political considerations have affected even the labeling of the conditions. Nonetheless, I have devised the following set of definitions (cf. Masters et al., 1982; Offir, 1982), which I find heuristically helpful in making differential diagnoses.

The orientations can be understood as variations of three underlying factors: gender identity, gender object choice, and gender role. By convention, definitions of sexual orientation assume that the gross biological anatomy of an individual defines the person's gender. Although it is well known that even biologically it is not possible to assign everyone easily to one of two genders, male or female (Fausto-Sterling, 1985, p.78), this assumption is still useful for understanding sexual orientation.

"Gender identity" is an almost ineffable but extremely persuasive subjective sense of gender. It is experienced as either male or female. It is very difficult to describe the subjective sense of being male or female and how it is known by an individual, but individuals do know it with an amazing strength of conviction. Even small children react strongly when their gender is misidentified, and do so at an age long before they have any sophistication about gender differences. It is rare to find a person who has any doubt about his or her gender identity. Masculinity and femininity in this sense seem to be something beyond simple convention.

"Gender object choice" refers to the gender of the persons who are most likely to provoke sexual arousal in an individual. Again, there are two categories: male and female. Gender object choice is a stable, intrinsic personality characteristic of sexual arousal preference and not of overt sexual behavior or fantasy. Although there are persons whose gender object choice is bisexual (i.e., they are intrinsically aroused by persons of either gender), most individuals are intrinsically aroused by only one gender (Bell, Weinberg, & Hammersmith, 1981; Klein & Wolf, 1985). The fact that only a few persons have an intrinsic bisexual orientation does not conflict with the fact that a large number of people occasionally have sexual fantasies or activities involving both sexes. The genitals respond to friction from either sex, and sexual impulses are easily attached to persons of either sex. Occasional sexual activity with or attraction to both sexes is common in college, where the usual canons of behavior are often questioned and are transgressed with reasonable ease. However, the therapist should be cautious about assuming that sexual activity with both sexes, especially in a college student, indicates a bisexual orientation. More often such behavior is the experimentation or current attraction of a heterosexual or homosexual person to someone unusual for his or her orientation.

"Gender role" refers to activities that are arbitrary with respect to sex but to which society, by convention, has assigned a gender. For example, our society designates smoking a pipe as male and wearing a dress as female, even though both can be done by either gender. To be a gender role, an activity must be arbitrarily assigned. Childbearing, for example, is not arbitrarily assigned; it is a gender function. Many aspects of child rearing, however, can be performed by either sex, and the designation of these activities as "female" is a matter of convention or convenience, not of necessity. The gender roles that most often come to the attention of the therapist are those of dress and grooming.

In summary, persons whose gender identity is dissonant with their anatomical gender are transsexual; persons whose gender object is persons of the same sex are homosexual; persons whose gender object choice is persons of the opposite sex are heterosexual; and persons whose gender role behavior in the realm of dressing and grooming is culturally inappropriate for their gender are transvestite.

Therapy with the Unsure or Unhappy Student

The first issue in therapy with students who are unsure of their sexual orientation is to realize how extremely difficult it is for them to cope with these strange anomalies in their lives, especially in light of the expectations of parents and peers. A clear diagnosis accompanied by acceptance is an indispensable aid therapists can provide these students. Students have often told their therapists that the most valuable aspect of their therapy was being given a name for their condition that allowed them to approach their situation with reason and thought. For example, a transsexual student had seen many professionals who gave him horrified looks, testosterone injections, and advice about dressing, grooming, and dating. He had even dated, married, and fathered a child to try to deny the reality of his life. The dignity he gained by being treated as a person with a recognizable orientation was therapeutic. He was finally able to bring his coping mechanisms to bear on real issues and solutions, and no longer had to fall back on a host of neurotic defenses against the shame he felt about not being the male that his parents and his previous professional helpers wanted him to be.

Sexual orientations can be and often are entirely independent of each other. A therapist must not assume that the presence of one orientation implies the presence of another; it is not clinically sound, and it is disrespectful to the student. A woman who is clearly attractive and conforms to all of the current conventions of female dress, grooming, and behavior may indeed be unambiguously and happily lesbian. Similarly, the male athlete who seems the epitome of campus masculinity may be transvestite *and* heterosexual. Lesbian women do not necessarily dress in male military fatigues and smoke cigars. Such women exist, but they are often heterosexual. Transvestite men do not necessarily eschew sports and prefer men as sexual partners. The presence of very unusual combinations does not necessarily imply the presence of major psychopathology. On the other hand, the therapist will also find stereotypical combinations. There are male and female homosexual transvestites, as well as transsexual homosexuals.

Since all of these conditions provoke disapprobation in the culture, students frequently have to be helped with feelings of self-hate and guilt. By treating the orientations respectfully as legitimate ways of living, the therapist can help restore self-esteem. However, the therapist should not underestimate the depth of a student's negative feelings concerning these socially unacceptable orientations.

Sexual orientations show as little susceptibility to change as do sexual impulses (Gonsiorek, 1982, p. 5). The goal with most students whose sexual orientations trouble them is to help them establish a constructive attitude to cope with the reality of their conditions and to avoid unrealistic objectives. A college student who enjoys dressing in the clothing of the opposite sex will be unlikely to outgrow that enjoyment. Finding persons of the same sex erotically attractive changes as seldom as does finding persons of the opposite sex attractive. However, students are not destined to follow their orientations slavishly; they have choices. Most persons who are aroused by members of the same sex can marry and live social and sexual heterosexual lives if they choose to do so, even though their orientation will rarely disappear.

Although changing sexual orientation is difficult at best, it is possible under certain circumstances. I am aware of three underlying causes or forms of sexual orientations, and which is present will determine the possibility of a change in orientation. The first underlying cause is "situational." This means that the behavior was forced by circumstances and was not initiated by an internal choice. A student who has attended only single-sex schools and has been sexually active is likely to have had homosexual experiences. The fact that the student was sexually active may have been due to a neurotic cause (such as a need to dominate or humiliate) or to a non-neurotic cause (such as a high sexual drive level), but the gender of the partner was determined entirely by the gender of those available. Transvestitism or transsexuality can also be situational. There are students whose parents dressed them in clothing of the opposite sex, treated them as if they were of the opposite gender, or both. One transvestite student's father had taken the boy as a child to bars dressed as a girl and made bets with others about the child's gender. He won his bets by taking his son to the men's room and showing the others the child's penis. The transvestitism stemmed from the approval and affirmation the child received from his father for appearing successfully as a girl.

Another cause of sexual orientations is "developmental." In the developmental form, the circumstances of the child's life are such that the child chooses an orientation because the orientation is rewarding and self-affirming. A stereotypical example is a boy known to his peers as a "sissy" or a "faggot," because he does not climb trees well, he cries when he falls down, he learns sewing easily, and he likes to read. Unlike the "tomboy," whose father will brag that his daughter can hit a baseball as far as any boy in the neighborhood, the boy's father will never brag that his son can knit as well as any girl. This boy will most likely be miserable and suffer low self-esteem. If one day he meets another boy who likes him—if that boy even loves and has sex with him, with all of the self-affirming rewards that a sexual relation can bring—this boy may declare himself a homosexual and find it to be intrinsically rewarding.

Both the developmental and the situational forms often become functionally autonomous, exist as if the condition were constitutional, and tend to be very resistant to change. However, students whose sexual orientation is due to either of these causes may be amenable to change if there is an intrinsic motivation to do so. This is the basis for the old prescription that a homosexual can change if he or she wants to do so.

The third form, the "endogenous" form, is less malleable than the other forms. There is growing evidence that some homosexual and transsexual persons' central nervous system functioning in the sexual control areas differs from that of nontranssexual and nonhomosexual persons (Glaude, Green, & Hellman, 1984; Seyler, Canalis, Spare, & Reichlin, 1978). As with some of the sexual appetites, it seems that these orientations may be "hard-wired." Whether they are present at birth or develop soon after, they may be the result of neurological structure and biochemical functioning rather than of personal choice. Consistent with these findings, some students tell therapists that they have "always known" they were homosexual, and others can state the day, month, and year in which they "discovered" it. Although this is not a litmus test, the sense of always having been homosexual may reflect the endogenous form. There is also clinical evidence that very early cross-gender identification occurs. I have examined a pair of genetically male fraternal twins, not yet 4 years old, one of whom stated clearly that he felt himself to be a girl and the other clearly that he felt himself to be a boy. Free-play situations with sex-typed toys and the interaction of the two brothers showed that they both accepted each other's gender self-assignments and that transsexuality was present at this early age.

In endogenous cases, little or nothing can be done to change the erotic attraction or the sense of gender identity. However, a person still has a choice of how to behave. A woman who is sexually attracted to other women can still marry, have children, and be a mother and a wife, even though she will still have sexual feelings for women. The choice for endogenous homosexuals is not whether they will experience sexual attraction to persons of the same sex (they will), but whether they choose to act on the attraction, and in what form.

Therapy with the Committed Student

Therapy with students who are reasonably firmly committed to their sexual orientation involves helping them to become better informed about their orientation and providing therapy for other problems they may have, while respecting their acceptance of their orientation.

The incidence of transsexuality is unknown but probably very low, with the male-to-female form outnumbering the female-to-male form by three to one. Nevertheless, I receive at least one call a year from some New England college counseling center that has a transsexual student asking for therapy. When a possible transsexual comes to a college counseling center that lacks an expert in the area, advice from or referral to an appropriate resource is indicated. A current list of available referral sources is maintained by the J2PC Information Services whose address is listed in the suggested bibliography at the end of this chapter.

Instances of transvestitism are more frequently encountered in the college counseling center, most often as a troublesome memory about which there is guilt rather than as a current behavioral orientation. Memories of past cross-dressing are best evaluated for their developmental meaning and dealt with as a psychotherapeutic issue. Current cross-dressing raises practical issues, since this behavior is not usually tolerated on campuses. Most cross-dressers are heterosexual, male, and interested in marriage and families. Raising the issue of talking with prospective girlfriends, and encouraging the person to anticipate managing his cross-dressing in practical situations, usually create a perspective conducive to productive problem solving.

The homosexual person is the "unusual" orientation most often encountered in the college counseling setting. Therapists who wish to provide service to committed homosexuals on college campuses today must recognize that there is a complex political atmosphere that may affect their success. On the one hand is the AIDS epidemic, which has increased homophobia in all sections of campuses and which fosters suspicion about those who purport to help homosexuals. On the other hand is the rise of gender study programs that involve students and faculty in critical and vigorous appraisals of traditional attitudes toward sexuality and, in particular, the attitudes of therapists toward treatment of homosexuals. I have heard individual therapists and even whole college counseling centers condemned by groups of students and faculty who believed that the therapists were less than rigorous in pursuing up-to-date knowledge about homosexuality. On a college campus a therapist can never know too much when dealing with homosexual students, and if a counseling center wishes specifically to aid the homosexual community, it must be as well informed about issues relevant to the gay culture as it is about therapeutic techniques.

As an example of how complex the current environment is, even the name used to label a homosexual orientation can evoke strong feelings among students that can alter the effectiveness and acceptance of a therapist. In the scientific literature, therapists will find different uses of the word "homosexual." The word was coined in the 19th century (Herzer, 1985) and simply means "same sex." The prefix "homo" is derived from the Greek word ὅμός, which means "one and the same," not the Latin word *homo*, which means "man." The word does not, therefore, technically distinguish between male and female. However, some current literature uses words that do distinguish between men and women—"lesbian" for women and "gay" for men, for example, in the organizational name *Gay and Lesbian Alliance*. In other literature, "gay" refers to homosexual persons with no gender distinction. Since many homosexual persons are deeply concerned about the word used to describe their sexuality, the therapist should respect an individual's preference.

Once in therapy, it is important to understand what each homosexual person expects. Among other issues, students may wish to explore possible lifestyles that acknowledge their homosexuality. Therapy can be helpful in exploring who should and has to know, when others need to know, and who can be helpful and how. It is not the job of the therapist to supply or advocate specific behavioral solutions to any question; the job is to aid students to understand their situation as clearly and accurately as possible, and to help students to be able to make choices themselves as realistically and effectively as possible.

A student's family can be most helpful in the "coming-out" process and in the longer run. Although family members may be shocked and even horrified when they first learn a child is homosexual, their love and caring for the student can usually be relied on to prevail unless there is already a serious disruption in the family. Contact with a student's family and family sessions are helpful. The student needs to understand that the family may have a "coming-out" problem of its own. It is one thing for parents to tell friends proudly that their daughter has a serious steady relationship with a man; it is another to announce with pride a relationship with a woman. Yet most family members have goodwill toward each other, and this can be marshaled if counseling includes them in an atmosphere of mutual caring and concern (Williams, 1987).

Occasionally a heterosexual student will experience homosexual impulses or have a homosexual experience. Similarly, a homosexual student may have heterosexual impulses or a heterosexual experience. Each wants to know what this means. Both cases may indicate the beginning of the emergence of a true orientation that has been masked for some reason. If this is true, a careful history will usually reveal some evidence of the orientation earlier in life. In most cases, what has occurred is a transitory event revealing that most people at some times have sexual feeling for persons of both sexes, and it does not suggest the emergence of a latent orientation. It is important to help a student understand that sexual orientations do not emerge suddenly and wholly formed without some history. If these students are concerned about conventionality, the heterosexual should not fear that he or she is turning into a homosexual or will become one because of a single act, and the homosexual should not take the experience to mean that he or she may really be heterosexual and the experience has rid him or her of homosexual impulses.

FINAL CONSIDERATION

This chapter has talked about therapy for sexual problems, but it is people who receive therapy, not problems. In doing therapy with students who have sexual problems, it is extremely important that the therapist not allow the sexual problem to define all of the therapy goals and directions. Students who have sexual concerns are real people with other problems, and they can use help for them. Even the best-intentioned therapist can easily be led into subtly downplaying other therapy problems. For example, homosexuals may have problems managing anger or dependency needs, quite apart from their concerns about sexual attraction. Many homosexuals were shy and tentative in peer group interaction during childhood, and they did not develop the interpersonal social skills that other children did. Diagnosis and treatment of their homosexuality will not compensate for the lost years of childhood social learning. The therapist who focuses only on sexual matters does a disservice to the whole person who is the patient. Above all, the therapist should remember that the presence of a sexual concern in a patient does not divorce that person from humanity, and that the most important therapeutic help is often obtained in areas other than the sexual.

SUGGESTED BIBLIOGRAPHY

Bell, A. P., Weinberg, M. S., & Hammersmith, S. K. (1981). *Sexual preference: Its development in men and women*. Bloomington: Indiana University Press.
Benjamin, H. (1966). *The transsexual phenomenon*. New York: Warner Books.
Feinbloom, D. H. (1976). *Transvestites and transsexuals*. New York: Delacourt Press.

Gonsiorek, J. C. (1982). *Homosexuality and psychotherapy.* New York: Haworth Press.

Gotwald, W. H., & Golden, G. H. (1981). *Sexuality: The human experience.* New York: Macmillan.

Green, R., & Money, J. (1969). *Transsexualism and sex reassignment.* Ann Arbor, MI: University Microfilms.

Harmatz, M. G., & Novak, M. A. (1983). *Human sexuality.* New York: Harper & Row.

J2PC Information Service. P. O. Box 184, San Juan Capistrano, CA 92693. Attention: Johanna M. Clark, (714) 496-5227.

Journal of Homosexuality. New York: Haworth Press.

Klein, F., & Wolf, T. J. (1985). *Bisexualities: Theory and research.* New York: Haworth Press.

Masters, W. H., Johnson, V. E., & Kolodny, R. C. (1984). *Human sexuality* (2nd ed.). Boston: Little, Brown.

McCary, J. L., & McCary, S. P. (1982). *McCary's human sexuality* (4th ed.). Belmont, CA: Wadsworth.

Offir, C. W. (1982). *Human sexuality.* New York: Harcourt Brace Jovanovich.

Koop, C. E. (1987). *Surgeon General's report on acquired immune deficiency syndrome.* Washington DC: U. S. Department of Health and Human Services.

Planned Parenthood Federation of America. (1984). *Basics of birth control.* New York: Author.

Strong, B., & Reynolds, R. (1982). *Understanding our sexuality.* St. Paul, MN: West.

REFERENCES

Alchhorn, A. (1955). *Wayward youth.* Evanston, IL: Northwestern University Press.

Bell, A. P., Weinberg, M. S., & Hammersmith, S. K. (1981). *Sexual preference: Its development in men and women.* Bloomington: Indiana University Press.

Blos, P. (1962). *On adolescence.* New York: Free Press.

Blos, P. (1979). *The adolescent passage.* New York: International Universities Press.

Brownmiller, S. (1976). *Against our will: Men, women and rape.* New York: Bantam.

Czinner, E. Z. (1970, January). The many kinds of rape. *Sexology,* pp. 12–15.

D'Augelli, J. F., & D'Augelli, A. R. (1977). Moral reasoning and premarital sexual behavior: Toward reasoning about relationships. *Journal of Social Issues, 33,* 46–66.

Engel, G. L. (1962). *Psychological development in health and disease.* Ann Arbor, MI: University Microfilms.

Fausto-Sterling, A. (1985). *Myths of gender.* New York: Basic Books.

Glaude, B. A., Green, R., & Hellman, R. E. (1984). Neuroendocrine responses to estrogen and sexual orientation. *Science, 225,* 1496–1499.

Gonsiorek, J. C. (1982). *Homosexuality and psychotherapy.* New York: Haworth Press.

Herzer, M. (1985). Kertbeny and the nameless love. *Journal of Homosexuality, 12,* 1–26.

Hopkins, J. R. (1977). Sexual behavior in adolescence. *Journal of Social Issues, 33,* 67–85.

Klein, F., & Wolf, T. J. (1985). *Bisexualities: Theory and research*. New York: Haworth Press.

Lorand, S., & Schneer, H. (1962). *Adolescents*. New York: Hoeber.

Masters, W. H., Johnson, V. E., & Kolodny, R. C. (1982). *Human sexuality*. Boston: Little, Brown.

McCary, J. L., & McCary, S. P. (1982). *McCary's human sexuality* (4th ed.). Belmont, CA: Wadsworth.

Notman, M. T., & Nadelson, C. C. (1976). The rape victim: Psychodynamic considerations. *American Journal of Psychiatry, 133*, 408–413.

Offir, C. W. (1982). *Human sexuality*. New York: Harcourt Brace Jovanovich.

Seyler, L. E., Canalis, E., Spare, S., & Reichlin, S. (1978). Abnormal gonadotropin secretory responses to LRH in transsexual women after diethylstilbestrol priming. *Journal of Clinical Endocrinology and Metabolism, 47*, 176–183.

Sutherland, S., & Scherl, D. (1970). Patterns of response among victims of rape. *American Journal of Orthopsychiatry, 40*, 503–511.

Williams, E. W. (1987). *From disclosure to acceptance: A complex and challenging journey for parents of gays*. Unpublished master's thesis, Smith College School for Social Work.

13

AIDS

RICHARD P. KEELING

Epidemiologists commonly conjure up the image of an iceberg to describe the epidemic of infection with human immunodeficiency virus (HIV). At the visible tip are people with the acquired immunodeficiency syndrome (AIDS), the ultimate clinical consequence of HIV infection. Beneath them are many other people who currently are infected by HIV but do not have AIDS. Some of these people have mild or moderately severe symptoms, called AIDS-related complex (ARC), or only chronically enlarged lymph nodes, called chronic lymphadenopathy syndrome (CLAS). But most infected people are at the very base of the iceberg: While harboring HIV, they are currently completely healthy.

The iceberg image describes the epidemiology of HIV infection on a college campus as well, with some important differences. Notably, the campus iceberg is even larger at its bottom, because few students will progress all the way through the various levels of infection to have visible AIDS while they are still in school. HIV may be latent for an average of 7–8 years before AIDS develops. Thus, in the traditional undergraduate institution, most people with AIDS will be older students, faculty, or staff members; in comprehensive universities, graduate and professional students will also be included. The great bulk of the clinical work of HIV infection and AIDS will concern students who are latently infected or mildly symptomatic, rather than students with serious disease—in other words, those with potential rather than actual illness.

In addition to the medical epidemic, an outpouring of print and broadcast media attention has kept AIDS in the public mind, addressing the medical problem in variably helpful, hurtful, or hysterical ways. The truly frightening medical and public health problem of AIDS has combined with this plethora of reports to generate and nourish another epidemic, an epidemic of fear, which has itself caused discrimination, disability, and death. Attitudes about sex, homosexuality, and intravenous drug use have added implications of darkness and immorality to the popular fear, and some thundering theological voices have blamed people with AIDS for their own illness. Taken together, these stigmatizing elements add a deeper, larger level beneath the campus iceberg: students who are afraid of or worried about HIV infection. Depending on the size and nature of the institution, then, college and university therapists will encounter relatively few students living with AIDS itself; some who have milder illness; more who are asymptomatically infected; and many more who are worried or afraid.

For any concerned student, AIDS creates and mixes several issues, including sexual behaviors and practices, approaches to intimacy, social and family relationships, psychological and spiritual needs, and adjustment to physical realities. These issues do not occur in isolation from pre-existing psychological problems or vulnerabilities (Forstein, 1987) or from ongoing developmental struggles. The great challenge of meeting the psychological needs of college students concerned about HIV infection is to integrate the specific issues of AIDS with the already demanding tasks of psychological maturation.

Given the complexity of these issues, students have a great need for information about AIDS. Information about HIV infection is readily available, but varies in quality and is perceived as unstable; students will often first want "the real facts." Just as counseling needs may underlie questions, questions may underlie concerns. The absence of adequate information provokes anxiety and fear, depression and denial; it can lead to both unsafe and overly cautious behavior. Unfortunately, some important information about HIV infection is not yet known, and the lack of clarity about such matters as the likelihood of eventually developing AIDS may complicate assessments of individuals' futures. Therapists can anticipate many questions, much repetition, and some frustration over limited answers (Macks, 1987).

In addition to information, students may need therapy to understand and manage their feelings about AIDS and to cope with psychological symptoms. They may have periods of crisis when problem sorting, identification of coping strategies, and enhancement of adaptive functioning are necessary. The question of organic neuropsychiatric disease caused by HIV may be raised because of certain behaviors or symptoms. Although there is much that is common in the experience of all students concerned about AIDS, certain groups have special needs. Gay men, for example, may find that AIDS has complicated the process of "coming out"; students who use intravenous drugs will have to address habituation and rehabilitation; and hemophiliacs must add this new concern to the many others related to their chronic illness.

Working with students who are concerned about AIDS places demands on therapists and can lead to problems in treatment. Although it may be satisfactory to send students to other sources for advanced or detailed information, therapists who are unfamiliar with basic concepts about HIV and AIDS may disappoint or frighten students. The overlap of psychological and organic brain syndromes in HIV infection requires that therapists be aware of the spectrum of presentations of HIV infection in the central nervous system (Holland & Tross, 1985; Wolcott, 1986), and that they have access to referral systems for evaluation of symptomatic students. The lack of complete information about AIDS may trouble therapists as well as clients. Therapists may be unable to deal with homosexuality or drug use in a nonjudgmental or comfortable fashion, and their unease will influence the success of the therapeutic relationship. When dealing with students known to be infected, therapists face their own feelings about chronic illness, loss, and death of clients. Thus college therapists must cope with their own concerns as they deal with students concerned about AIDS, as must mental health professionals who care for AIDS patients in other settings (Horstman & McKusick, 1986).

Students with concerns about HIV infection and AIDS may present to the therapist with virtually any psychological symptom; therapists must appropriately respond to both the specific issues concerning AIDS and to the more general need for assessment, evaluation, and therapy of psychological discomfort (Faulstich, 1987). The sections that follow present some specific management guidelines for students in each of several categories of concern.

HEALTHY STUDENTS

Students who fear they have been or might eventually be infected by HIV comprise the vast majority of the campus population concerned about AIDS. These students may or may not have any significant personal risk of infection; their worries about "catching AIDS" may be an appropriate reaction after a rational assessment of risk behavior, an irrational reaction derived from confusion and ignorance, or some combination of the two. These worried students therefore need information, which can reduce fear and provide the resources for preventing future infection.

Although most college students have reasonably accurate knowledge about the transmission of HIV, they commonly are mistaken about key details. It is therefore wise to go beyond their initial question or expressed concern about AIDS, and probe for further concerns. A useful question to ask is this: "Why are you concerned about being infected?" In the safe setting of a therapist's office, students may gradually disclose their uncertainties and questions, and the therapist can correct their misinformation.

Dealing with Realistic Possibilities of Infection

A key educational and counseling message for healthy students is to avoid infection by engaging in low- or no-risk behaviors. The therapist should provide or reinforce information about safer practices; assist students in assessing their own risk of infection; work with them to develop assertiveness so that they can protect themselves in relationships; remind them about the possible negative effects of alcohol or other drugs on judgment in intimate situations; and confront the developmental influences of peer pressure and disavowal of risk ("it can't happen to me"). A therapist may be quite directive in encouraging risk-taking students to take precautions, and in reminding those whose behavior may create risks for others of their obligations and responsibilities.

Worries about contracting HIV infection and about practicing safer behaviors need to be explored in the context of other personal issues. For example, a woman's tearful frustration about her inability to get her boyfriend to wear condoms during intercourse may coexist with her own ambivalence about sexual activity or with anger at her dependence on the relationship. The immediate need may be for clarification of the value of the relationship and development of concrete strategies for dealing with her boyfriend. In follow-up, the therapist can explore the relationship between her self-concept and sexual expression; she may feel isolated and worthless when not in a sexual relationship. Over the longer term, it may be possible to help her define a more comfortable way to explore intimacy. A gay man reveals that he cannot seem to practice safer sex; it eventually turns out that he is often intoxicated before and during sexual activity. The therapist, after reinforcing information about the effect of alcohol on judgment, may work with the student to establish behavioral goals that exclude alcohol from potentially sexual settings, and then may pursue questions of self-esteem and alcohol dependency (Flavin, Franklin, & Frances, 1986). A male student who initially expresses his concern about being infected by his girlfriend eventually admits to having anonymous homosexual encounters; although he always wears a condom with the girlfriend, he has not taken adequate precautions with the men. Since he finds homosexuality unacceptable, he has difficulty in acknowledging these relationships sufficiently to plan for safety. The therapist will have to deal with this student's denial and guilt in order to promote consistent safety. The ability of any student to adopt reliably safer behaviors depends on self-confidence, self-esteem, and communications skills. Part of the therapeutic plan may thus include group workshops on such topics as assertiveness, communications, and stress management.

HIV Antibody Testing

A difficult question for the student worried about AIDS concerns HIV antibody testing. Although students will usually receive formal pretest and posttest counseling elsewhere in conjunction with the testing procedure, the decision of whether to pursue testing may be explored first with the college therapist. In some cases, the possibility of testing is the dominant issue in therapy; in others, it arises during the course of discussion. Dealing with antibody testing requires an understanding not only of the significance of the test's results, but also of its limitations and hazards. Blanket recommendations about testing are useless. What is required is a detailed individual assessment of two risks: first, of infection, and second, of testing. The risk of infection is assessed by reviewing the student's sexual experience, use of intravenous drugs, history of blood transfusions, and current behaviors; this discussion may be completed by others outside of therapy. The risk of testing relates to both the social hazards of testing—such as the possibility of discrimination resulting from the accidental or malicious disclosure of test results—and the psychological aftermath of the procedure (Green, 1986). A therapist should not accept a student's cavalier statement that "I can handle it." On the contrary, a series of questions should pursue important answers: "Suppose your test came back positive: What would you do? To whom would you turn for support? Whom could you safely tell? What do you think you would do differently then? Would you wish you hadn't been tested?"

Self-destructive behavior may occur following a positive test result. Most students foresee a future bright with potential and anticipate a long and healthy life uncluttered by serious problems; the limitations suggested by a positive test dramatically change this picture. "It was like the collision of two huge air masses in the summertime, one very warm and the other cold and foreboding," said one student. "They told me my test was positive, and nothing has been the same since." When the first contact is made by a student already in crisis, the therapist must intervene to establish the student's level of functioning, identify his or her coping skills, and assess the risk of self-destructive behavior. Obviously, either students in crisis should be discouraged from immediately taking the test, or they should receive intensive counseling if they go ahead with it.

It is important that neither therapist nor student see a negative result as an ultimate resolution or the elimination of worries. Students with negative tests may feel licensed to continue whatever behaviors they had pursued prior to testing, irrespective of risk; some will embrace the mythology that they are somehow "immune" to HIV. Accordingly, a negative test result should be seen as a step in therapy as opposed to a goal in itself. The therapist's important questions will include not just "How do you feel about having this negative test?", but also "What does this make you think about your previous sexual behaviors?" and "What will you do differently now that you know your test is negative?"

Fears of Casual Contagion

Some students fear casual contagion. They worry about being infected by a roommate, a mosquito, a toilet seat, or a food service employee. Certainly, the therapist's first response should be to provide information and reassurance; on the other hand, it is likely that students who reach a therapist's office suffering from anxiety, panic, or obsession about casual contagion have other issues needing attention. These fears may obscure deeper prejudice against gay people or drug users, or the influence of rigid religious or moral convictions. Sometimes these feelings stem from ambivalence and shame about a student's own sexual feelings, behaviors, or interests. The fact of covert homosexual encounters, for example, may not surface for several visits. A student's fear of "catching AIDS" from his gay roommate may, in fact, represent a reaction to unacceptable homoerotic attraction to the roommate. The therapist's approach to these students should go beyond education to inquiring why the concern exists and exploring what beliefs or experiences are relevant to the concern. The greatest challenge is often to get the student to agree to a second visit, so that deeper issues can be addressed more thoroughly.

HEALTHY STUDENTS
WHO ARE SEROPOSITIVE

Students who have positive HIV antibody tests have important adjustments to make and critical needs to be met. A positive test imposes limitations on potential. Many students initially will interpret the test result as a "death sentence," seeing it as a promise of their eventually having AIDS and dying. Their world seems turned upside down; all of the invincibility and invulnerability of youth comes crashing down with this single piece of data. Seropositive students struggle to re-establish control, preserve hope, and identify an acceptable way to live with this new information. In the process, they reconsider academic life, re-evaluate career goals, review relationships, and reassess priorities. "It was a time of hyperuncertainty," recollected one student.

Seropositive students may contact a therapist before they thoroughly understand the significance of the positive test. It is thus important to assess their level of information and to provide clarification and education. Unfortunately, much is unknown about the significance of positive results: How likely is it that a seropositive person will develop AIDS and die? How much time is there? Are there things that can be done to lower the chances of developing AIDS? Both therapist and client must accept ambiguous answers as the client begins to get used to the idea of the positive test, and living with uncertainty will become an important skill for the student later. The therapist has the difficult role of trying to keep the student in a middle position between denial of the possibility of eventual serious illness and a dysfunctional state because of worry about that possibility.

Fears

Seropositive students harbor fears, many of which are realistic. Dominant among them is the fear of transformation from health to disease, from asymptomatic seropositivity to AIDS itself, and ultimately from life to death. This fear can truncate career choices, confuse plans for graduate or professional school, and affect current and future relationships. Students struggle with deciding what current efforts and expenditures are worthwhile and meaningful in the face of an uncertain future. The therapist can help these students sort out priorities in life and move toward a workable outlook. It is particularly helpful to emphasize that decisions made today are not binding tomorrow. Continuing for the present in graduate school, for example, does not obligate one ultimately to finish the degree. Looking far to the future, seropositive students may foresee not only the ultimate outcome of AIDS, but also the process involved: the vision of disability, dependency, impoverishment, and isolation that arises not only produces great sadness, but conflicts with the ongoing developmental tasks of separation from parents, building autonomy, and establishing identity. The therapist can allow for ventilation of these fears, provide support for the strengthening of coping skills, and encourage the maturation of a sense of personal identity and value.

Seropositive students will also probably fear rejection—by parents, friends, roommates, and siblings. Stories of the painful rejection of seropositive people are everywhere. The possibility will seem particularly acute for gay men whose disclosure of seropositivity is contemporaneous with "coming out" (Forstein, 1987). The fear of rejection related to one or both secrets may delay disclosure, so that students isolate themselves from people who could provide support and understanding. The fear of rejection also may be great enough to interfere with a student's willingness to disclose seropositivity to a sexual partner, thereby potentially placing the partner at risk of infection. These threats of rejection may make seropositive students captives of their fears. Therapists should help them reach out by encouraging them to make initially limited disclosures to friends, and to discuss their concerns in settings where rejection will not occur, such as support groups for seropositive people. Therapists must also reinforce the need to protect others even when disclosing to them is painful.

Worry about Physical Symptoms

The fear of eventual transformation to AIDS often leads to hypervigilance about physical symptoms and biological rhythms and to serious upset concerning minor complaints or variations from normal (Forstein, 1987; Miller, Green, Farmer, & Carroll, 1985). Students aware of the possibility of Kaposi sarcoma will see it in every bruise, and every sneeze and cough raises anxiety about *pneumocystis* pneumonia. Therapists can help by encouraging students to identify a health care provider with whom they can develop a trusing relationship, so that questions are answered expeditiously and accurately (Forstein, 1987); over time, most seropositive students return to a calmer acceptance of physical variations as they acquire experience with their condition. A therapist's observation that most seropositive students feel the same fears at first is often very reassuring.

Anxiety

At the everyday level, seropositive students face the hourly clash of hope and fear. The emotional strain of alternating fears and hopes undermines confidence and may lead to depression and despair (Miller, 1986). The excitement of a new acquaintance, for example, may lead quickly to despair about the limited potential of the relationship. Students may respond to these conflicts by denial ("I just can't believe anything is really going to happen; I've got to live my life as if nothing is wrong") or by depression ("What's the point? Nothing I do will really matter, anyway"). Some, caught halfway between, experience anxiety and may express their psychological discomfort in apprehensiveness, irritability, or agitation. They may evidence physiological signs of anxiety, hyperventilation, or panic attacks when confronted with conflictual situations. The therapist should seek to unravel attitudes and beliefs underlying conflict, to promote gradual acceptance of the realities involved in seropositivity, and to help the student define reasonable shorter-term goals. The treatment of anxiety in the college setting commonly involves a cognitive approach emphasizing rational discussion to undermine negative, anxiety-provoking thinking; the use of anxiolytic medication for short periods may sometimes be helpful, especially when sleep is disturbed (Miller, 1986).

Anger and Guilt

Seropositive students may feel and express anger in different ways, depending on gender, family patterns, ethnicity, and cultural norms. Anger at being seropositive and infected will be joined by anger at external events, such as encounters with unsympathetic health care providers or the compromise of confidential information. Students may feel anger at God, at the persons who they believe transmitted HIV to them, or at society in general for its attitudes (Gold, Seymour, & Sahl, 1986). The therapist can work to help students to channel anger constructively—perhaps by suggesting alternate vehicles for energy, such as working with a volunteer AIDS service organization—and to eschew inappropriate or destructive anger, such as that which exposes other people to risk of transmission of the virus. The therapeutic goal is ventilation of anger without penalty, coupled with attempts to find a constructive outlet for the energy.

As they feel anger toward people who may have infected them, seropositive students feel guilt about people they may have infected. Their sense of guilt may be augmented if their behavior has not been consistent with family or religious values that prohibit premarital sexual intimacy or homosexuality. Many will lament "disappointing my family" by getting infected.

Sadness and Depression

Taken together, many of the reactions discussed above define a pervasive sense of loss and grief. Students' thoughts are dominated by their actual or potential loss of life, health, physical appearance, ability, career, academic degree, relationships, marriage, childbearing, social success, and self-esteem. The work of the therapist is to accept these fears, acknowledge the pain involved, and help the student marshal old and new coping skills. Depression itself may respond to increasing physical activity, planning social contacts, focusing on class work, and returning to known sources of relaxation and enjoyment (music, movies, dancing, sports, reading). The use of antidepressant medication is seldom necessary (Miller, 1986), but may be helpful when students have pre-existing vulnerabilities to depression or when vegetative signs are clear. Where available, support groups for seropositive people may provide additional assistance (Gold et al., 1986).

STUDENTS WITH LIMITED CLINICAL MANIFESTATIONS

Students with the early development of constitutional signs, lymphadenopathy, or minor recurrent infections typical of CLAS or ARC deal with the same fears as seropositive students, but in an accentuated and accelerated fashion. The timetable seems shorter; the possibility of terminal illness looms larger. The therapist's role at this stage is to provide support as students experience their fears, encouragement as they decide how best to use their energies, and assistance as they adjust to the limitations of chronic illness. Serious questions of academic continuation will arise and require sensitive handling.

It is during the time of ARC or CLAS that therapists will need to be especially vigilant for evidence of the organic neurological disorders associated with HIV. Neuropsychiatric illness may be the first evidence of symptomatic AIDS (Berger, Moskowitz, Fischl, & Kelley, 1987). The majority of people with ARC or AIDS eventually have neurological manifestations of infection, ranging from frank dementia (AIDS dementia complex), to subtle changes in cognition and mood, to deficits in coordination, movement, or sensation (Carne & Adler, 1987; Holland & Tross, 1985; Wolcott, 1986). The psychomotor retardation of depression may mimic the early signs of dementia; the occurrence of headaches and odd neurological symptoms may puzzle therapist and consultant alike. Whenever any question of organic neuropsychiatric disease exists, the therapist should refer the student for neuropsychiatric evaluation.

STUDENTS WITH FULL-BLOWN AIDS

The multiple losses, changes, and adjustments associated with AIDS will touch young people especially deeply. The anticipation of death and disability are real: "It's breathing down my neck now." Each student with AIDS seems to have his or her own hierarchy of losses and fears. The loss of good health, childbearing potential, independence, or good looks may seem most critical at any given time. The therapist can help by identifying the most pressing concerns and helping the student sort out which ones need therapeutic attention. Psychiatric symptoms at this stage always raise the possibility of the existence of underlying HIV infection of the central nervous system (Berger et al., 1987).

For college and university therapists, full-blown AIDS creates the necessity to deal in an immediate way with fears of death and dying. Helping students work through stages of preparation for death is unfamiliar work; since most students will have had to leave school before the final stages of illness, it will also be rare. Support groups can be valuable in anticipatory grief work. It is important to anticipate and respond effectively to the possibility of suicide; the rate of suicide among people with AIDS is much higher than that of the general population. Suicide seems to be more likely to occur if accompanied by multiple losses; intimate involvement with another person who has died of AIDS; lack of a social and financial support system; or increased dependency, pain, amd loss of control of bodily functions (Goldblum, 1987). In the face of a diagnosis of full-blown AIDS, some students have raised the issue of "being allowed" to commit suicide to permit what they believe will be death with more dignity. These requests raise complex legal, ethical, and moral dilemmas for the therapist (Goldblum & Moulton, 1987; Miller, 1986).

Medical, social, and economic realities will often dictate that students with AIDS leave school. The departure may bring a greater sense of loss and termination, and may signal the end of the therapeutic relationship. However, therapists may help by maintaining some kind of communication with students after they leave and by making referrals for further therapy.

STUDENTS CONCERNED ABOUT OTHERS

Students may benefit from therapy when significant persons in their lives have AIDS. Interventions may focus on (1) dealing with the illness, (2) grieving, and (3) addressing students' worries about the risk of contagion. Many of the same concerns felt by those with chronically ill relatives or friends will be heard in the voices of these students, but there are new concerns as well because of the stigmatization, secrecy, discrimination, and fear associated with AIDS. For example, a student who would otherwise ask for support from friends in the case of a seriously ill brother may be afraid to do so if the brother's illness is AIDS.

Therapists' work must start, again, with education—about AIDS itself; the meaning of certain symptoms, tests, or events; and the progression of disease and dying. It is important that students understand transmission of HIV, for they may be fearful for their own safety in dealing with sick persons. Therapists may recommend short published brochures or essays on maintaining compassionate relationships with people with AIDS (Beckham, Palacios, Patti, & Shernoff, 1988). Students may need to ventilate their anger or guilt about their relationship with the sick persons. As the illness progresses, they may need assistance in working through stages of grief; though the process may be greatly complicated by the stigma of AIDS, therapists can help them move toward a peaceful, affirmative view of the dying or lost persons (Shearer & McKusick, 1986). In some areas, therapists have the option of referring concerned students to a support group for people who care or grieve for persons with AIDS.

REFERENCES

Beckham, D., Palacios, L., Patti, V., & Shernoff, M. (1988). When a friend has AIDS. In S. Alyson (Ed.), *You CAN do something about AIDS* (pp. 69–71). Boston: Stop AIDS Project, Inc.

Berger, J., Moskowitz, L., Fischl, M., & Kelley, R. (1987). Neurologic disease as the presenting manifestation of the acquired immunodeficiency syndrome. *Southern Medical Journal, 80,* 683–686.

Carne, C. A., & Adler, M. M. (1987). Neurological manifestations of human immunodeficiency virus infection. *British Medical Journal, 293,* 462–463.

Faulstich. M. E. (1987). Psychiatric aspects of AIDS. *American Journal of Psychiatry, 144,* 551–556.

Flavin, D., Franklin, J., & Frances, R. (1986). AIDS and suicidal behavior in alcohol-dependent homosexual men. *American Journal of Psychiatry, 143,* 1440–1442.

Forstein, M. (1987). AIDS anxiety in the "worried well." In M. Helquist (Ed.), *Working with AIDS: A resource guide for mental health professionals* (pp. 83–107). Berkeley: University of California Press.

Gold, M., Seymour, N., & Sahl, J. (1986). Counseling HIV seropositives. In L. McKusick (Ed.), *What to do about AIDS* (pp. 103–110). Berkeley: University of California Press.

Goldblum, P. (1987). Suicide: Clinical aspects. In M. Helquist (Ed.), *Working with AIDS: A resource guide for mental health professionals* (pp. 161–166). Berkeley: University of California Press.

Goldblum, P., & Moulton, J. (1987). AIDS-related suicide: A dilemma for health care workers. In M. Helquist (Ed.), *Working with AIDS: A resource guide for mental health professionals* (pp. 157–160). Berkeley: University of California Press.

Green, J. (1986). Counseling HTLV-III seropositives. In D. Miller, J. Weber, & J. Green (Eds.), *The management of AIDS patients* (pp. 151–168). London: Macmillan.

Holland, J. O., & Tross, S. (1985). The psychosocial and neuropsychiatric sequelae of the acquired immunodeficiency syndrome and related disorders. *Annals of Internal Medicine, 103,* 760–764.

Horstman, W., & McKusick, L. (1986). The impact of AIDS on the physician. In L. McKusick (Ed.), *What to do about AIDS* (pp. 63–74). Berkeley: University of California Press.

Macks, J. (1987). Meeting the psychological needs of people with AIDS. In M. Helquist (Ed.), *Working with AIDS: A resource guide for mental health professionals* (pp. 1–28). Berkeley: University of California Press.

Miller, D. (1986). Psychology, AIDS, ARC, and PGL. In D. Miller, J. Weber, & J. Green (Eds.), *The management of AIDS patients* (pp. 131–150). London: Macmillan.

Miller, D., Green, J., Farmer, R., & Carroll, G. (1985). A "pseudo-AIDS" syndrome following from fear of AIDS. *British Journal of Psychiatry, 146,* 550–552.

Shearer, P. & McKusick, L. (1986). Counseling survivors. In L. McKusick (Ed.), *What to do about AIDS* (pp. 163–172). Berkeley: University of California Press.

Wolcott, D. (1986). Neuropsychiatric syndromes in AIDS and AIDS-related illnesses. In L. McKusick (Ed.), *What to do about AIDS* (pp. 32–44). Berkeley: University of California Press.

14

Anorexia Nervosa and Bulimia Nervosa

RANDOLPH M. LEE

Most psychotherapists who work with college students would agree that the disorders or symptom patterns that have shown the most dramatic increase over the past decade are the eating disorders: anorexia nervosa and bulimia nervosa. Relatively rare on college and university campuses as late as the early 1960s, primary anorexia nervosa can be diagnosed in 0.25–0.50% of college-age women, and primary bulimia nervosa in 5% according to conservative (though wide-ranging) estimates (see, e.g., Andersen, 1985; Garfinkel & Garner, 1982; Johnson & Connors, 1987; Mitchell & Eckert, 1987). Approximately 90% of cases are women; among males with diagnosed eating disorders, more are bulimic than anorectic. Clearly, eating disorders have become a significant problem on most college campuses, and they confront the college psychotherapist with an abundance of challenging and complex issues.

Although there are obviously differences between anorexia nervosa and bulimia nervosa, there are also significant similarities with regard to referral, diagnosis, psychodynamics, and treatment. In this chapter I describe a treatment approach that is essentially applicable to both anorexia and bulimia. Of course, it is important to recognize that treatment planning must be adapted to the individual patient, and there should be differences in treatment between some anorectic and bulimic patients, just as there should be differences in treatment among different anorectic individuals. But the psychodynamic aspects of anorexia nervosa and bulimia nervosa are sufficiently similar that treatment of both in a college environment can be meaningfully described together.

Although other disorders involving food and eating also confront the college psychotherapist (e.g., obesity), the focus in this chapter is exclusively on anorexia nervosa and bulimia nervosa. Also, although as many as 10% of these patients are male, for the sake of simplicity the female pronouns "she" and "her" are used in referring to these individuals.

Anorexia nervosa and bulimia nervosa are each symptom complexes—patterns of symptoms that typically occur together and represent consistent themes or conflicts, such as identity, control, suppression of affect (especially anger), and ambivalence about maturity. These symptom complexes and the underlying conflicts have biological, societal, interpersonal, and individual components; effective treatment must address each of these aspects. A brief description of each follows.

The importance of the biological aspect of anorexia or bulimia is demonstrated by the health risks from starvation, cardiac damage, tooth and bone decay, and laxative and diuretic abuse (to mention but a few), which make medical monitoring and coordination an important part of therapeutic planning. At the same time, other physical concomitants of the disorders (loss of menstruation, emaciation, exhaustion, etc.) often have to be dealt with in the course of psychotherapy. Although these issues are relevant to treatment of eating disorders in any context, they are often magnified in the college environment, where parents are usually not around to monitor health changes and peers may have neither the influence nor the motivation to alert anyone to potential health crises in a student. The therapist, then, is often in the difficult position of being *in loco parentis* as well as therapist—a conflict fraught with transferential and defensive implications.

The societal aspects of eating disorders are particularly significant in the college environment. There is virtual unanimity among researchers that one of the major reasons for the increase in eating disorders is the societal pressure to be thin. This aspect of our society is well documented (e.g., Bruch, 1978; Garfinkel & Garner, 1982; Schwartz, Thompson, & Johnson, 1982) and needs no repetition here. It hardly requires a major leap of logic to recognize that a college campus, with its great density of adolescents, is a ripe environment for a magnification of this pressure and provides additional problems in the identification and treatment of these individuals.

The individual and interpersonal components of eating disorders entail a complex chain of consequences, involving early conflicts and psychodynamic precursors of the problem, the current manifestation of these conflicts, and the effect of these manifestations on other people. Although this chain exists in greater or lesser measure in any emotional disorder, we shall see that it takes on some unique and potent dimensions in anorectic and bulimic patients. Furthermore, one of the perplexing and therapeutically troublesome aspects of eating disorders is that the symptoms of anorexia or bulimia may reflect a relatively mild dysthymia or other neurotic pattern, a more pervasive characterological problem, or a full-blown psychotic disorder, even though the initial presentation and appearance of the patient may be quite similar in all three cases.

CRITERIA AND TERMINOLOGY

The significant increase during the past decade or so in the number of patients presenting with eating disorders has led to terminological and diagnostic confusion. Different criteria and terminology (e.g., "bulimarexia," Boskind-Lodahl, 1978; Boskind-White & White, 1983) have appeared in various sources. Furthermore, the increased public attention to eating disorders has itself had a direct effect on the diagnostic criteria of the disorders by facilitating earlier recognition and identification of affected individuals. The third edition of the *Diagnostic and Statistical Manual of Mental Disorders* (DSM-III; American Psychiatric Association, 1980) requires, among other criteria, "weight loss of at least 25% of original body weight" (p. 69). But public and media attention has become so widespread, and so many anorectic women are identified before their weight loss has reached the DSM-III criterion, that the revised third edition (DSM-III-R; American Psychiatric Association, 1987) reduces the criterion to 15% and uses that figure only as an example of "minimal normal weight for age and height" (p. 67). Similarly, DSM-III lists the diagnosis of Bulimia, while DSM-III-R changes it to Bulimia Nervosa, with substantially revised criteria to reflect current patterns. Additional confusion arises in that DSM-III-R excludes from the diagnosis of Bulimia Nervosa "a person of average weight who does not have binge eating episodes, but frequently engages in self-induced vomiting for fear of gaining weight." Likewise, a woman with "all of the features of Anorexia Nervosa . . . except absence of menses" is not diagnosed as having Anorexia Nervosa. Both cases are diagnosed as Eating Disorders Not Otherwise Specified (p. 71).

The rapid increase in the prevalence of these disorders (particularly among college-age individuals), the sociology of their growing public attention, and the large amount of research being undertaken have thus created some understandable confusion that is not likely to subside immediately. Because of this confusion, it is important to establish a common frame of reference in discussing these disorders. Although DSM-III-R is not without flaws, it does provide a useful framework, and therefore in this discussion I use its criteria:

1. The diagnosis of Anorexia Nervosa requires refusal to maintain normal body weight with a weight maintenance at least 15% below normal. At the same time, the patient feels an intense fear of gaining weight or becoming fat and disturbances in the way she experiences weight, size, or shape. Finally, the diagnosis requires the absence of at least three consecutive menstrual periods (American Psychiatric Association, 1987).

2. The diagnosis of Bulimia Nervosa requires recurrent episodes of binge eating with a sense of loss of control over eating during the binges, regular use of either self-induced vomiting, laxatives or diuretics, dieting or fasting, or vigorous exercise. Also required is a minimum of two binge episodes per week over a period of at least 3 months and excessive concern with body shape and weight (American Psychiatric Association, 1987).

The DSM-III-R has the advantages of providing a common reference point for this discussion and reflecting the changing pattern of eating disorders in our society. Its major disadvantage is its focus on symptoms to the exclusion of dynamics. The college psychotherapist is cautioned that effective treatment is dependent not only on correct diagnosis of the eating disorder, but also on the pattern and intensity of the underlying psychopathology.

One final issue should be mentioned in the context of symptoms. Given the extensive publicity and awareness of eating disorders on college campuses today, the college psychotherapist must be cautious not to "overdiagnose" eating disorders, thereby perhaps missing important but unrelated pathology. Many college students who occasionally engage in self-induced vomiting are not truly bulimic; many who periodically engage in severe dieting are not anorectic. Particularly in a college environment, these behaviors may be transient attempts to "lose a few pounds," or they may be manifestations of mild anxiety. Alternatively, these symptoms may be semiconscious ways of getting attention or providing a rationale for going to the college mental health service, since symptoms of an eating disorder are an "acceptable" reason to their peers (or themselves). Careful initial evaluation sometimes reveals that eating disorder symptoms mask other pathology that simply could not be faced.

For example, Lauren, a 19-year-old sophomore, presented with bulimic symptoms, saying that she could not stop forcing herself to vomit after eating dinner with her sorority sisters. The purging, she said, did not occur while she was at home, but had persisted for over 3 months during the spring semester. By the end of the second session, she was able to identify and acknowledge the severe anxiety and guilt she felt over her sexual attraction to one of her sorority sisters.

As she began to work in therapy on her guilt and anxiety, the vomiting symptoms stopped completely after three sessions.

THEORETICAL OVERVIEW

It is important to consider the developmental context of anorexia nervosa and bulimia nervosa. These disorders usually emerge symptomatically in adolescence but represent conflicts that originated in early childhood. In psychodynamic terms, the symptom complex of both anorexia and bulimia represent a desperate attempt by the individual to maintain or regain a sense of control and independence over herself and her world by visible, rigid control of her body. A number of authors have described the presymptomatic picture of the anorectic or bulimic individual (e.g., Bruch, 1978; Levenkron, 1985), and there exists reasonable consensus among most psychotherapists about the general pattern. Let us consider this theoretical picture in some detail.

Prior to the manifestations of anorectic or bulimic symptoms in adolescence, the behavioral pattern of the young woman is appropriately described by Levenkron (1978) as that of "the best little girl in the world." Although there are, of course, great variations, typically she is a relatively well-educated girl from an upper-middle-class family; she is often the eldest child and less often an only child of parents who present an external picture of relative stability. Both her parents are probably quite intelligent and achievement-oriented. In fact, there may be a subtle competition between her parents with regard to achievement, although it rarely emerges in overt conflict. Her father may compensate for his possible perception of himself as second best by looking for external sources of support and validation. Thus, not only is his home frequently painted and his grass always carefully mowed, but he may like to show off his beautiful (thin!) wife and children. He may report with obvious pleasure that his daughter got four A's last term and has the lead in the school musical. Conflicts of any kind are dealt with internally, with as little outward display as possible. As Bruch (1978) notes, "these girls come from homes that make a good first impression. Everything a girl can need for her physical well being and intellectual development has been provided" (p. 23).

Both parents are loving and are very eager for their daughter to succeed, a fact that they convey in subtle ways. In contrast to a parent who angrily demands to know why there are B's on the grade report, the parents of the presymptomatic daughter are more likely to say, "Honey, it makes us so happy to tell our friends about your wonderful grades!" Because of her great desire to please and her keen ability to pick up subtle cues about what people want from her, the young girl complies fully with her parents. She satisfies their needs for success and is never a problem. She hides her "bad" feelings; does not cry; helps her mother with the baby without question or (conscious) jealousy; needs very little discipline; and generally helps her family to stay outwardly successful, calm, harmonious, and loving—until she becomes symptomatic.

These pleasing and compliant behaviors grow out of conflicts about control, separateness, autonomy, dependence, and nurturance—conflicts that typically begin before the second year of life, when the child is beginning to get a sense of herself as a separate person. These conflicts may be due to particular inadequacies in mothering. The child's mother may have had difficulties being emotionally nurturant because of her own conflicts and concerns; she may have had difficulty accepting her daughter's separateness because of her own insecurities (see, e.g., Rizzuto, Peterson, & Reed, 1981). Often, the nurturing process was for some reason not rewarding to the mother, so she turned to more visible forms of support. In other words, she may have valued behaviors in her daughter that demonstrated the success at mothering she could not feel, and she may have gradually, subliminally conveyed these needs and conflicts to her daughter.

Bruch (1973) describes similar patterns as etiologically significant. She suggests that a failure to develop automony because of overcontrol and/or intrusiveness may lead to an oversocialized, caretaking, obedient, compliant mask as a defense against intrusion. This pattern, Bruch believes, leads to ego deficits that emerge later in adolescence, a time of life that requires increasing independence—something the child cannot tolerate.

Thus, the girl has learned, as Levenkron puts it, that "in order to get love, I must avoid needing love" (1985, p. 235). As she is growing up, she is often sought out by her family for advice ("Where shall we go today?", "What shall we have for dinner?"). This reinforces her sense that she is pleasing and caretaking, but it also reinforces her belief that she should not bother her parents with her own needs, since she is being "good" for not having any! She comforts herself by ordering her external world through rigid control. She wears a mask, or a "full-time persona" (Levenkron, 1985, p. 237), to cover the inner feelings of dyscontrol that she cannot express. She has learned to feel organized, in control, able to take care of her family, and able to avoid "disruptive" emotions (such as anger, resentment, and sadness). She has learned to be perfect.

These psychological factors may manifest themselves in any number of ways. One of the most important reasons why they sometimes present as eating disorders is the current sociocultural emphasis upon thinness and bodily attractiveness as criteria of "perfection." Although the underlying dynamics are far from new, the emphasis upon thinness and dieting in recent years has played a significant role in determining the symptoms.

For years, this pattern may go along quite smoothly. The girl does well, meeting the subtle needs and demands of her parents while feeling protected as the good child of loving parents; seemingly, she is fully in control. The onset of the eating disorder symptoms typically occurs at a time of major change in the girl's life—a change that requires independence on her part and thus upsets her precarious balance of control and protection. The change may be puberty itself, bringing with it awareness of bodily changes and sexual development. It may be graduation from high school, the beginning or breakup of an adolescent love affair, the beginning of college and consequent separation from her family, serious illness in herself or a member of her family, or death of a loved one. Or it may be a superficially innocuous event that triggers a strong flood of emotion, which she cannot experience directly but instead transfers to her body image.

For example, Melissa was an actively anorectic 19-year-old sophomore who recalled that her first real diet, and the initiation of her compulsive starvation, occurred while she was vacationing on the Maine coast with her mother and brother. Her father had been away on business and arrived at the cabin 2 weeks into the vacation. After greeting his wife and son, he turned to Melissa, who was standing in a bathing suit, and "affectionately" exclaimed, "Hi, thunder thighs!" She lost 38 pounds that summer.

Because the girl's strength and control have been so tenuous and so dependent upon her ability to keep her life perfect and ordered, any loss of control or difficulty in coping with changes is frightening and overwhelming. An obsessional diet or self-induced vomiting become immediate means of regaining control, methods in which she retains total mastery. As the diet (or vomiting) continues, she develops a new measure of success and control that is not dependent on the wishes and demands of others. She is, in her own eyes, really free for the first time, not having to answer to anyone. She sees herself as confronting the world and directly acting for herself, not her parents. Appeals to gain weight (in the case of the anorectic) or to stop bingeing and vomiting (in the case of the bulimic) simply increase her resolve. She has unconsciously found a way to stop having to please her parents, and even to express her anger at them and others. But she is doing more than just expressing long-suppressed affect at her family; she is also expressing her own drive for selfhood—her own identity—even though in a self-destructive fashion.

It is at this point, facing these issues of control and intense anger, that the college psychotherapist must begin to work.

REFERRAL AND PRESENTATION ISSUES

Referral for treatment of patients with eating disorders is frequently quite different in a college health service than in other settings, for a number of reasons. The younger adolescent who is living at home is frequently brought for help by her increasingly worried parents, or she is referred by her pediatrician or family practitioner following a general medical examination. The college student, however, is ofter away from home, typically living in a dormitory environment where no one may notice her continued weight loss or her increasingly frequent and clandestine vomiting.

Even more complicated and problematic is the fact that, for a while, college peers may support and even envy their anorectic friend's ability to lose weight and be "so good about dieting." The bulimic woman's peers may provide attention and support for her ability to eat as she pleases without gaining weight. They are, of course, unaware of her trips to the bathroom following each meal to purge herself of the food. In one extreme case, Cathy, a bulimic 20-year-old junior, had made a careful study of virtually all the public bathrooms on campus and could tell which ones were most likely to be vacant at any given time of day. Based on this, she planned which direction to walk after meals to minimize the likelihood of interruption during her vomiting purges.

Another factor that makes the referral process more complicated in the college environment is that many students with eating disorders, particularly anorectics, are campus "stars." These "best little girls" have grown into very competent athletes (especially in track and cross-country); excellent performers in drama, music, and dance productions; and academic successes. Eating-disordered students are usually over-represented on dean's lists and among those graduating with honors.

Anorectic students are almost never self-referred. Most frequently they are referred by an athletic coach or a faculty advisor or through the college health service, where they have gone because of some (usually related) medical problem. In some cases, friends are successful in getting an anorectic student to appear at the mental health service, often by literally coming with the student to the session. This practice may be very helpful in establishing initial rapport.

Bulimic students are more likely than anorectic students to seek help on their own, sometimes acknowledging that they have an eating disorder, other times presenting other problems and concerns without mentioning the bulimic symptoms at all. In many cases the bulimic is so fearful, ashamed, and embarrassed by her symptomatic behavior that she will go to great lengths to hide it from everyone. Jeanette, for instance, reported in therapy that she was so embarrassed by her compulsion to binge that she would go to bed at the same time as her roommates and lie awake until they had gone to sleep. She would then crawl across the room and into the hallway where she would rummage through the trash in search of discarded pizza crusts, since she was too fearful of discovery to hide food in her room.

Whereas the anorectic student often sincerely believes that she does not have a problem and therefore needs no help, the bulimic is so painfully aware of her problem, and often so disgusted by it, that she simply cannot confide in anyone. She is sure that any revelation will lead to public ridicule and rejection and to the total dissolution of the shaky facade of self-esteem that she has struggled to erect.

PRETREATMENT: THE EARLY SESSIONS
AND MEDICAL MONITORING

For both the anorectic and the bulimic student, the early sessions are crucial, perhaps even more so than in other problems in college psychotherapy. Because the student is often invested (consciously or unconsciously) in the denial of her symptoms, the therapist must be able to establish rapport quite quickly, to convey concern and awareness of the problems facing the student, and yet to do so without confronting the student's denial so much that she does not return. This is particularly troublesome with the anorectic student, whose symptoms are ego-syntonic. She sees no reason to change eating patterns that provide her with attention; that at least initially affirm her looks and figure; and that give her a growing sense of control and power over herself and against those who would, in her eyes, run her life.

For the bulimic, it is also important not to confront the denial too early, but not because the symptoms are ego-syntonic. Rather, the reason is the intensity of shame and humiliation she feels. The therapist must express concern but must be careful not to humiliate the patient into a defensive retreat.

The first question to be addressed, of course, is that of the student's medical condition and physical health. Regardless of professional affiliation, theoretical orientation, or treatment approach, the college psychotherapist must recognize that these conditions have serious, potentially fatal physiological concomitants. The bulimic student can (and usually does) appear quite healthy, and the anorectic student in the relatively early stages may simply appear stylishly slender. Nevertheless, the range of potential problems is vast, and the importance of early and periodic medical monitoring cannot be overstated. Medical correlates of starvation, purging, and laxative abuse are well documented (Brownell & Foreyt, 1986; Garfinkel & Garner, 1982). Medical monitoring is particularly significant in the college environment, especially when the student is away from home. If her family does have a regular family practicioner, he or she is not likely to be close enough to provide ongoing monitoring. Even if the family physician is available, the association that the physician has with the patient's family may obviate any kind of effective relationship with the student. Furthermore, the college therapist may be seen as another person in collusion because of his or her communication with the family practitioner.

The more desirable model is for the nonmedical psychotherapist to have an established relationship with a professional, preferably within the college environment (such as through the college medical service). This individual can perform an initial physical examination, coordinate laboratory testing, and provide regular weigh-ins and follow-up examinations, whose frequency should be related to the severity of the symptoms.

Many therapists believe that more direct involvement in a patient's health, and especially her weight, is important. Some have scales in their offices and begin each session by weighing the patient. However, this practice imbues the psychotherapy session with an anxiety-provoking "challenge" and sets up exactly the same struggle for control that the individual has faced at home. It might be argued that such a transferential battle permits a working through of the struggle in the session, but in my opinion it raises the level of denial and affective suppression without allowing effective resolution of the conflicts.

In addition to initiating therapeutic rapport and discussing the necessity of medical monitoring, the early sessions are the time to establish the ground rules for treatment in the college mental health service. The issue of ground rules can be tricky. They must be established early in the course of treatment, yet their introduction before the student is willing to acknowledge her problem can impede or eliminate an effective working alliance. The early discussion of ground rules not only is important medically, but also demonstrates that the therapist does indeed know what he or she is doing; the patient will not be left to flounder in the confusion that she already feels (although she could never admit this at the time). Although ground rules may vary, I have found the following to be effective, expressed orally and modified as necessary: (1) The student agrees to an initial physical examination (including blood and other laboratory testing as recommended by the medical professional) and to regular weigh-ins and/or checkups, as recommended; (2) the student gives authorization for the psychotherapist to communicate with the medical professional about the medical monitoring; and (3) the psychotherapist agrees to maintain confidentiality (in accordance with state and federal law and professional ethics) regarding the treatment, and to provide treatment on an outpatient basis as long as the student is not at medical risk that requires hospitalization. We also explain to the student that her parents will not be notified without her consent (assuming she is of legal age), and that although they do not need to be involved in the treatment, we may decide, if she agrees, to involve them later to some extent.

This point represents a departure from some other approaches to eating-disordered patients, and deserves elaboration. Although parental interaction in early childhood is significant in the later development of eating disorders, it is important to develop treatment strategies that do not require current parental involvement. One obvious reason is that the college psychotherapist often does not have the student's family close at hand and so cannot easily involve them. Also, since many college students have effectively left home, planning to return again only occasionally at holidays, the need to deal with current parental issues is less pressing. Of course, there remains the need to deal with psychodynamic issues involving parents.

TYPOLOGY OF EATING DISORDERS

Before beginning the actual treatment process, the college psychotherapist must make an assessment of the level of psychopathology in the student, since a relatively mild neurotic pathology and a severely disturbed psychotic-like pathology may present relatively similar initial symptom patterns, either in bulimic or anorectic form. One of the most frequent mistakes with eating-disordered students arises from underestimation of the level of psychopathology. Because these students are well practiced at pleasing others and maintaining effective, affable personas, and because often they are bright, they are frequently better able to mask their disturbances than students coping with, say, dysthymia or anxiety. Despite their facade of sophistication, many of these students have poor ego strength and employ relatively primitive defenses such as splitting.

Denise, a college junior, was an honors English major. She was also an accomplished vocalist and actress, winning the lead in several musicals and ensemble performances. Yet she was actually a quite severely disturbed anorectic. Although emaciated, she complained about her "pregnant" stomach. She had reduced her food intake gradually, and now would eat only "white" foods; other colors, she felt, were bad. She had virtually no sense of herself as a separate person, alternating between being totally fused with her boyfriend and then with her parents. When one was "good" the other was "bad," and vice versa. She literally could not report a feeling that was hers, saying instead, for example, "What should I feel?", or parroting a phrase used by her mother or her boyfriend, often expressed through teary whining very much like that of a young child.

Treatment of the eating-disordered student depends on her level of disturbance. Although the severity of disturbance falls along a continuum, two general types can be identified.

The first type—the ego-intact student—can form at least reasonably effective interpersonal relationships. She has some sense of herself as a separate entity, though she is often unable to function separately. When her manifest identity is challenged, she experiences anger and avoidance, but she stays relatively well organized in regard to ego functions. This patient seems to choose among elements of several reasonably functional "selves" (the compliant and dutiful daughter, the somewhat rebellious child, etc.). She is often aware of her intense need to please and of the dangers of doing so, yet finds herself unable to avoid acting this way. She is both compliant and manipulative. For example, she might gain 10 pounds in 2 weeks "for the therapist" if asked to do so, but she would then immediately lose the weight again. Overall, this student is far from emotionally healthy and is therapeutically difficult, but her ego structure is at least partly engaged in containing external stress.

The second type—the ego-fragmented student—functions with a much less intact ego structure and more primitive object relations. She has little or no sense of herself as a separate object. Her identity at a surface level is bound up in a sense of herself as good, successful, and thin, but even this tenuous identity crumbles when she is pushed past simply being compliant. She is almost totally a mask, with almost nothing behind it. Her focus is on controlling internal stress and the threat of immediate disintegration. It is as if she is desperately holding together a very fragile personality organization that threatens to disintegrate with the slightest conflict. Whereas the ego-intact student copes largely with external stress and its internal neurotic elaborations, the ego-fragmented student holds off a psychotic decompensation. Wheras the ego-intact patient may gain weight "for the therapist," the ego-fragmented anorectic simply cannot gain the weight without total disorganization. Most important, whereas the symptomatology for the ego-intact patient is the manifestation of a neurotic conflict, the eating disorder for the ego-fragmented patient may actually be her highest level of functioning, allowing her to stay in touch with the external world, deal with its social pressures, and permit limited but ongoing relationships.

Denise, in the example given above, is an example of the ego-fragmented type; she had virtually no sense of herself as a separate object. The following example demonstrates how the symptoms of a less severely disturbed, ego-intact patient manifested a neurotic conflict triggered by early sexual abuse. Alice, a sophomore, had been bulimic on and off since becoming sexually active at the age of 16. For months her symptoms would almost completely subside, and then for weeks or months the bingeing and purging would occur almost daily. Her basic ego structure was intact. After several months of psychotherapy, she was able to talk about an uncle who, between the time she was 9 and 11, lay on top of her and simulated intercourse, then forced her to masturbate him. Her vague awareness of her own arousal triggered extreme guilt, and she was able to recognize in therapy that the bingeing created a sensation of abdominal pressure similar to the experience of having her uncle on top of her. Her violent, self-abusive purging emerged as a way of re-enacting the abusive situation and neurotically alleviating the associated guilt.

Although an extended discussion of assessment is beyond the scope of this chapter, we should mention that standard projective tests reveal several clear distinctions between ego-intact and ego-fragmented students. For example, figure drawings from ego-intact patients tend to be infantilized and childlike, almost as if drawn by a 5-year-old. The drawings of ego-fragmented patients tend to be more psychotic, sometimes with bodies separated from heads, ghostlike features, and severe distortions. Rorschach protocols also show some striking differences. Ego-intact protocols appear more neurotic, with identity and boundary issues predominating; ego-fragmented protocols appear disintegrated and more characteristic of schizophrenic thought. The literature in this area is growing rapidly (see, e.g., Shapiro, 1986).

PSYCHOTHERAPY

Although there are important differences in the treatment of anorectic and bulimic students, and in the treatment of ego-intact and ego-fragmented students, many aspects of the process are essentially the same. Inasmuch as both anorexia nervosa and bulimia nervosa are symptom complexes that have similar etiological and psychodynamic elements, it follows that the stages of therapy are more or less parallel. In this discussion, the assumption is made that students are both medically and psychologically stable enough to be seen on an outpatient basis in the college mental health service. Futhermore, it is assumed that students' primary symptom complex involves the eating disorder, not, say, a major depression or a dysthymic disorder with some secondary anorectic or bulimic symptoms. Treatment of these latter students may be similar in ways, but is not directly discussed in this chapter.

Early Treatment Issues

I begin with an elaboration on early treatment issues in light of the two types of eating disorders. As I have suggested, the primary focus of the early sessions must be on establishing rapport and trust. The therapist must bear in mind that this student has not really been able to trust anyone for most of her life. In the ego-fragmented (more severely disturbed) patient, object-relations deficits have been substantial, and therefore the therapist working with this type of young woman must be prepared for a long period of resistance. The student sees any attempt by the therapist to establish a relationship through friendliness or support as an intrusion, a hostile or controlling gesture designed to manipulate her into eating or stopping the binge–purge cycle. By contrast, in the ego-intact patient, the establishment of the early relationship can become almost a game. Since her anger and need for control are more on the surface, she frequently attempts to engage the therapist in a manipulative battle of words and wills. She at once avoids, deflects, and pleases, telling the therapist the things she knows he or she wants to hear. The therapist at this point seems to be nothing more than another parent who will do whatever is necessary in order to get her to submit regarding food and eating. She sees herself as finally having freed herself from the controlling forces of her past; she has discovered something that no one can force her to do, no matter what, and this resolve has become the keystone of her distorted sense of herself. For this reason, the therapist must avoid being parental—explaining how much she is hurting herself by starving or bingeing and purging, or telling her that he or she wants to help her be able to eat "normally," or even telling her that she needs help. Doing so diminishes the likelihood of success.

The task of these early sessions is to convey a willingness to understand the student, a respect for her need for control, and an understanding that her perceptions are indeed the way she sees things; she is not lying or kidding or trying to be stubborn. The therapist must also convey that the goal is not to force her to gain weight or eat normally—indeed, it is not to force her to do anything—but to help her feel more at peace with herself. This approach, important with either the ego-intact or the ego-fragmented patient, will frequently elicit complaints about others (parents, coaches, doctors, friends, etc.), all of whom, she reports, will not leave her alone when she is quite able to take care of herself.

Thus, a delicate balance is required. The patient wants to be reassured that the therapist can be of help. She does not want to be left alone with her inner confusion and chaos. At the same time, given her difficulty in accepting nurturance or intimacy from anyone, she needs to be sure that the therapist is not going to "take over." Being caught like this between Scylla and Charybdis is almost always extremely frustrating for the therapist. From the beginning, the patient tells the therapist what he or she wants to hear, yet withdraws with scornful contempt and subtle ridicule if the therapist believes it. If the therapist confronts the manipulative (and often unconscious) compliance, the patient denies and again withdraws, protecting herself from transferred parental intrusion. Heads she wins, tails the therapist loses!

The college psychotherapist faces these problems even more than the private practitioner. Because the psychotherapist is an employee of the college, the student may perceive him or her as a controlling authority, which damages the therapeutic relationship. This transference issue is magnified when the therapist is also active on campus as a faculty member, speaker, or trainer of resident assistants. It is, therefore, of extreme importance that the confidentiality of the relationship be discussed fully and completely early in the therapy process. It may well make sense to define "rules" with regard to these roles. For example, it is virtually always unwise to allow a bulimic or anorectic student to enroll in a course taught by the college psychotherapist during the time of treatment. Although this transference issue applies to college psychotherapy generally, the eating-disordered student's heightened concerns in regard to control and autonomy, and the danger of underestimating such a student's level of psychopathology, lend these considerations increased significance.

The final issue with regard to early treatment concerns the activity level of the psychotherapist. Although the patient seems vigorously determined to maintain her sense of order and control and to resist any intrusion by the therapist, she is also a frightened little girl underneath, afraid that she will "blow it." Having had to "take care of things" in her family while growing up (in the case of the anorectic), she will be overwhelmed now if the therapist also looks to her for direction. With the ego-intact patient, this can reduce the effectiveness of the therapeutic alliance. With the ego-fragmented anorectic, the result can be decompensation and more rapid retreat into food avoidance. It is important, therefore, that the therapist be relatively active, verbal, and involved, especially in the early sessions. Placing the primary responsibility for leading the session on the student not only places her in the position of having to please the therapist (since that is her way of relating), but it also confronts her with the frightening realization that she is still alone and even her therapist needs her to take charge.

Of course, the therapist's activity must be supportive and reflect issues that the student is willing and able to discuss. Asking questions, pressing for elaboration, and encouraging verbalizations are all appropriate interventions. In these early sessions there should be little or no confrontation, especially concerning eating or the expression of emotions. These areas need not be avoided, particularly if they are raised be the patient, but applying pressure will probably lead to quick termination of psychotherapy.

Course of Therapy

The central task of therapy is to help the anorectic or bulimic student to understand how her control of her physical body (which has now become dyscontrol) represents a distorted attempt to defend against the depression, confusion, disorganization, and anxiety that she feels as a consequence of low self-worth. These students need to recognize, as Bruch (1985) puts it,

> the extent to which they have always done what they had thought they were supposed to do, repressing their genuine development. As a matter of fact, the encouraged "good" behavior can be recognized as an important source of maldevelopment. Faked and make-believe expressions and reactions are praised as if they were genuine, with the result that the ability to differentiate between genuine and pretended feelings does not develop. The task of therapy is to help patients discover their genuine selves, and what is valid about themselves. (p. 15)

Various theoretical orientations have been used to treat eating-disordered patients. Although the literature suggests that classical psychoanalysis is not usually effective, modified psychoanalytic approaches have been used with success (e.g., Wilson, 1983). Some therapists, most notably Levenkron (1985), employ a "nurturant–authoritative" model or a systems perspective (Minuchin, Rosman, & Baker, 1978; Root, Fallon, & Friedrich, 1986), whereas a growing number of professionals (e.g., Agras, 1987; Garner & Bemis, 1985; Weiss, Katzman, & Wolchik, 1985) believe that cognitive–behavioral techniques are required to change the eating pattern, especially with bulimic students. Garner and

Garfinkel (1985) provide an excellent survey of approaches to psychotherapy with these patients.

Regardless of approach, the special circumstances of the college environment influence the course of therapy. In the college setting, the course of therapy—after the pretreatment stage discussed earlier—can be divided into four stages; of course, the stages in practice are overlapping and not mutually exclusive.

Stage 1—Relationship Development

Following the preliminary work of treatment, the first stage of therapy, relationship development, involves an extension and deepening of these early treatment issues. The anorectic or bulimic student takes a much longer time than other students to recognize that the therapist is indeed her ally and not a deceptive agent of her parents or the college. She needs to be listened to, taken seriously, and valued, and this process is neither quick nor easy.

Particularly with the ego-fragmented patient, powerful countertransference feelings almost inevitably emerge. The frustration, anger, and feelings of helplessness, impotence, and failure that eating-disordered individuals elicit can be overwhelming. So often, for example, the student seems to be developing a working therapeutic alliance. She starts talking about feelings and how much better she is doing, yet with consistency and determination she continues to lose weight or to binge and purge. The passive–aggressive manipulation that so angers and frustrates others now comes out in full force toward her therapist, triggering countertransferential rage in even the strongest psychotherapist's ego. On a primitive level, the psychotherapist feels, "How can she do this to me when I'm trying so hard, with all my clinical experience and empathy, to help her?" It is important for the psychotherapist to realize that it is not just countertransference creating the intense feelings; the patient's extensive projective identification clearly triggers the anger and frustration.

As suggested earlier, the patient will tell the therapist what he or she wants to hear. Is the therapist interested in dreams? The eating-disordered patient will report (probably quite accurately and honestly) some intense, symbolic, and salient dreams. If the therapist presses for expression of feeling, he or she will be rewarded with crying, rage, or exuberance. If it is intellectual insight that the therapist subtly asks for, the student (who may have read as much about her disorder as the therapist) may interpret her behavior *ad nauseam*. Again, she has been successful at being compliant; she is the epitome of the Woody Allen character Zelig in the film of the same name. As Cohler (1977) points out, therapy with an anorectic "leads to intense emotional reactions in the therapist, perhaps the most intense encountered in any therapeutic relationship" (p. 353).

Staying with the patient emotionally; continuing to provide consistent, noncondescending, affirming attention; being honest and direct; and setting firm limits usually permit the gradual emergence of a trusting relationship in the ego-intact patient, and at least a working alliance in the ego-fragmented patient.

Stage 2—Affect

The eating-disordered student, particularly the ego-fragmented patient, does not know what she is feeling. She can recognize internal states, almost as sensory fragments, but she cannot put them into words. For this reason, the therapeutic process at this stage involves the identification of internal emotional experiences and their differentiation from physiological states and experiences. In the more severely disturbed student, this process can take months as she learns to discriminate, for example, the sensation of tightness in her stomach from the associated feelings of anger or anxiety or sadness. Ultimately, the goal of this stage is not only to allow the student to experience her emotions, but to connect these feelings to events and people, now and in the past.

We can see here one reason for accurate assessment of the level of severity. In the ego-intact patient, too little confrontation about feelings can lead to failure. She can tolerate being shown her manipulation; in fact, this confrontation is necessary in order for her to feel understood and accepted. She starts therapy with a sense of herself, and the threat of ego disintegration is not severe. The ego-fragmented individual, however, cannot deal with confrontation; too much of it, in fact, leads to failure. She needs time to identify and accept herself as a feeling individual before she can cope with the effect those feelings have on others, and vice versa. Her projective defenses simply cannot be bulldozed when there is little or nothing to replace them.

Stage 3—Reality

As the eating-disordered student gains increasing familiarity (if not always comfort) with her feelings, and as she learns to individuate her internal feeling states from other experiences (a task of far greater magnitude in the ego-fragmented person), she is increasingly able to confront reality distortions that have been so central to her functioning. This third stage comes sooner in the ego-intact patient, though there is a danger of assuming that she can handle these reality confrontations before she is ready. The issues in this stage involve both cognitive and perceptual distortions. Examples of the former are as follows: "I am either fat or I am thin"; "Life is black or white"; "I am totally chaste or promiscuous"; "My weight is the best measure of my self-worth"; "I must be perfect or no one will like me"; "Others' expectations for me are more important than my own"; and "My parents are beyond reproach in all matters." The perceptual distortions primarily center on the anorectic's view of herself as fat, even when she is physiologically emaciated. She actually does not see herself as thin, and believes that the calories in a normal meal will make her fat. These perceptual distortions cannot be confronted until well into the therapeutic process, following considerable progress in the first two stages.

Stage 4—Dynamics

Although the dynamics of the eating disorder unfold gradually throughout the therapeutic process, and discussions about family issues, control, anger, self-respect, and self-esteem appear in all stages, there is usually a period near the conclusion of therapy when the dynamics become the central therapeutic focus. At this point, if the therapy has been relatively successful, the student is within the normal range of weight and is eating more or less normally. She has improved in recognizing feelings and expressing them appropriately. She has a generally solid sense of herself and of the boundaries between herself and others. Her reality testing is improved, and she does not suffer from the cognitive and perceptual distortions that characterized her earlier functioning. As therapy now moves toward termination, the remaining issues involve further exploration of long-repressed or internalized feelings; recognition of the way those repressed feelings have influenced current behavior and relationships; and strengthening of her sense of identity and separateness.

OTHER ISSUES OF COLLEGE
PSYCHOTHERAPY WITH EATING DISORDERS

Use of the Academic Calendar

One of the anomalous aspects of doing psychotherapy in a college environment is the necessity of operating within the academic calendar. Psychotherapy with students does not usually fit neatly into two 13- or 14-week semesters; the pace and continuity of therapy are therefore not as smooth as in a private practice setting. The disruptions of vacations, particularly summer breaks, can have a profound effect on the kind of psychotherapy that may be undertaken, as well as on the therapeutic relationship. This issue is of particular relevance with the eating disorders. To some extent, the college psychotherapist must simply endure these interruptions and accept the fact that the calendar may disrupt, and sometimes prolong, treatment. At the same time, however, the therapist can, to a degree, anticipate and utilize the breaks to advantage.

Jean, for example, was struggling with the relationship phase of therapy when Christmas vacation arrived and she was to return to her home 1,500 miles away. Recognizing that the complete cessation of contact for 4 weeks would set the process back considerably, the therapist encouraged her to keep a diary as if she were writing to the therapist. Not only did this approach keep the relationship from regressing, but the student was actually able to become more comfortable with her own feelings through the less directly confrontational mode of writing, and was able to discuss some subjects she had previously kept from the therapist.

Of course, with an ego-fragmented patient, or where there is any indication of health risk, it is necessary to make a referral to a psychotherapist who can see the student over the summer. Although this is far from ideal, it is better than no contact whatsoever or mere phone or mail contact with the college therapist. In the best of circumstances, the second psychotherapist has had experience with eating-disordered patients and is willing to provide the college therapist with a full report at the end of the summer. Several organizations maintain national referral services for psychotherapists who specialize in eating disorders; this is an advantage when the therapist is not able to provide a knowledgeable personal referral.* Many of the same issues apply to termination. The psychotherapist working with college students must recognize the constraints and potential advantages of the calendar and make adjustments in the treatment plan accordingly. The important point is that the calendar need not always be a drawback, but can be a useful therapeutic tool.

---

* Several such national organizations are the Center for the Study of Anorexia and Bulimia (CSAB), 1 West 91st St., New York, NY 10024, (212) 595-3449; American Anorexia/Bulimia Association (AABA), 133 Cedar Lane, Teaneck, NJ 07666, (201) 836-1800; the National Association of Anorexia Nervosa and Associated Disorders (ANAD), Box 271, Highland Park, IL 60035, (312) 831-3438; and Anorexia Nervosa and Related Eating Disorders, Inc. (ANRED), P.O. Box 5102, Eugene, OR 97405, (503) 344-1144.

Parental Noninvolvement

The absence of direct involvement by parents in the treatment presents some potential problems. The parents may have a subtle, and often unconscious, need to retain the status quo with their daughter; they may be unable to deal with her growing up. To the extent that such dynamics exist in either parent, there may be direct or indirect sabotage of the psychotherapy. Sabotage may be quite direct, such as telling their daughter not to continue psychotherapy at college, or it may be more subtle, such as continuing to reinforce the disordered behavior while their daughter is at home.

Sometimes problems may arise even when parents' intentions are good. For example, Elise had battled anorexia nervosa for several years during high school and had undergone inpatient and outpatient psychotherapy, with only termporary change. She came to college, which was several hours away from her home, weighing a relatively stable 72 pounds and standing 5'1". Although she was initially eager to live away from home and go to college, she had always been extremely dependent on her parents and was immature for her age. Her parents felt that being away from home might be good for her, and they were quite strong (and well-meaning) in encouraging her to stay at school, even when she decided that she wanted to return home. During a phone call when Elise tearfully asked to come home, her father told her that she should stay at school and try to work things out unless she was at medical risk. Taking this cue, she began immediately to lose more weight, dropped to 64 pounds, and was hospitalized at home within 2 weeks.

Had Elise's parents had close, ongoing contact with either the college therapist or a private therapist, they might have avoided this mistake. Certainly, the college psychotherapist can arrange such consultation for parents near their home. However, the close coordination of the various treatment components is lacking. Thus, though there are advantages to developing treatment strategies at a distance from parents, distance also creates special problems.

Psychopharmacology

There is growing evidence that antidepressant medication and other forms of psychopharmacological intervention are sometimes beneficial in the treatment process of eating disorders. Garfinkel and Garner's (1987) recent book provides a good description of much of this recent work. The college psychotherapist is encouraged to evaluate the appropriateness of psychotropic medication (or psychiatric consultation for such evaluation) in working with eating-disordered students.

Mistakes

A number of therapeutic mistakes can be made even by competent therapists in working with these patients. Some of the most common therapeutic errors are being therapeutically inactive, focusing prematurely on weight and eating issues, being manipulated (especially into believing that the patient is doing better than she is), playing a parenting role, and getting into battles over control. The therapist cannot avoid these errors all of the time, but he or she can minimize them by constantly attending to the myriad of deflections and highly effective strategies that the student will throw directly in the path of her own road to health.

FINAL THOUGHTS

Even more poignantly and forcefully than other problems facing college psychotherapists in the 1980s, anorexia nervosa and bulimia nervosa represent challenges that demand attention to a delicate balance (or, more appropriately, a delicate imbalance) of societal, psychological, and biological forces in young women who are trying desperately to gain some autonomous sense of themselves. The process of psychotherapy with these individuals is a frustrating, demanding, yet often rewarding engagement, the dimensions of which are still evolving. Even at this writing, the patterns are beginning to shift. The incidence of bulimia is apparently increasing at a faster rate than that of anorexia, and the number of cases of compulsive exercising is also increasing.

Patterns of psychotherapy parallel patterns of social change. This statement is true in any therapeutic context and with any emotional disorder, but it is arguably nowhere more true than in the college environment, and particularly with regard to eating disorders. The effective college physician can successfully and consistently diagnose mononucleosis, treat strep throat, or set a fractured tibia without reference to the social attitudes and values of the student population. The college psychotherapist's effectiveness, however, depends not only on knowledge and understanding of psychotherapeutic theory and technique, but also on awareness of and adaptability to current cultural attitudes and expectations.

The college community provides an environment quite different from a private practice, and effective psychotherapy in this environment demands attention to a number of dimensions. For example, the college psychotherapist must pay attention to his or her degree of involvement in the college community, the balance between the image of a "friend" or "teacher" and that of an objective psychotherapist, and the ways in which he or she establishes community rapport between the psychotherapy service and students, faculty, and administrators. Not paying attention to these issues can reduce the therapeutic effectiveness of otherwise skilled therapists. Although these issues are important in all aspects of college psychotherapy, they are particularly relevant as college psychotherapists struggle for increasing understanding and effective treatment of eating disorders.

REFERENCES

Agras, W. S. (1987). *Eating disorders: Management of obesity, bulimia, and anorexia nervosa*. New York: Pergamon Press.

American Psychiatric Association. (1980). *Diagnostic and statistical manual of mental disorders* (3rd ed.).Washington, DC: Author.

American Psychiatric Association. (1987). *Diagnostic and statistical manual of mental disorders* (3rd ed., rev.). Washington, DC: American Psychiatric Association.

Andersen, A. E. (1985). *Practical comprehensive treatment of anorexia nervosa and bulimia*. Baltimore: Johns Hopkins University Press.

Boskind-Lodahl, M. (1978). The definition and treatment of bulimarexia: The gorging/purging syndrome of young women (Doctoral dissertation, Cornell University, 1977). *Dissertation Abstracts International, 38*, 717 A.

Boskind-White, M., & White, W. (1983). *Bulimarexia: The binge/purge cycle*. New York: Norton.

Brownell, K. D., & Foreyt, J. P. (Eds.). (1986). *Handbook of eating disorders*. New York: Basic Books.

Bruch, H. (1973). *Eating disorders: Obesity, anorexia nervosa, and the person within*. New York: Basic Books.

Bruch, H. (1978). *The golden cage*. Cambridge, MA: Harvard University Press.

Bruch, H. (1985). Four decades of eating disorders. In D. M. Garner & P. E. Garfinkel (Eds.), *Handbook of psychotherapy for anorexia nervosa and bulimia* (pp. 7–18). New York: Guilford Press.

Cohler, B. J. (1977). The significance of the therapist's feelings in the treatment of anorexia nervosa. In S. C. Feinstein & P. Giovachini (Eds.), *Adolescent psychiatry: Vol. 5. Developmental and clinical studies*. New York: Jason Aronson.

Garfinkel, P. E., & Garner, D. M. (1982). *Anorexia nervosa: A multidimensional perspective*. New York: Brunner/Mazel.

Garfinkel, P. E., & Garner, D. M. (Eds.). (1987). *The role of drug treatments for eating disorders*. New York: Brunner/Mazel.

Garner, D. M., & Bemis, K. M. (1985). Cognitive therapy for anorexia nervosa. In D. M. Garner & P. E. Garfinkel (Eds.), *Handbook of psychotherapy for anorexia nervosa and bulimia* (pp. 107–146). New York: Guilford Press.

Garner, D. M., & Garfinkel, P. E. (Eds.). (1985). *Handbook of psychotherapy for anorexia nervosa and bulimia*. New York: Guilford Press.

Johnson, C., & Connors, M. E. (1987). *The etiology and treatment of bulimia nervosa*. New York: Basic Books.

Levenkron, S. (1978). *The best little girl in the world*. New York: Warner Books.

Levenkron, S. (1985). Structuring a nurturant–authoritative psychotherapeutic relationship with the anorexic patient. In S. W. Emmett (Ed.), *Theory and treatment of anorexia nervosa and bulimia* (pp. 234–245). New York: Brunner/Mazel.

Minuchin, S., Rosman, B. L., & Baker, L. (1978). *Psychosomatic families: Anorexia nervosa in context*. Cambridge, MA: Harvard University Press.

Mitchell, J. E., & Eckert, E. D. (1987). Scope and significance of eating disorders. *Journal of Consulting and Clinical Psychology, 55*, 628–634.

Rizzuto, A.-M., Peterson, R. K., & Reed, M. (1981). The pathological sense of self in anorexia nervosa. *Psychiatric Clinics of North America, 4*, 471–487.

Root, M. P. P., Fallon, P., & Friedrich, W. N. (1986). *Bulimia: A systems approach to treatment*. New York: Norton.

Schwartz, D. M., Thompson, M. G., & Johnson, C. L. (1982). Anorexia nervosa and bulimia: The sociocultural context. *International Journal of Eating Disorders, 3*, 20–36.

Shapiro, A. L. (1986). Anorexia nervosa: An empirical and clinical exploration of some psychological issues (Doctoral dissertation, New York University, 1985). *Dissertation Abstracts International, 47*(4), 1744B.

Weiss, L., Katzman, M., & Wolchik, S. (1985). *Treating bulimia: A psychoeducational approach*. New York: Pergamon Press.

Wilson, C. P. (Ed.). (1983). *Fear of being fat*. New York: Jason Aronson.

15

Ethnic and
International Students

ALEJANDRO M. MARTINEZ
KAREN H. C. HUANG
SAMUEL D. JOHNSON, JR.
SAM EDWARDS, JR.

College therapists who work with ethnic and international students must distinguish individual dynamics from culturally generated ones. Theoretically, most of us readily acknowledge that cultural influences are a vital force in determining life patterns, intrapsychic development, belief systems, and coping styles. Yet when we are faced with ethnic students in our clinical work, these theoretical understandings can become blurred. The difficulty stems in large part from the complexity of ethnicity and culture. Ethnic groups differ from the mainstream in complex ways; the various ethnic groups show great variability among themselves; and individuals within a given group also vary greatly. This complexity raises a challenge to us as clinicians: How can we work successfully with individuals who are significantly different from ourselves?

An assumption throughout this chapter is that one need not learn a whole new therapeutic modality when working with ethnic and international students. ("Ethnic" refers here primarily to Asian-American, black, and Latino students born in this country; "international" refers primarily to students from Third World countries.) Rather, one must step back and view in a new light that which is usually taken for granted in the therapeutic process—for example, norms about disclosing personal information. This chapter highlights the different and unexpected ways in which culture and ethnicity influence the therapeutic process.

In particular, we point out some problems that all ethnic groups tend to share, examine problems that pertain to particular groups, and consider the following aspects of treatment: referral, assessment, communications, ethnic background of the therapist, and structuring of therapy.

PROBLEMS OF STUDENTS

How ethnic and international students deal with higher education and its many intellectual, social, and personal challenges depends in general on their relative degree of immersion in mainstream American culture versus their own culture of origin. Those who predominantly identify with either culture are less likely to experience major identity or self-concept problems than are those who feel torn between both cultures. The former may sometimes find themselves in situations of cultural conflict, but the issues do not appear intrinsic to their psychological integration. In contrast, those who experience discordance between two sets of cultural values often experience powerful and debilitating stress.

The cultural conflicts can be basic. For example, many non-Western world-views are rooted in the concept of interconnection between mind and body, between parent and child, and between neighbor and neighbor (Hsu, 1955; Lee, 1960). Along with these ideas is an emphasis on maintaining harmonious interpersonal relations. Unlike the mainstream culture, in which striving for autonomy and independence is paramount, these cultures value harmony, togetherness, and unity. Cultural differences are also expressed in mundane ways, such as clothing styles; tastes in food, sports, and entertainment; and dating practices. Because of all these differences, ethnic and international students caught between cultures often feel torn. Should they strive to maintain their own values and practices? Doing so means feeling isolated from the mainstream culture, but abrogating their own culture may engender guilt, leave them feeling rootless and lonely, and provoke opposition from family and friends. Thus students often have serious cultural conflicts on both intrapsychic and interpersonal levels. Even simple decisions can evoke discomfort. Should a Japanese student eat rice or a sandwich for lunch? Should a student from India wear a sari or Western attire?

Meanwhile, members of the mainstream culture may also react to minority students in problematic ways. At the extreme, mainstream persons may exhibit blatant racism, as happened to an Indian student who overheard his roommate's parents derisively joke about him, "Maybe he can't even speak English." On a more subtle level, mainstream students may simply betray ignorance or indifference or clumsiness in their efforts to reach out.

Cultural factors can also be significant when they are used by students in defensive or self-defeating ways. For example, a female Mexican student indicated that it was culturally inappropriate to challenge authority figures. Although in fact it is culturally normative in her native country to be respectful toward elders, she had taken a cultural norm and made it into an inflexible rule that justified her lack of assertiveness. Similarly, a Chinese-American student justified her lack of academic effort by explaining that competitiveness was against her culture. She used her background to rationalize her self-defeating behavior.

Black Students

Providing psychotherapy to black students can be a complicated experience for therapists on college campuses. Most white therapists and even many black therapists do not fully appreciate the complexity of racial identity, or the many social, economic, and cultural factors that contribute to black student development. As a consequence, they may fall into the trap of simplifying black students' issues, responding as if all blacks shared the same personality characteristics and set of problems. A corollary of this mistake is to overemphasize the significance of race and treat everything that black students bring up in treatment as a "black" concern. Yet a "color-blind" approach that denies racial concerns and treats blacks solely according to universal principles of human development is equally misguided and can also undermine a therapist's credibility. Therapists must strike an appropriate level of concern for racial group issues if they are to be effective with ethnic groups in general and black students in particular.

One effective way to conceptualize variability among blacks is in terms of racial identity development, a theory put forth by several black psychologists (Cross, 1971; Thomas, 1971). These authors hypothesize that blacks experience identity transformations, involving shifts in attitudes toward other blacks and toward whites, as part of their overall psychological development. These identity transformations, which a student may not be fully aware of, are stimulated by influential social experiences, such as going to college. The stage of racial identity students are in—or may be struggling with—helps determine their adjustment to college and responsiveness to psychotherapy. Four (or sometimes five) stages have been identified (Carter, 1986; Hall, Cross, & Freedle, 1972; Parham & Helms, 1981, 1983).

In the first stage, "pre-encounter," students have not accepted or "encountered" themselves as black. They think of the world in white terms; deny their racial heritage and hold themselves and other blacks in low regard; idealize and perhaps identify with whites; and tend to be anxious and have low self-esteem. Although students who are squarely in this stage are rare on most college campuses, therapists will find students who have not completely moved beyond this developmental level. Therapists' task with such students is to help them accept themselves as black and, by extension, to foster their self-acceptance in general.

The "encounter" stage, which comes next, involves an emerging black identity. Students at this level tend to have an uncritical attitude toward other blacks and a confused and critical attitude toward whites. This stage may be succeeded by the "immersion–emersion" stage, in which students struggle to eliminate all vestiges of the pre-encounter perspective and to clarify the implications of their new black identity. Their stance toward blacks has evolved into idealization, and toward whites into denigration and rejection. With a black student at this stage, the therapeutic task for the white therapist is to see whether a therapeutic relationship is possible, and if not, to make a referral to a black therapist. Treatment needs to expand such students' essentially narrow and defensive world-view, which in its own way can be as limiting as the pre-encounter perspective, and to enable students to emerge from the social withdrawal that is a concomitant of their attitudes.

Finally, in the "internalization" stage, students have accepted their blackness and are self-confident about their identity. At the same time, they view whites realistically and tolerantly. The problems these clients present in psychotherapy do not tend to concern racial identity as such, but pertain to other aspects of black life or to the kinds of concerns that trouble students of all backgrounds.

An example of how racial identity can enter into the therapy process, and how a culturally sensitive therapist can deal with it, is the case of Jason, a black student at a predominantly white college. Bright, motivated, and an athlete in track, Jason had previously worked well with Al, his white therapist, but one day at the end of his sophomore year he seemed more distant than usual. When Al asked whether something was bothering him, Jason was initially evasive, then eventually said that he had received a D+ in a course on behaviorism and that the white professor, during a personal conference, told him that there was nothing that could be done to raise the grade. Asked to say more about his feelings, Jason replied, "I'm not sure I can talk to *you* about it." Al asked, "What's wrong? We've always been able to talk before." "I just don't feel you can help me with this one," said Jason.

Sensing the problem, Al asked, "Does this have something to do with my being white?" Jason replied in the affirmative. He then went on to add that the professor, hearing about Jason's plans for graduate school, had said, "I don't see any problem here at all. Blacks have never made any contribution of significance to psychology, and you [Jason] aren't any threat to alter that pattern." "That made me furious," Jason said loudly. "Anyway, this crap has got me thinking that you just can't trust white people worth a damn! I realize now that I'm black and I just have to take care of me and the people I know I can trust—black people."

Such experiences of racial conflict or racism can move black students to recast their racial identity; in Jason's case, it propelled him into the encounter stage. It is then critically important for therapists to allow these students "space" to embrace a new identity, to confront the conflicts associated with becoming black, and to renegotiate their relationships with whites. Al's response to Jason's outburst was empathic and nondefensive. He made it clear that he was willing to continue working with Jason, but he stressed that Jason if he wished could speak to a black therapist, who also worked at the counseling center. Al added, "I'd still like you to let me know how things turn out, and if there's anything I can do to be of help, please let me know." Thus Al acknowledged Jason's right to reject a white's offer of assistance as part of this student's effort to achieve a higher level of racial identity development.

In addition to racial identity, other dimensions of black students' experience and other concerns they have may be identified. Some students are, or feel, academically unprepared because of their previous school experiences for the volume, complexity, and pace of work at college or for the competitive academic norms that prevail there. A black freshman, for example, found that he felt unready for the tests, lectures, and homework he encountered at his predominantly white, prestigious university. Frightened that he could not "catch up" to his white classmates, and feeling burdened by an inner sense of responsibility to be a good example for his race (many blacks feel that in failing they let down the whole black community), he felt depressed and contemplated suicide. Fortunately, he volunteered for academic assistance and voluntarily came to the counseling center for psychological support before acting on his suicidal impulses. Many black students, obeying an internalized mandate that they must be strong, conceal their academic and emotional problems and never seek help. They then end up dropping out of school without notifying anyone of their plans to leave.

Socioeconomic concerns often trouble those black students who are from low-income families and disadvantaged neighborhoods. Part of their problem is simply to pay the bills. Even with financial aid packages, they may be barely able to cover expenses at college, and the frequent necessity to work part-time while attending school may divert time and energy needed for studies. The other part of the problem is adjusting to living with predominantly middle-class classmates. The contrast in financial circumstances and modes of behavior may cause them to feel embarrassed, humiliated, or resentful, particularly if their racial identity has not fully developed.

Finally, black students at college face the same concerns as anyone else. Can they fit in with peers? Will they find a niche within society? Can they speak up in class? These concerns, and others like them, often have a special twist because of race and racial identity development. Fitting in with peers, for example, can be especially difficult for those students who both are black and also have personal insecurities stemming from their family upbringing; these factors in combination cause some black students to experience themselves as outsiders on campus. Fitting in may be hard, too, if blacks discover that the black community at college is less supportive and united than they had hoped for or had experienced in their hometowns. Some segments of black students remain strangers to one another, deliberately passing one another by on campus. Doubts about career, universal among college students, may be intensified for blacks because they lack role models within certain professions. Fears about participating in class discussions, another common theme in college psychotherapy, may be accentuated for blacks because of sensitivity about their speech. A freshman explained that he didn't talk in class because his speech was "too heavy with blackness."

Asian-American Students

For Asian-American students, four domains of concern can be highlighted: (1) socializing, (2) dating, (3) academic pressures, and (4) degree of verbal communication.

With regard to the first issue, the mainstream student's college party is usually an ambiguous situation that includes a fair amount of alcohol consumption and physical contact. This mode of socializing is often uncomfortable for more traditional Asian-American students; the format, structure, and customary behaviors of such parties are not characteristic of their socializing patterns. There is simply no Asian equivalent to the cocktail party, for instance. The consumption of alcohol and high level of physical contact are generally considered inappropriate in Asian households (except for particular celebrations), and discouraged for youths. However, since parties are the most generally accepted and occasionally the only readily available forum for making friends, the discomfort may significantly conflict with the wish to participate. Indeed, some Asian-American students seeking counseling services present with the seemingly simple yet thorny problem of feeling unable to "make friends" because of unfamiliarity with this form of mainstream socializing. Complicating the problem, some Asian-American youths narrowly focus on academics in high school and therefore come to college unfamiliar not just with parties, but with all aspects of socializing.

For example, a Japanese-American freshman was attending a prestigious California university that had a social reputation of friendliness and ease. A devoted student in high school who had never socialized much, he had arrived on campus expecting to make friends easily. Instead, he found himself unable to think of anything to say in social situations. At breakfast, he found himself listening to everyone else, too hesitant and unsure of himself to speak up, and in the dorm he rarely initiated conversation for fear of rejection. In particular, he felt embarrassed by the physical contact, the hugging that he observed between others and longed for himself. Much of the initial work in therapy focused on helping him to label his feelings and hidden expectations for instant popularity. Later his confusion and concerns about Western behavior, such as hugging, were dealt with. The therapy validated his cultural experience and familial values and helped him realize that his conflicts had an understandable basis; they were not simply due to personal inadequacies. At the same time, the therapist concentrated on skills training, enabling him to "fit in" better when he so chose. At the end, the treatment focused on integrating his conflicted feelings concerning emotional and physical closeness, and on differentiating his own wishes from outside expectations, so that he could act in ways that felt comfortable to him.

Associated with socializing is the issue of dating and sexual mores. Traditional Asian cultures discourage casual physical contact and explicitly forbid premarital sex. Since such behavior has historically been associated with the Caucasian mainstream in the minds of many Asian parents, Asian-American youngsters are often discouraged from interracial dating. Asian parents often impress the virtues of chastity on their children and encourage them to emphasize academics over dating, whereas mainstream students often reverse these priorities. The result is often a significant degree of conflict for Asian-American students. For many, conflicts over parental disapproval of dating partners can be intense, often with the parents threatening to disown the child (the threat is rarely carried out). Quite often, those youths who do shift toward more liberal values and participate in forbidden activities feel tremendous guilt and have to expend considerable psychic energy defending against this feeling. On the other hand, those who adhere to the traditional ways often feel socially alienated and invalidated.

One young Chinese/Japanese-American woman sought treatment for a variety of issues, including a conflict over her boyfriend. She felt attracted to him and enjoyed his company, though she did not love him. Since her cultural upbringing would not allow her to enjoy the intimacy for what it was, she felt intense guilt over the relationship. She attempted to defend against the guilt by talking herself into believing she loved the man. She also reacted by vacillating in her dealings with him between intimacy and conflict. The therapy focused on helping her to differentiate genuine feelings from defenses. Although such issues are not uncommon for any college student, the difference for Asian-American students is that the guilt can be particularly intense and isolating.

Academic pressures pose a complexity of problems for many Asian-American students. First, many arrive at the university with a studious orientation, only to find a new "fun self" at school, which engenders identity conflicts. Second, many find it difficult to balance the competing needs for achievement and socializing; they feel guilty when socializing and feel a sense of "missing out" when studying. Third, many Asian-American students receive consistent and concerted performance pressures from parents who are anxious for their children to become physicians, engineers, or entrepreneurs. To earn less than straight A's or to change to "soft" majors is often tantamount to filial treason in their families. Selecting a major can be a metaphor for separation and individuation from the parental system, and, similarly, choosing a different career path has serious implications for parent–child relationships. In treatment, therefore, emphasis should not necessarily be placed on facilitating students' ability to confront and individuate from their parents. This would probably go counter to cultural standards and ultimately create greater distress. Instead, counselors should aid students in clarifying their own values and wishes in the context of family and cultural expectations. Sometimes, students find that a compromise is the most fruitful solution.

Verbal expression is the fourth area of difficulty often cited by Asian-American students. Whereas the mainstream culture emphasizes verbal assertiveness, Asian cultures generally value reserve and restraint. Classroom discussion, usually led by a non-Asian instructor, is therefore often experienced as intimidating by Asian-American students. As a result, many of them feel introverted and inhibited in the classroom (Sue & Kirk, 1972). Similarly, Asian-American students in social situations often complain of verbal inhibitions around Caucasian friends. In addressing this issue in treatment, it is important to consider how current and personal historical factors contribute to the situation. One student, for instance, noted that she felt insecure in her classroom discussion because the instructor regularly cut her off. In her case, the current situation interacted with pre-existing cultural inhibitions and reverberated with her early childhood victimization by racist peers. Work with this woman focused on addressing her pain, examining the childhood adaptiveness of her reserve, and mobilizing her current anger at being cut off during discussions.

Latino Students

Latinos (a term we prefer to "Hispanics," which sometimes carries negative political connotations) share some of the concerns that black and Asian-Americans have, but historical and contextual differences make their experience distinct. Many Latino students are members of communities that have been targeted by overt prejudice and discrimination. These communities generally have lower personal and family incomes, have fewer years of education, are overrepresented in low-paying occupations, and are underrepresented in higher education, compared to Asian-Americans and mainstream Americans. In general, they are characterized by an impoverished quality of life and reduced opportunities for advancement.

Given this backdrop, entering academia is commonly a source of stress for Latino students, challenging their sense of individual, familial, community, and cultural identity. Although mainstream students have to separate from families as well, their end goal is integration into the community and larger society; for Latino students, education represents a sharper break from family and community. These students typically have significant community support to attend a university, and they represent a source of pride for their parents. Yet involvement in mainstream institutions entails a process of enculturation in which their families' values are underrepresented within the university's social and intellectual arenas. Not surprisingly, many Latino students feel ambivalent about involvement at college. The stress of making the transition from the family to the institution is often intensified and complicated by the dearth of Latino role models who have achieved success through continued education. Latino students can see what they are leaving, but do not know where their college experience will lead. In addition, when they go home they must face the reaction of their families to the personal changes that are being brought out by the educational experience. It is not unusual for family members to "test" a student to see whether he or she is still part of the family.

At the same time, these students frequently experience tremendous pressure for academic success. Being pioneers in higher education, they often perceive themselves as test cases. Their performance will determine whether the institutional door will remain open for others from their communities. Yet this task is difficult because their precollege preparation is frequently inferior to that of their mainstream peers. Latino students may also doubt their abilities. If they have been admitted to the university through affirmative action, they may have feelings of not fully belonging. This insecurity and self-doubt may be compounded by instances of racism and the recognition that the institution is insensitive to the intellectual heritage of their own culture. As a reaction, some students develop militant views; others withdraw and isolate themselves from the persons and resources that could help them succeed.

Latino students also encounter genuine acceptance and concern from majority-culture peers, staff, and faculty, which sometimes can cause its own problems. How do they learn to respond differentially to well-meaning versus rejecting mainstream persons? How do they learn the difference between genuine friendliness and patronizing treatment?

Other issues are frequently encountered with Latino students. Those who believe in traditional male and female sex roles or in traditional religious teachings may find their beliefs and practices challenged in the classroom and by their peers. Those who come from families that have been divided because of economic and political circumstances—who may have some family members in the United States and others in perhaps Mexico, El Salvador, or Puerto Rico—must deal with concerns of separation and sense of identity.

International Students

In certain respects, international students have the same problems as American-born ethnic students. However, as foreigners, they often face additional conditions that require adjustment. First, they must adjust to American values and ways. Unlike American minority students, they do not tend to feel internally conflicted about American culture; their basic identification is with their native culture. However, various aspects of the American experience—sexual practices, social conventions, material wealth, the relatively unstructured atmosphere in classes, perhaps racial prejudice—may come as a shock. Second, they usually have to adjust to English as a second language, which makes coursework more difficult and complicates relations with professors and peers. Third, reduced socioeconomic status is an issue for those who come from a privileged class in their own country.

Many international students have had to make significant personal compromises to study in the United States. Some come without their immediate families; others are unable to go home for years. Separation from home may engender loneliness, guilt, and perhaps conflict about where to settle after college. Those who come with their families have to deal with the stress of their families' adjustment to life here.

TREATMENT

Referral Issues

Ethnic and international students tend to underutilize counseling services. One reason is that they prefer to seek help from individuals they know. Rather than call an anonymous secretary to schedule an appointment with a stranger, many prefer to contact someone who is known to them, however vaguely. In addition, many of these students feel more comfortable and empathically understood by someone from a similar background. Although many majority-culture therapists may empathically understand the experience of these students, the students themselves must experience such therapists as empathic. When students' problems are related to cultural conflicts, initial rapport is often best established with a culturally similar therapist.

These students tend to enter the treatment system in less formalized ways than the usual explicit request for an appointment. Rather than saying "I am depressed and need therapy," they tend to make casual and oblique overtures. A student may approach a therapist in an informal gathering, presentation, or workshop and in the course of conversation nonchalantly say, "I'm not sure about problem X and I'd like to stop by to talk with you sometime." Although the overt statement sounds casual, suggesting that the person is requesting a casual conversation, implicitly this is a request for psychotherapy. Being aware of the duality of such communications and the stigma these students often attach to seeking "real therapy," therapists should not respond by stating, "You want therapy." Instead, they should arrange to meet with these students, maintaining an unspoken understanding of the purpose of the session. Furthermore, at the first meeting the usual intake questions should be minimized and the filling out of forms should be de-emphasized in order to put these students at ease. After rapport has been established, the relationship can be re-examined and redefined as needed.

Ethnic and international students frequently avoid seeking treatment until a crisis occurs. According to their values, personal problems should be handled privately by an individual and within the family. As a result, some of these students try to handle their problems on their own as long as possible, and they enter treatment or are compelled by others to seek treatment only as a last resort. Often the state of crisis then combines with their traditional feelings of shame or embarrassment about psychotherapy to result in a rather affectively charged entry into treatment. The wish to handle problems on their own often persists while therapy proceeds, resulting in ongoing ambivalence about treatment.

Another reason why ethnic and international students may not initially utilize psychological services is that they are attending to other dimensions of their problem. Psychological services or the counseling center does not seem to them the obvious place to get help. This means that these offices must have effective links with other departments. For example, international students experiencing academic difficulties may first contact their academic advisor or the foreign student advisor, even though the academic difficulty stems from problems for which a psychological intervention is appropriate. If the academic advisor or foreign student advisor is familiar with the counseling center, a referral can then be made.

Assessment Issues

Ethnic and international students' problems may be difficult to assess. For one thing, many of these students come from backgrounds where feelings and psychological issues are not openly discussed, and so they may have a difficult time now expressing the psychological basis of their concerns. Communication issues loom large with ethnic and international students—a topic we explore in depth in the next section.

A second reason why assessment may be difficult is that these students' problems are complex; external pressures may be intricately interwoven with psychopathological issues. For example, a black unmarried mother of two children spent the majority of the time in her sessions angrily discussing her financial problems and the unpleasant meetings she had with her financial aid administrators, who "act like they are taking money from their own pockets to give to me." Her concern for her children and her financial problems were genuine. But as the therapy progressed, it became apparent that this woman's reality-based concerns were interacting with her psychopathology; she was an antisocial personality. The task of assessment—and ultimately therapy—was thus to recognize and respond appropriately to all sources of her difficulties.

Communication Issues

Ethnic and international students have exceedingly diverse linguistic backgrounds. Some only speak English; others are bilingual; and still other have limited facility in English. Those who are bilingual tend to carry out some verbal exchanges in English and others in their native tongue, so that their vocabulary in neither language offers them the range of expressiveness available to monolingual speakers of either language. Often bilingual students may find feelings and personal thoughts easier to express in their native tongue than in English. To add to this linguistic complexity, some students use somewhat different meanings for corresponding words in English and their native languages. There are also variations within a language—for example, black English—that affect meanings and norms of expression. Students' particular linguistic backgrounds can subtly influence their communications with therapists.

Therapists therefore often have to make certain accommodations to students' linguistic backgrounds. For example, an Iranian student who presented with depression was unable while conversing in English to get in touch with his feelings. He was asked to play during the session an audiotape of his mother, speaking in Farsi, made just before her death. Only after listening to her voice in his native tongue was he able to talk more about his feelings in relation to her and her death.

An interesting problem arises when the client and therapist share two languages. The choice of language used in the therapeutic interaction then tends to carry meaning, since ethnic students commonly use their native tongue with friends and English when dealing with perceived outsiders. Furthermore, English is often linked with obsessional defenses and represents a form of resistance to affectively charged material, particularly among international students. A student from Mexico, for example, elected to have therapy in English, even though she was more fluent in Spanish. Only when the therapy was switched to Spanish, at the therapist's suggestion, was she able to plumb important issues such as feeling rejected by her mother and feeling deprived in general while growing up. Also significant are language shifts that may take place during the course of a session, suggesting shifts in mood, feelings of closeness to the therapist, and degree of resistance. Bilingual therapists therefore need to be sensitive to the choice of language made by both them and their bilingual clients.

An additional communication problem in therapy can occur because other cultures have their own norms about asking and transmitting information. Thus therapists' questions intended to be straightforward may be interpreted by clients as rude and intrusive, while direct answers to these questions may be regarded as unacceptable. Therapists therefore have to be sensitive to how they couch questions and must be understanding about indirect replies.

Given the taboos against verbal disclosure among many of these students, attention to nonverbal behavior is crucial, particularly during the first session—the time when many of these students decide to continue or drop out. For example, a therapist's walking the client to the threshold at the end of a session indicates to traditional Chinese-American students an invitation to return. Not doing so subliminally communicates a rejection. Handing out business cards with name and title is also of critical importance, since it conveys credibility and legitimacy.

Another source of misunderstanding in therapy occurs because of semantic difficulties. Sometimes clients are unfamiliar with an English concept. For example, the question "Are you feeling depressed?" may not be understood by some international students. "Are you feeling happy?" or some equivalent may be required instead. The semantic difficulties can also lead to subtle misunderstandings by therapists. In reviewing an adult Brazilian student's relationship with her grown children, a therapist commented that her continual reference to them as "my children" was suggestive of a continued perception of them as children. The client clarified that she had been using the term as an accommodation to English and to the therapist. She explained that in Portuguese, "*mis hijos,*" or "my children," was technically appropriate to describe "grown children." Similarly, a Brazilian man came to psychotherapy concerned with his current family situation, particularly with his relationship to his 3-year-old daughter. In discussing her, he would typically refer to her as "the child" (as in "the child is demanding a lot of my time"). This might have easily been misinterpreted as an unusual and somewhat depersonalized way to refer to his daughter. However, since "*la nina*" or "the child" connotes affection, the student was merely providing a literal translation of the Portuguese term.

Particularly for bilingual students who are not fluent in English, the act of communicating in English can be highly stressful and give rise to mispresentation of their problems. Students must organize their personal experience in a more formal manner than they may feel comfortable with, resulting in disruptions of fluency, cognitive organization, and psychological integration. Such disturbances are not simply related to linguistic competence. Rather, the demands of expressing themselves in a second language may constitute a distraction that impairs cognitive functioning. It is as if there is an intermediary in the session. First, they have to organize their ideas, feelings, and images into words (in the first language), and then they must translate the concepts and words into English; correspondingly, they have to hear what the therapist is saying in English and translate it to the first language.

Ethnic Background of the Therapist: Transference Implications

One question with any type of client is who is the most appropriate therapist or counselor. Is it someone from the same background? We are all familiar with the medical student who is only comfortable speaking with a psychiatrist because the psychiatrist alone knows what the medical student experience is "really" like. With ethnic and international students, there are arguments for and against therapists from the same background.

On the one hand, some of these students simply feel that it is inappropriate to speak of certain issues (such as racism, discrimination, ethnicity, and identity) with white therapists. Having therapists from the same background may enhance rapport and promote students' willingness to disclose material. Students then perceive their therapists as sensitive and responsive to their unique sociocultural attributes. Therapists of a similar background to ethnic and international students may also help change the perception that counseling is only for "Americans" or white students. In addition, since the faculty members at most universities and colleges are predominantly white males, Caucasian male therapists may be perceived as symbols of judgment and control, whereas therapists from the same background permit these students to feel free to be themselves. An international student had requested a change of therapist to one who could speak her language. Several sessions later, she said that the greatest benefit of the change was that she felt freer to make mistakes and admit to insecurities without the typical judgment she experienced from "Americans."

On the other hand, some clients prefer therapists whose background differs from their own, particularly if they want to deal with material that would be embarrassing to share with individuals of the same background. For example, it can be easier for students to talk about lacking a strong affiliation to their culture and values if they are seeing counselors who are not of their background. A gay male Latino student was offered the option to see a Latino therapist; the student strongly objected. He expected to find the same homophobia in the therapist that he had found in his Latino community, whereas he felt that Caucasians were more tolerant of homosexuality. Similarly, a female Latino graduate student felt a great deal of apprehension on being assigned a Latino therapist. She found ethnic men to be oppressive, while white men seemed to be more open to equal relations between men and women. In this case, initial work with a white male therapist and later with a Latino therapist made it possible for significant work to take place in her relationships with ethnic males (including her father). In addition, students who are uncomfortable with the white majority may best be helped by "confronting" white therapists with their feelings of anger, helplessness, and anxiety. Finally, clients may object to therapists from the same background because they perceive them as too closely identified with the institution, or as role models who are too intimidating, or as persons likely to overidentify with students or deny identification altogether.

Thus we cannot always predict beforehand whether it helps to have therapists from the same or different cultural background as clients. What we can say is that therapists' ethnic background always carries meaning to clients; it is a source of transference reactions. Therapists should be attentive to these meanings and encourage their exploration in treatment. At the same time, therapists must be alert to their own countertransference reactions based on clients' ethnic backgrounds. Do they judge clients as less intelligent, or more disturbed, or less treatable, or less capable of an insight-oriented approach, on the basis of the clients' backgrounds? Does a student's value system, or tendency to speak with an accent, blind a therapist to the student's true problems and potential?

Structuring of Therapy

Ethnic and international students are generally unfamiliar with psychotherapy. Therefore, therapists should explain the nature of the process and the goals of treatment to them at the start. Therapists should explain that resolving personal conflicts, some of them unconscious, can bring relief from suffering—an idea that is unfamiliar to many of these students. Therapists also must be prepared to take an active stance. The usual procedure of waiting for clients to present their problems will probably lead to awkward, anxious silences, since these clients have often been culturally conditioned to avoid expressing personal problems, particularly to respected authority figures such as therapists. Others may not share information without encouragement because they believe that it is dangerous to share information in the United States. Perhaps their families have come to the country illegally and have to be silent in order to remain.

Given that many ethnic and international cultures are centered around personal relationships, it is not surprising that clients from such cultures often ask personal questions of their therapists. Clients often do so in an attempt to establish a sense of communality with therapists. Rather than interpret such questions as defenses or as a search for clues about how to behave, it can be quite appropriate to simply give direct answers. Sharing credentials and social information, such as place of birth and marital status, helps to foster rapport with the client.

For example, a young Chinese-American woman sought treatment because of uncontrollable fits of crying. She was suffering from an adjustment reaction with depressive and anxious symptoms, following the news that her sister would probably soon die of brain cancer. When asked about her family history, she explained that her parents were quite traditional since they were from Asia, and that she experienced some conflict as the result of their differences in acculturation. She then asked, "Are your parents immigrants?", to which the Chinese-American therapist responded, "Yes, I know what it's like." Following this, the client continued with her description, apparently satisfied that the therapist could empathize with her experience. Had the therapist followed the more orthodox technique of asking her the reasons for her questions and her feelings at the time of asking, the empathic connection would probably have been damaged and the client offended.

SUMMARY

The therapeutic issues raised by ethnic and international students are complex, inasmuch as these students differ from mainstream students in general respects; the various ethnic groups differ among themselves; and individuals within each group vary. Furthermore, some issues students bring to therapy pertain to their ethnic background, and others do not. A key general issue for these students is cultural conflict. Students who do not strongly identify with either the mainstream or their own culture may find themselves torn in regard to values, tastes, goals, and practices. Another general issue for all ethnic and international students is to deal with the many reactions to them that mainstream students exhibit.

Several issues tend to apply particularly to a given group. Racial identity development stands out as a key theme among black students. Asian-Americans commonly have concerns centered around socializing, dating, and academic pressures. Many Latinos experience strong ambivalence about involvement in college. International students typically have to adjust to a new culture, language, and set of life circumstances.

The therapy of these students is not radically different from that of mainstream students, but certain modifications are recommended. Since these students enter treatment less readily than mainstream students, therapists need to encourage them to come, and should be flexible in setting up the original therapeutic contract. Assessment requires paying close attention to reality-based concerns as well as to psychopathological and developmental issues. Among communication issues, therapists must recognize students' semantic difficulties, the significance of their using English versus their native language in sessions, their difficulties in translating their experiences into English, and their taboos against self-disclosure. The ethnic background of therapists evokes transference responses for these students; meantime, therapists have countertransference reactions to the students in return. Finally, therapists often have to provide more structuring for these students at the start of treatment.

REFERENCES

Carter, R. T. (1986). *The relationship between black American students' value orientations and their racial identity attitudes.* Unpublished manuscript, Southern Illinois University.

Cross, W. E. (1971). The negro to black conversion experience: Toward a psychology of black liberation. *Black World, 20* (9), 13–27.

Hall, W. S., Cross, W. E., & Freedle, R. (1971). Stages in the development of black awareness: An empirical investigation. In R. L. Jones (Ed.), *Black psychology* (pp. 156–165). New York: Harper & Row.

Hsu, F. L. K. (1955). *Americans and Chinese: Two ways of life.* New York: Henry Schuman.

Lee, R. H. (1960). *The Chinese in the United States of America.* Hong Kong: Hong Kong University Press.

Parham, T., & Helms, J. (1981). The influence of black students' racial identity attitudes on preference for counselor race. *Journal of Counseling Psychology, 28,* 250–257.

Parham, T., & Helms, J. (1983). Relationship of racial identity attitudes to self-actualization and affective states of black students. *Journal of Counseling Psychology, 32,* 431–440.

Sue, D. W., & Kirk, B. (1972). Psychological characteristics of Chinese-American students. *Journal of Counseling Psychology, 19,* 471–478.

Thomas, C. (1971). *Boys no more.* Beverly Hills, CA: Glencoe Press.

16

Returning Students

ELIZABETH A. JOHNSON
ALLAN J. SCHWARTZ

Returning students, who are sometimes called "nontraditional students" or "re-entry students," make up a diverse group whose education has been interrupted for some time and who are older than the traditional college student (Magoon, 1980; Mitchell, 1979). Returning students differ from traditional students on such factors as background, maturity level (Papier, 1980), and sex, with larger numbers of women than men returning to school (Mitchell, 1979; Weinstein, 1980). The literature suggests that the number of returning students has greatly increased in recent years (Magoon, 1980; Parks, 1981), and, in fact, the Carnegie Council on Policy Studies on Higher Education (1980) has projected that by the year 2000, 50% of all college undergraduates will be older than 22.

Returning students resume their formal education with goals of improving their economic status and advancing their careers, and with expectations of general self-improvement (Christian & Wilson, 1985; Erickson, Kimmel, Murphy, & Newcomer, 1976; Papier, 1980). At college, however, they encounter distinctive problems and concerns. Three clients seen at a university mental health service serve as good examples. One student had left her position as a vice president at a financial institution to pursue a doctoral degree. A single person in her early 40s with well-defined career goals, she felt that despite holding one advanced degree she would need to complement her existing education and experience with additional training and formal credentials, in order to compete successfully and attain her career goals in her male-dominated profession. However, having previously met her needs for companionship almost exclusively through interactions with her colleagues at work, she now felt particularly deprived in the school setting, where virtually all her fellow students were two decades younger than she. She also found herself less fluent than her classmates in some of the technical academic skills that were most emphasized in her curriculum.

A second client had been trained and employed as a special education teacher prior to and during the early years of her marriage and then discontinued her career when she began her family. At about age 30, when her younger child reached school age, she began doctoral studies in an allied field. In returning to school, she relinquished a considerable measure of the satisfaction that she had enjoyed from child-centered contacts with other suburban mothers. In addition, she now confronted the triple challenge of fulfilling the full-time (i.e., residency) requirement of her doctoral program; working to partially underwrite the cost of her studies; and fulfilling the demands of her parenting, homemaking, and marriage responsibilities.

A third client found that the marriage into which she had somewhat uneasily entered as a teenage undergraduate had unraveled as she pursued her own career and achieved a new level of personal autonomy and maturity. Once she divorced, the traditional assumption of economic semidependence that had informed her earlier decision to marry no longer seem viable, and so she resumed her formal education several years later. At this point she was forced to juggle the multiple demands made on her time by full-time study, her wish to consolidate a new marriage and begin a family, and the need to support herself economically.

Such problems and concerns are typical of older students who return to college. Some of these problems directly involve the experiences they encounter at college; others are indirect consequences of returning to the status of student; and still others stem from these students' developmental stage. Meanwhile, returning students, like traditional students, also suffer from a variety of individual problems quite apart from their college experience. Thus, returning students require special consideration as a therapeutic population.

A FOUR-DIMENSIONAL APPROACH

Several approaches to counseling and psychotherapy for returning students have been developed. One approach, geared specifically to women students, advocates a practical, problem-solving orientation (Dickstein, 1984; McGraw, 1982; Wheaton & Robinson, 1983). Interventions focus on helping clients find practical solutions to institutional challenges and to responsibilities in their day-to-day lives. A second approach employs a systems orientation, analyzing the individual student's role within the structure and needs of the institution. Interventions are designed to encourage students to accept their personal strengths while attributing the causes of their distress to the characteristics of the situation rather than to personal inadequacy (Roach, 1976; Wheaton & Robinson, 1983). Another approach, which also has a pragmatic orientation, employs a meld of individual psychotherapy and broad-based social support (e.g., Claus, 1986). By providing career counseling, support groups, and advice in addition to traditional psychotherapy, this approach tends to improve returning students' chances for academic success and reinforce their ability to control their environment and their lives.

The strategy we propose in this chapter draws on these and other therapeutic approaches in attempting to help returning students master their distinctive challenges. In general, we advocate a comprehensive approach that (1) invites affective growth, (2) facilitates cognitive awareness, (3) replaces maladaptive patterns of behavior, and (4) builds self-esteem. Accordingly, four distinguishable but interrelated dimensions are addressed within the therapeutic relationship. We offer below examples of interventions associated with each of these dimensions.

Affective growth can be facilitated in several ways. One method is simply to encourage the expression of emotion. Emotional catharsis detoxifies intense emotions and helps clients value their emotional selves. In addition, accurately empathic interventions that focus on clients' feelings assist them in identifying and differentiating their feelings. Affective growth is also facilitated by encouraging clients to be specific and detailed when relating past and current events. This practice, especially when applied to emotion-laden events, puts clients "in" the described situation; they remember the events more clearly and re-experience the feelings of that time. A related technique is informal role playing with key figures in clients' lives. For example, a returning student is encouraged to "tell your professor what you would say if you didn't have to worry about the consequences," and is then surprised by the powerful emotions that emerge.

Cognitive awareness can be facilitated by summarizing and organizing the material that clients present, restating it in a more coherent fashion that defines one or more themes. Clients begin to hear these themes as this process is repeated again and again. A related method involves drawing explicit parallels and identifying patterns in clients' relationships and behaviors. A therapist might say to a client, "It seems that your reaction to your professor is similar to what you have felt about your mother in the past." To assist the client in developing these perspectives, the therapist can teach and model a point of view that continually links past experiences, present situations, and events in the therapy itself. Cognitive awareness can also be increased by providing information, dispelling myths, and suggesting where and when to obtain more information. Finally, cognitive awareness is facilitated by directly explaining the process of therapy and the ways in which therapeutic change occurs.

Behavior, including maladaptive learning patterns, can be changed through a number of techniques. The therapist can consciously model clear communication and good interpersonal skills; such modeling is especially important, since inadequate social skills are frequently a presenting complaint of returning students. Maladaptive learning patterns can be modified by reinforcing desired behaviors and teaching clients to self-reinforce. Another method is to promote skills development, such as through assertiveness training, relaxation protocols, or time management techniques. Assigning homework related to these programs increases transfer of learning and thus enhances behavioral change. It is also helpful to structure therapy to keep motivation high. This can be achieved by emphasizing the therapist's status as an expert, reinforcing positive expectations about treatment, and planning success experiences for the client. These elements increase the chances of therapeutic success and increase the extent of desired change.

Building self-esteem can also be facilitated in many ways, such as by exhibiting confidence in oneself as a therapist while also showing and explicitly expressing respect and liking for a client. Accurately empathic interventions by the therapist enable the client to feel understood and valued, enhancing the client's sense of self in a less specific, more all-encompassing way. A therapist who is comfortable being a support or buffer for the client enhances the client's sense of personal power and self-confidence, while a client–therapist relationship that is based on acceptance and trust also strengthens the client's self-esteem. Finally, giving an objective assessment of the client's performance and abilities can improve the self-esteem of self-critical clients.

The same goals of affective growth, cognitive awareness, behavioral change, and enhanced self-esteem also apply, of course, to traditional students. However, we believe that the broad-gauge approach we have presented is particularly appropriate for returning students because of the multiple sources of their problems. One must beware with these clients of attributing difficulties to a single causative factor and thereby applying a one-dimensional therapeutic program. For example, an older student's complaint about feeling different or isolated on campus may stem partly from the student's personal history and therefore call for certain measures, such as modifying a negative self-image. At the same time, objective conditions on campus *do* cause older students to feel different and isolated; therefore, the therapist may also want to acknowledge this fact and encourage the student to search outside the institution for appropriate companionship. A sensitive therapeutic approach requires attending to returning students' needs along all four dimensions.

Deciding when to apply a particular intervention is a matter of clinical judgment, not hard-and-fast rules. The decision partly hinges on individual differences: Some returning students need an approach relatively weighted toward behavior, others need an emphasis on affect, and so forth. The decision must also be guided by the moment-to-moment shifts within the therapeutic hour. In our experience, a flexible response rather than a consistently applied concentration on one dimension best serves the needs of the returning student population.

In the sections below, we illustrate how treatment interventions are applied. The majority of the material is taken from sessions with three female clients, different from those described above, who were seen in a university mental health service for a contractual, time-limited psychotherapy lasting 12 weeks. The material is organized according to the main sources of their problems.

FEELING ISOLATED AND DIFFERENT

Among the chief problems older students face when they return to college is feeling different or isolated, feeling that they do not fit in (Frost, 1980). These feelings come about because they often live off campus, because other students may ignore them (and perhaps vice versa), and because in fact they are different in many ways from traditional students. In addition, for some returning students, as for traditional students, the sense of being different may have been a lifelong concern.

In helping students with this concern, the therapist may want to take a behavioral tack, encouraging them to make social contacts on or off campus. Empathic responses designed to boost self-esteem also can be therapeutic, as we see with Ann (not her real name), a 32-year-old single woman:

> ANN: The people who are in my classes—they are all very much younger than me.
> THERAPIST: That must really add to the loneliness in a way.
> ANN: I think so. . . . I mean there are some very nice people in the classes, but the fact is, if you are older and you have worked for 15 years, you have a different perspective; which means that you don't actually feel terribly close to people who, um, you know, are very much younger.

THERAPIST: You need some people who really understand what you're going through and who will be there with you through this time.

In a later session, Ann brought up her concerns again:

ANN: I mean, I'm overwhelmed with [my] discontent and the frustration. It just seems so utterly ridiculous: My constant companions [are] all totally 10–15 years younger than me.

THERAPIST: I guess it's hard right now to remember all of the times in your life when you have found new friends somehow.

The therapist's responses in the first instance were empathic, addressing Ann's wish for a connection, validating her feelings, and inviting her to feel close to the therapist. As such, these responses were geared toward both the affective and self-esteem dimensions. The therapist might also have made an even more explicit invitation to a therapeutic connection: "Here you have someone who can be that support for you." Doing so, however, would require measuring the meanings for the client and the therapeutic risks of encouraging such dependency.

In the second exchange, the therapist again sought to increase Ann's self-esteem, this time by reminding her of past successes. This is an example of providing clients a more objective, positive view of themselves. The therapist reinforced Ann's expectancy for change by demonstrating confidence in her ability to overcome her isolation.

In addition to feeling isolated on campus, returning students may not necessarily have support from outside; if anything, significant others may become an additional stressor (Benjamin & Levy, 1979; Dickstein, 1984). Since support from multiple sources is essential to returning students (Kirk & Dorfman, 1983; Mardoyan, Alleman, & Cochran, 1983), therapists need to attend to this issue, as illustrated in these excerpts with Carolyn, a divorced woman in her late 30s:

CAROLYN: And if you would expect anybody to [support you], it would be your family. You suspect that strangers aren't going to know your life story, but to some point you expect or hope that your family understands at least.

THERAPIST: Say, "I really need your support. I can't do it by myself."

CAROLYN: I can't do it by myself. Help me! (*Cries*)

At a later point in treatment, Carolyn mentioned other sources of support:

CAROLYN: . . . Women have a very difficult time during the school year. Women are not overall supported like the male students are. . . . They [school authorities] need to help the women students focus better. I think that students coming here would feel more like staying here if some of that took place. I think it's hard when you lose fellow students because you build up not only your relationships; you build up study partners. One of my best friends left last week and I won't see her again for a long time. . . .

THERAPIST: Nobody seems to care that you lost someone very important to you.

CAROLYN: Nobody cares.

THERAPIST: You look sad.

CAROLYN: I guess I really miss her.

The therapist's efforts with this client were directed toward the affective dimension. In the first instance the therapist initiated a role play, which was familiar to Carolyn and therefore enabled her to have a cathartic response. In the second intervention, empathic reflection of Carolyn's feelings allowed her to identify and experience them fully.

Since returning students tend to feel isolated from younger classmates and also have academic doubts, support from professors is seen as important:

ANN: . . . People in the department don't treat new students more with kid gloves. They don't have that awarenss that we are older than everybody else, are plunked down and are suddenly a total stranger. Maybe our mind is not totally focused on the work.

THERAPIST: I guess they don't give enough credit to how lonely and scary it is.

ANN: I don't really see what they could do and how, but if they just kind of displayed an awareness that it was there, instead of immediately expecting us to forge ahead.

THERAPIST: What would you say to them, if you could really let them know how you felt?

ANN: I need more awareness from you, I have to have more. . . . Ha! That is the story of my life.

Ann responded to the first intervention, a feeling-oriented empathic statement, by ignoring the affect identified by the therapist. (This intervention would have been enhanced by " . . . how lonely and scared *you* are.") Noting Ann's response, the therapist was more directive in encouraging emotional insight in the second intervention, which encouraged expression of feelings and suggested a brief role-playing experience. Ann responded by discovering a parallel between her current experience and her past history.

CHANGE OF STATUS

Another common concern for returning students is their change of status. They often exchange the role of an authority for that of a subordinate, and many times a dwindling paycheck and large loans add to their sense of diminished status, as Carolyn explained:

> CAROLYN: Part of the problem with this school is that they have this view of students as a certain age and they come in a certain package . . . and boy, when you walk into that and all of a sudden this person [the professor and advisor] is making you feel very small, you feel like a kid again.
>
> THERAPIST: You tend to forget your past success and status as a businesswoman and the fact that you have years more experience than these youngsters.

And again:

> CAROLYN: I'm almost 38 years old . . . but giving everything up; I'm giving up a salary, a paycheck; and kind of going back down the ladder was a big thing to do.
>
> THERAPIST: Your strength let you take that risk; and maybe that same strength will help you cope with how hard it all is now.

In the first instance, the therapist sought to increase Carolyn's self-esteem. The therapist allied herself with Carolyn, showing liking and respect for her, expressing faith in her, and drawing her attention to past successes. In the second exchange, the therapist sought to strengthen Carolyn's confidence in being able to bring about change. The therapist acknowledged the client's present distress while suggesting that she had the capacity to bear and alleviate that distress.

Associated with the change in status is an increase in dependency—or a change to a new form of dependency. Unlike traditional students, who are in the process of separating from parents, returning students have by and large achieved independence from their families of origin. Most are used to being treated as independent adults, though some older women students have subordinated their own needs to those of others and may not have completely resolved dependency issues or developed their own identity. Now as returning students they must adjust to the dependent (even infantilizing) role of student, which requires compliance and submission of self to the evaluation of others (Mardoyan et al., 1983). For many this is an uncomfortable, conflict-ridden role. Related to this conflict, it has been reported that many re-entry students feel that as mature adults they should not need to ask for help, such as by going to therapy (Brandenberg, 1974).

Ann described her feelings about the student's role as follows:

ANN: In terms of the kind of lifestyle I have here, I'm very help-less and dependent. There's particularly something in being a student—it's kind of a relationship of weakness. I think that is the cause of the conflicts with the professors, because those are the only people around me who are my age and the kind of people that I'm used to associating with.

THERAPIST: Returning to a dependent, childlike position, like that of student, seems to have resulted in your feeling like a child in all parts of your life. I think much of your current frustra-tion may be due to this regressive atmosphere that you are in.

Carolyn stated related feelings:

CAROLYN: I should be taking care of myself. I've made a mess. As an adult with a child, I shouldn't have created a situation that it's difficult for us to live in financially. Obviously this isn't the way somebody my age conducts themselves. I'm supposed to be independent but I'm not.

THERAPIST: Once you're used to living independently, returning to the dependent role of student that makes you into a child again feels very uncomfortable. What you label as something wrong with you could also be seen as due to the circumstances of being a returning student.

In these instances, the therapist sought to enhance self-esteem and invited cognitive growth. The therapist validated the clients' affective experience, but reframed their explanations by introducing a perspec-tive that shifted some of the "blame" from them personally. This per-spective enabled Ann and Carolyn to identify and discard myths they had embraced about returning to school—myths that typically under-mine returning students' self-esteem.

Interventions in regard to change of status also begin to identify patterns in the students' development that, when more fully addressed, will bring increased personal understanding. For example, accommodation to a subordinate or dependent role is made more conflictful when an individual was humiliated as a child for being dependent. Identifying a history of such experiences and linking that history to the current school situation provides clients with an understanding of their current distress. However, it is especially important with returning students when considering historical or "genetic" factors to affirm the reality of their difficult current circumstances.

JUGGLING MULTIPLE ROLES

Returning students have to manage a variety of roles as they seek to balance responsibilities between school and home (Karr-Kidwell, 1984). They have to attend to financial needs (Claus, 1986; Erickson *et al.*, 1976), child care responsibilities (Benjamin & Levy, 1979; Tittle & Denker, 1975), recreational needs, and relationships with spouses and friends outside the school setting, while they also fulfill school-related obligations. In seeking to coordinate these roles. they understandably tend to long for freedom from time-consuming university rules and regulations (Ferguson, 1966; Mardoyan *et al.*, 1983). In general, going back to school requires more compromises and adjustments in their already well-defined lives than is required of traditional students, as this excerpt illustrates:

ANN: It can't be just work. Maybe when you're 20 you can just work. Basically I find studying appreciable and sufficient reason to be here now, but it can't be a be-all and end-all. . . . Life is going on, and all the other things I enjoy and that are important to me still have to be there. Music, poetry, spring, all sorts of things. But I can't do those things and still pass my classes.

THERAPIST: It's important to fit those treats in. In fact, before next week I'd like you to make up a list of at least 10 things you can do to treat yourself. The activities should take less than an hour each and be easily accessible to you.

Afraid of failing, Ann felt that she needed to study 24 hours a day in order to reach her goals, but in doing so she was neglecting herself in other ways. The therapist prescribed a homework task in a confident, unambivalent tone that conveyed permission for Ann to break her maladaptive pattern. Ann's later pleasure at achieving this task reinforced her new behavior. In addition to its behavioral dimension, the therapist's comment had a cognitive component in that it implicitly educated Ann about effective study skills—a theme that later could be taken up explicitly.

The goal of helping older students juggle multiple roles also emerged with Melissa, a 43-year-old wife and mother of three:

> MELISSA: I think there is a better way, or that there is some other way that the family can get organized. . . . I mean, we're still sort of newcomers at this whole ball game, with the mother not being there full-time, and I think we need to learn some organization skills.
>
> THERAPIST: It sounds like we may want to spend some time on helping you set priorities and learn how to best manage time in order to balance all of your responsibilities and needs.

The therapist here endorsed Melissa's view that the complexity of her life rather than some personal inadequacy was causing her difficulties. Doing so enhanced her self-esteem. The therapist also presented herself as an ally who could help Melissa achieve more effective time management; this strategy was designed to keep Melissa's motivation high and enhance the likelihood of therapeutic success. It should be noted that the therapist's comment was directed simultaneously at the client's self-esteem, cognitive awareness, and behavior. Such comments that are addressed to several dimensions at once can be particularly effective within a brief treatment paradigm.

Carolyn too needed assistance in balancing roles, specifically in combining her studies with meeting her 6-year-old son's needs:

> CAROLYN: It's harder now, because when I'm in a class I can't get out to go for him. I always try to budget my time around classes so if something comes up with my son and I have to meet with his teacher, I schedule it when I'm not in a class. It's different than when you're working, because my job was such that I could come and go.
>
> THERAPIST: Now it's more like a juggling act.
>
> CAROLYN: So now it's more juggle. . . . Life wasn't as complicated at 20 as it is at 37. . . . I can barely do the laundry and go to the grocery store. Forget about dishes or anything else.
>
> THERAPIST: I wonder if you are aware of all of the child care options and household assistance options in this area. Let me tell you about some of them.

Once again, the therapist's responses demonstrated a flexible approach that helped the client along several dimensions. The first response, an empathic paraphrase, prompted Carolyn to provide further detail about her struggle. The therapist then addressed the cognitive and behavioral dimensions by providing information. As with Melissa, attention was directed toward the here-and-now, toward supporting Carolyn's efforts to find ways out of her current dilemma. Interventions directed at the affective dimension also could have been employed, if necessary—for example, if feelings of fear and anger were causing symptomatic behavior, or if Carolyn were having an emotional response to the therapist's comments.

Managing multiple roles can also engender ambivalence and guilt, especially in older women students. Although developmental theorists have suggested that at midlife many women want to reduce responsibilities to their families and concentrate on self-development and growth (Traupmann, 1982), women still feel obligated to their families and therefore guilty when they take time away from home (Dickstein, 1984; Weinstein, 1980). Thus returning to college creates a conflict in needs between nurturing and achieving, as this excerpt with Carolyn, the divorcee, illustrates:

CAROLYN: My family would have been happier . . . if I had married and had three children and lived in suburbia and been a housewife. My life didn't go that way and I don't have any problems, I don't feel guilty about that, but I think that I want them to be proud of who I am.

THERAPIST: If only you could make both them and you happy.

CAROLYN: Yeah. Do I take care of everyone else or do what I want to do?

THERAPIST: It's quite a bind. No wonder going to school can feel so uncomfortable. The more you succeed in what you want to do, the further you move from what they expected.

Similarly, Melissa described her feelings as follows:

MELISSA: I have always loved school, and I would really like to be able to do what I can do with school and continue to do that. I don't want to not be able to do that because of logistics that have to do with my family, and I don't want to not be able to do that because of wondering what other people will think if I keep going to school and am not the classic mother. I need to know that I can do it and not be a bad person or a bad mother.

THERAPIST: You're saying, "It's impossible to please everybody."

MELISSA: Yeah, I'm so mad. It's just too complicated.

THERAPIST: I can't do this.
MELISSA: I can't do this. I won't do this! (*Yells.*)

The therapist's accurate reflections here, it will be noted, led to cognitive awareness and expression of feeling.

ACADEMIC CONCERNS

Returning students have self-doubts and fears about not making it in the academic milieu (Astin, 1976; Erickson *et al.*, 1976; Papier, 1980). Researchers have attributed their fear to lack of self-confidence (Grabowski, 1972; Kirk & Dorfman, 1983), fear of failure (Arfken, 1981), and guilt and anxiety (Wheaton & Robinson, 1983). One has to remember that some returning students left school originally because of academic problems, and that most others, even if originally successful, have not dealt with academic pressures for years. Carolyn's testimony is not unusual:

> CAROLYN: I was never terribly good [at this subject] to begin with. So, for me to study as intensely as I did, to go over and over and read the stuff and try to compact it in, I mean there wasn't any more that could be squeezed in. By the time I got to the exam . . . I was hysterical. I just cried. I couldn't do it. . . . Letting go and letting down and walking away from it and feeling, "Okay, you know it's a hopeless situation, just do the best you can," are difficult kinds of things to do.
>
> THERAPIST: I guess it's hard to convince yourself that letting down some, building in relaxation time, and even studying a little less will actually help you do better on tests.

And during another session:

> CAROLYN: I go through a stage where I feel so hopeless, I will never know all of this, you've got to be kidding, this is ridiculous. Through some of these episodes sometimes I cry. . . . It's too much. Much of the time I don't think I can do it.
>
> THERAPIST: You seem to forget how well you did the last time you were in school, and how successful you've been in most anything you've tried throughout your life.

In cases like these it is useful to dispel the myth, as the therapist did here, that endless study maximizes academic performance. Another helpful tack is to remind the client of past successes; here, this communicated the therapist's confidence in Carolyn and mobilized her own confidence. As always with clients who experience strong negative feelings, it is also wise to convey empathic understanding of these clients' inner experience while at the same time pointing the way toward a more realistic interpretation of events. Accordingly, the therapist might have said to Carolyn, "When your full efforts don't seem to be good enough, it's hard to convince yourself that you can succeed," or "You've been feeling so helpless and overloaded, it's no wonder you forgot how well you did in the past."

Academic concerns are often rooted in self-concept issues that have their origin in early family relationships. This excerpt illustrates the unearthing of these issues, as the therapist first placed the academic fears in a wider context and then made the connection between current fears and early experiences:

MELISSA: Yeah, I'm scared of that whole thing of what I am— whether I can do the work.

THERAPIST: It sounds like you're scared about doing well in your work, but the fear goes deeper than that. Maybe you even get afraid of whether you're okay as a person.

MELISSA: I don't know. Probably equally scary are the thoughts of really screwing up the family . . . or not really having a contribution to make in what other area I tried. I think those are equally scary. I would not want to go through more school or get out into being a counselor without having there be some redeeming social value there. . . .

THERAPIST: "Can I really do this?" and "Am I doing the right thing?" That sounds like your mother talking.

MELISSA: I guess so. It was *so* important to get good grades and to be a good girl. How can I get her to shut up?

Another aspect of academic concerns is a sense of time urgency, which prompts the wish to finish school quickly (Grabowski, 1972; Kahnweiler & Johnson, 1980). Although there is a realistic component to this concern, therapists can help place it in perspective for panic-stricken clients. In the following vignette, the therapist simply responded to the affective component of the client's statements:

MELISSA: If I decide to do doctoral work, there is no way it can just be slow and easy. I mean, considering my age, I just can't poke along and do this over a number of years. . . . [I need to] get out with a reasonable amount of time left to do something with it.

Therapist: I wonder how that feels, to have yet one more pressure sitting on you?

Melissa: It's too much. Sometimes I feel like I just can't do it. I may be a middle-aged woman, but I still want a mother.

DEVELOPMENTAL CONCERNS

Most returning students are women in their 30s (Hovey, 1988). As such, they are at a different stage of life from that of the traditional undergraduate, who wrestles with the developmental issues of separation from family, formation of identity, and establishment of intimate relationships with peers. Of course, these issues often apply to older students as well. Returning women students may be struggling to separate at last from their families of origin or from restrictive marriages. Housewives who have been overdependent on their husbands, or returning students of either gender who are dissatisfied with their jobs, may return to college to establish a new career identity and thereby redefine their personal identity. Single, divorced, or unhappily married returning students may also still be wrestling with the fundamental developmental crisis of intimacy versus isolation; perhaps at college they can find a partner, or so involve themselves academically that they have less need of one.

But beyond these typically late adolescent issues lies another cluster of concerns pertinent to these students' stage of life. Older students are more likely than traditional students to have parents who are deceased, ailing, or in need of assistance. The challenge for older students is to mourn the loss of parents or respond appropriately to parents' changing needs. Older students may also have marital problems. Their children may be a source of concern, or they may be troubled by childlessness, their failure to fulfill in the usual way the task Erikson (1950) calls "generativity." Many have gone through a painful divorce, been laid off from a job, encountered the "empty nest" syndrome, or recovered from a disease or psychological disability—changes that have perhaps inspired their return to school. College is seen as a haven, an escape, a means toward betterment.

Unlike the concerns previously discussed in this chapter, none of these problems is engendered by the college experience. However, they inevitably have an impact on returning students' adjustment to college. In responding to these concerns, therefore, therapists must keep a dual perspective. Attention must be paid both to these personal problems and to their effect on studies. If a woman has recently divorced, for example, the therapy necessarily must concentrate on all the personal implications of this most stressful event. At the same time, attention must be paid to the woman's studying, attendance at class, test performance, and so forth, all of which are at risk in the aftermath of her divorce.

CONCLUSION

Although we have not highlighted their strengths, returning students bring certain assets to the psychotherapeutic enterprise. More mature than traditional students, they tend to possess a developed sense of self and have a clear sense of goals for therapy and their lives. At the same time, however, their lives are generally more complex than those of traditional students. They tend to feel different and isolated at college; they have to adjust to a change of status; they must juggle time-consuming and sometimes conflicting roles; they experience academic self-doubts accompanied by pressures to finish school quickly; and they have particular concerns associated with their developmental stage.

Effective therapy requires responsiveness to this special cluster of needs. In this chapter we have espoused a four-pronged approach designed to foster affective, cognitive, behavioral, and self-esteem changes. But we have not formulated rules governing when to emphasize a given therapeutic goal. Rather, we have tried through use of examples to give a sense of effective therapeutic responses. Perhaps the most important aspect of working with returning students is flexibility on the part of the therapist. Sensitivity to their specific needs is the surest therapeutic guide.

REFERENCES

Arfken, D. E. (1981). A lamp beside the academic door: A look at the new student and his needs. *Viewpoints, 120.*

Astin, H. S. (1976). Continuing education and the development of the adult woman. *Counseling Psychologist, 6,* 55–66.

Benjamin, E., & Levy, J. A. (1979). *Barriers to educational opportunities for re-entry women in private universities.* Evanston, IL: Program on Women, Northwestern University.

Brandenberg, J. B. (1974). The needs of women returning to school. *Personnel and Guidance Journal, 53,* 11–18.

Carnegie Council on Policy Studies on Higher Education. (1980). *Three thousand futures: The next 20 years in higher education.* San Francisco: Jossey-Bass.

Christian, C., & Wilson, J. (1985). Reentry women and feminist therapy: A career counseling model. *Journal of College Student Personnel, 26,* 496–500.

Claus, J. K. (1986, April). *Adult students in community college: Learning to manage the learning process.* Paper presented at the 70th Annual Meeting of the American Educational Research Association, San Francisco.

Dickstein, L. J. (1984). Psychiatric issues of women college students today. *Psychiatric Annals, 14,* 653–660.

Erickson, L., Kimmel, E. W., Murphy, M. T., & Newcomer, W. J. (1976). Back to school: The older-than-average student. *College and University, 51,* 679–692.

Erikson, E. H. (1950). *Childhood and society.* New York: Norton.

Ferguson, M. A. (1966). Adult students in an undergraduate university. *Journal of College Student Personnel, 7,* 345–348.

Frost, M. E. (1980, September). *Toward understanding the needs of college students who delay entrance.* Paper presented at the 88th Annual Convention of the American Psychological Association, Montreal.

Grabowski, S. M. (1972). Educational counseling for adults. *Adult Leadership, 20,* 266.

Hovey, S. (1988, May). College degree programs for working adults. *On Campus* (magazine of the American Federation of Teachers), pp. 8–9.

Kahnweiler, J. B., & Johnson, P. L. (1980). A midlife development profile of the returning woman student. *Journal of College Student Personnel, 21,* 414–419.

Karr-Kidwell, P. J. (1984, May). *Re-entry women students in higher education: A model for non-traditional support programs in counseling and career advisement.* Paper presented at the Women and Work Symposium, Arlington, TX.

Kirk, C. F., & Dorfman, L. T. (1983). Satisfaction and role strain among middle-age and older re-entry women students. *Education Gerontology, 9,* 15–29.

Magoon, T. M. (1980, November). *Student life and the task of counseling in colleges and universities in the 1980s* (Research Report No. 17-80). Paper presented at the Counseling Seminar, Japan Association of Student Counseling, Tokyo.

Mardoyan, J. L., Alleman, E., & Cochran, J. R. (1983). Adapting university counseling centers to meet the needs of an older student body. *Journal of College Student Personnel, 24,* 138–143.

McGraw, L. K. (1982). A selective review of programs and counseling interventions for the reentry woman. *Personnel and Guidance Journal, 60,* 469–472.

Mitchell, G. N. (1979). *The new majority: The educational needs of present and future women students of the California community colleges.* Sacramento: California Community and Junior College Association.

Papier, S. N. (1980). Counseling for the re-entry woman. *Viewpoints, 120.*

Parks, D. R. (1981). *Life-cycle developmental theory as a tool for college counselors.* Charlottesville: Center for the Study of Higher Education, University of Virginia.

Roach, R. M. (1976). Honey won't you please stay home. *Personnel and Guidance Journal, 55,* 86–89.

Tittle, C. K., & Denker, E. R. (1975). *Re-entry woman: A selective review of the educational process, career choice, and interest measurement.* Albany: New York State Education Department, Bureau of 2-Year College Programs.

Traupmann, J. (1982, March). *Midlife women in continuing education: A comparative study.* Paper presented at the 66th Annual Meeting of the American Educational Research Association, New York.

Weinstein, L. (1980). *The counseling needs of re-entry women: Field evaluation draft.* Washington, DC: Association of American Colleges, Project on the Status and Education of Women.

Wheaton, J. B., & Robinson, D. C. (1983). Responding to the needs of re-entry women: A comprehensive campus model. *National Association of Student Personnel Administrators Journal, 21*(2), 44–51.

Index

essential to please parents & withhold her anger
or they will withdraw their love + support
caught in between need to be true to herself
and need for their approval + love

fear of self-assertion
Stifle drive toward selfhood, squelching self
in effort to please emotionally ungiving parents
- cultivate false self, neglecting genuine personality development

p. 21
make the most of opening sessions - st. may not come back
therapist may need to be tactfully active -
work to create an encouraging, safe, effective ambience